30th Hemophilia Symposium

Hamburg 1999

Editors: I. Scharrer, W. Schramm

Presentation:

HIV Infection and Epidemiology in Hemophilia
Gene Therapy in Hemophilia A and B
Therapy of Hepatitis C
Inhibitors in Hemophilia
Long-term Results after Joint Replacement
Pediatric Hemostasiology
Case Reports

Scientific board:
I. Scharrer, Frankfurt/Main
W. Schramm, Munich

Chairmen:
H. H. Brackmann (Bonn); R. Burger (Berlin); L. Gürtler (Greifswald)
L. Hovy (Frankfurt/Main); W. Kreuz (Frankfurt/Main); E. Lechler (Cologne)
H. Lenk (Leipzig); E. O. Meili (Zurich); I. Pabinger (Vienna)
H. Pollmann (Münster); I. Scharrer (Frankfurt/Main)
W. Schramm (Munich); R. Seitz (Langen)

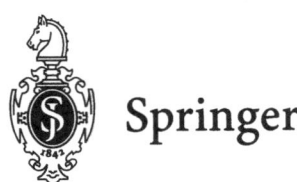

Springer

Professor Dr. med. INGE SCHARRER
Hemophilia Center, Dept. of Internal Medicine
University Hospital
Theodor-Stern-Kai 7
D-60590 Frankfurt am Main
Germany

Professor Dr. med. WOLFGANG SCHRAMM
Dept. of Hemostasiology
University Hospital
Ziemssenstr. 1a
D-80336 München
Germany

Mit 107 Abbildungen

ISBN 978-3-540-67677-5

Library of Concress Cataloging-in-Publication Data
30th hemophilia symposium : Hamburg, 1999 / editors, I. Scharrer, W. Schramm.
    p. cm.
    ISBN 978-3-540-67677-5   ISBN 978-3-642-18240-2 (eBook)
    DOI 10.1007/978-3-642-18240-2
    1. Hemophilia--Congresses. I. Title: Thirtieth hemophilia symposium. II. Scharrer, I.
    III. Schramm, W., 1943-IV. Title.
    RC642 .A15 2000
    616.1'572--dc21

© Springer Verlag Berlin Heidelberg 2001
Originally published by Springer Verlag Berlin Heidelberg in 2001

The use of general descriptive names, registered names, trademarks, etc. in this publication does not imply, even in the absence of a specific statement, that such names are exempt from the relevant protective laws and regulations and therefore free for general use.

Product Liability: The publisher cannot guarantee the accuracy of any information about dosage and application contained in this book. In every individual case the user must check such information by consulting the relevant literature.

Typesetting: cicero Lasersatz, 86424 Dinkelscherben

Printed on acid-free paper   SPIN 10772308   21/3130   5 4 3 2 1 0

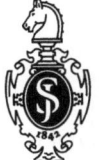

Springer-Verlag Berlin Heidelberg GmbH

Contents

VIII. Research Cooperation

IX.a Poster: Hemophilia

IX.b Poster: Thrombophilia

IX.c Poster: Molecular Biology

IX.d Poster: Pediatrics

IX.e Poster: Case Reports

IX.f Poster: Hemorrhagic Disorders

IX.g Poster: Diagnostic Problems

List of Participants

ACKERMANN, K., Dr.
Klinik und Poliklinik für Kieferchirurgie/Klinikum der Ludwig-Maximilians-Universität, D-München

ALISCH, A., Frau
Abt. f. Transfusionsmedizin, Universitätsklinik Eppendorf, D-Hamburg

AMANN, B., Dr.
Städt. Kliniken Dortmund, Med. Klinik, D-Dortmund

ANDERS, O., Prof. Dr.
Klinik und Poliklinik für Innere Med. der Universität Rostock, D-Rostock

ANGSTWURM, M., Dr.
Abt. Hämostaseologie, Med. Klinik Innenstadt der Ludwig-Maximilians-Universität, D-München

ARENDS, P., Dr.
Arzt für Kinderheilkunde, A-Güssing

ASBECK, F., Prof. Dr.
I. Med. Klinik, Städtisches Krankenhaus, D-Kiel

AUERSWALD, G., Dr.
Professor-Hess-Kinderklinik, Zentralkrankenhaus St.-Jürgen.-Str., D-Bremen

AUMANN, V., Dr.
Zentrum für Kinderheilkunde, Med. Fakultät, Otto-von-Guericke-Universität, D-Magdeburg

AYGÖREN-PÜRSÜN, E., Dr., Frau
Zentrum der Inneren Med., Hämophilieambulanz, Klinikum der J.-W.-Goethe-Universität, D-Frankfurt/Main

BACHHUBER, R.
Bluter Betreuung Bayern e. V., Med. Klinik Innenstadt der Ludwig-Maximilians-Universität, D-München

BAHLE, R., Dr., Frau
 Kinderärztin, D-Neubrandenburg

Balleisen, L., Prof. Dr.
 Abt. Hämatologie und Onkologie, Innere Med., Evangelisches Krankenhaus,
 D-Hamm

Barthels, M., Frau Prof. Dr.
 D-Hannover

Bau, J., Dr., Frau
 Abt. Transfusionsmed. und Transplantationsimmunologie,
 Universitätskrankenhaus Eppendorf, D-Hamburg

BAUM, G.
 Bundesministerium für Gesundheit, D-Bonn

BAUMGARTNER, CH., Dr.
 Facharzt für Kinder und Jugendliche, CH-Gossau

BECK, CH., Frau Dr.
 Ärztin für Kinderheilkunde, D-Berlin

BECK, K.-H., Dr.
 Abt. Transfusionsmed., Klinikum der Albert-Ludwigs-Universität, D-Freiburg

BECK, E.A., Prof. Dr.
 Arzt für Hämatologie, CH-Lugano

BEECK, H., Frau Dr.
 Inst. für Transfusionsmed. und Immunhämatologie, Klinikum der Stadt
 Ludwigshafen, D-Ludwigshafen

BEESER, H.P., Prof. Dr.
 Inst. für Qualitätsmanagement und Standardisierung in der Transfusionsmed.
 und Hämostaseologie, D-Teningen

BENEKE, H., Dr.
 Sektion Hämostaseologie, Abt. Innere Med. III, Med. Universitätsklinik, D-Ulm

BERGER, H., Dr.
 Hämostaseologie/Med. Klinik III, Westpfalz-Klinikum GmbH, D-Kaiserslautern

BERGER, K., Frau
 Abt. Hämostaseologie, Med. Klinik Innenstadt der Ludwig-Maximilians-
 Universität, D-München

BERGMANN, F., Frau Dr.
Gemeinschaftslabor, Dr. Keeser und Prof. Arndt, D-Hamburg

BERNIEN, B., Frau
Abt. Transfusionsmed. und Transplantationsfimmunologie,
Universitätskrankenhaus Eppendorf, D-Hamburg

BERTHOLD, B., Dr.
Hämophiliezentrum, Klinik für Innere Medizin I, Klinikum Neubrandenburg,
D-Neubrandenburg

BIEWENER, A., Frau
Abt. Hämatologie und Onkologie, Labor, Med. Hochschule Hannover,
D-Hannover

BINDER, F., Dr.
Herz- und Gefäßklinik, Rhönklinikum, D-Bad Neustadt an der Saale

BLATNY, J., Dr.
Faculty Children's Hosp., J.G.Mendela, Hematology, CZ-Brno

BLAZEK, B., Dr.
FNsP Ostrava, Children's Dept. - Hematology, CZ-Ostrava - Poruba

BÖTTCHER, D., Prof. Dr.
Abt. Innere Med., Krankenhaus Bethesda, D-Wuppertal

BRACKMANN, H.-H., Dr.
Inst. für Experimentelle Hämatologie und Transfusionsmedizin der Universität,
D-Bonn

BRAUN, U., Frau Dr.
Deutsche Hämophiliegesellschaft, D-München

BREUER, W.
IGH, D-Bonn

BROCKHAUS, W., Dr.
Abt. für Hämostaseologie, Hämatologie und Angiologie,
Klinikum Nürnberg Süd, D-Nürnberg

BROCKMANN, M.
Abt. Transfusionsmed., Transplantationsimmunologie,
Universitätskrankenhaus Eppendorf, D-Hamburg

BRUHN, H.D., Prof. Dr.
I. Med. Klinik, Klinikum der Christian-Albrechts-Universität, D-Kiel

BUDDE, U., Prof. Dr.
Gemeinschaftslabor Dr. Keeser und Prof. Arndt, D-Hamburg

BURGER, R., Prof. Dr.
Robert-Koch-Institut, D-Berlin

BUX-GEWEHR, I., Frau Dr.
Inst. für Hämostaseologie und Transfusionsmed., Heinrich-Heine-Universität,
D-Düsseldorf

CALATZIS, A., Dr.
Abt. Hämostaseologie, Med. Klinik Innenstadt der Ludwig-Maximilians-
Universität, D-München

CERNA, Z., Dr.
FN Plzen-Bory, Hematology, CZ-Plzen-Bory

CLAUSEN, N., Dr.
Barnafdelningen, Skejby Hospital, DK-Aarhus

CVIRN, G., Mag.
Universitäts-Kinderklinik, A-Graz

CZWALINNA, A., Dr.
Abt. Hämophilie/Med. Poliklinik, Med. Hochschule Hannover, D-Hannover

DICATO, M.A., Prof. Dr.
Département Hématologie, Service de Médicine Interne,
Centre Hospitalier du Luxembourg, L-Luxembourg

DIEPOLDER, H., Dr.
Med. Klinik II, Klinikum Großhadern, D-München

DOCKTER, G., Prof. Dr.
Kinderklinik, Universitätskliniken des Saarlandes, D-Homburg

DODOJACEK, R., Dr.
Universitäts-Kinderklinik, A-Graz

DOMSCH, CHR., Dr.
Abt. Hämostaseologie, Med. Klinik Innenstadt der Ludwig-Maximilians-
Universität, D-München

DORLINGSCHAW, O., Frau Dr.
Klinik und Poliklinik für Innere Medizin IV, Medizinische Fakultät
der Martin-Luther-Universität Halle-Wittenberg, D-Halle

DORNDEY, A., Dr.
Deutsche Angestellten Krankenkasse (DAK), D-Hamburg

DULICEK, P., Dr.
Hämatologische Abt., I. Med. Klinik, Universitätskrankenhaus, CZ-Hradex Králové

EBER, ST., Prof. Dr.
Abt. Hämatologie, Kinderspital Zürich, CH-Zürich

EBERL, W., Dr.
Kinderklinik, Städtisches Klinikum Holwedestraße, D-Braunschweig

EHRENFORTH, S., Frau Dr.
Zentrum der Inneren Med., Hämophilieambulanz,
Klinikum der J.-W.-Goethe-Universität, D-Frankfurt/Main

EICKHOFF, H.H., Dr.
Orthopädische Klinik, St.-Josef-Hospital, D-Troisdorf

EIFRIG, B., Frau, Dr.
Abt. Onkologie/Hämostaseologie, Med. Klinik, Universitätskrankenhaus
Eppendorf, D-Hamburg

ERNST, R., Dr.
Facharzt für Kinderheilkunde, D-Münster

ESCURIOLA ETTINGSHAUSEN, C., Frau Dr.
Zentrum der Kinderheilkunde, Klinikum der J.-W.-Goethe-Universität,
D-Frankfurt/Main

ETZLER, J., Frau
WFH Information Clearinghouse, c/o Med. Klinik, Klinikum Innenstadt,
D-München

FAESSLER, H., Dr.
FMH Medicina interna, CH-Chiasso

FALGER, J., Frau Dr.
Universitätsklink für Kinderheilkunde, A-Wien

FASEL, Dr.
Zentralinst. für Med. und Chem. Labordiagnostik, Universitätsklinik
Innsbruck, A-Innsbruck

Fischer, M., Prof. Dr.
Zentrallaboratorium, Krankenhaus der Stadt Wien-Lainz, A-Wien

FLEISSNER, S., Frau
Abt. Hämostaseologie, Med. Klinik Innenstadt der Ludwig-Maximilians-
Universität, D-München

FRANKE, ST., Frau
Zentrum der Inneren Med., Hämophilieambulanz,
Klinikum der J.W.Goethe-Universität, D-Frankfurt/Main

FRANKE, D., PD Dr.
Schwerpunkt für Gerinnungsstörungen und Gefäßkrankheiten, D-Magdeburg

FREGIN, A.H.E.
Inst. f. Humangenetik, Biozentrum, Universität Würzburg, D-Würzburg

FRICK, U., Frau Prof. Dr.
Inst. für Klinische Chemie der Ernst-Moritz-Arndt-Universität, D-Greifswald

FUCHS, A., Frau
Hämophilieambulanz, Universitätsklinik für Innere Medizin I, A-Wien

FÜRST, W., Dr.
Vorarlberger Gebietskrankenkasse, A-Dornbirn

GALLISTL, S., Dr.
Zentrallabor, Universitäts-Kinderklinik, A-Graz

GAMPER, A., Dr., Frau
Kinderspital und Infektion, Allg. österr. Landeskrankenhaus, A-Salzburg

GARTENERNE, K., Dr., Frau
Bluttransfusionsdienst, H-Szombathely

GASTPAR, H., Prof. Dr.
D-Neusäss

GEHLHAAR, K.-D.
Blutspendedienst, Zentralinstitut Springe, D-Springe

GEIB, R., Frau Dr.
Kinderklinik, Saarbrücker Winterbergkliniken, D-Saarbrücken

GEIDEL, K., Frau
Abt. Transfusionsmed., Transplantationsimmunologie,
Universitätskrankenhaus Eppendorf, D-Hamburg

GENSER, N., Dr.
Universitätsklinik für Kinderheilkunde, A-Innsbruck

GIERISCH, M., Frau Dr.
Universitätsklinik für Kinder und Jugendliche, D-Erlangen

GÖBEL, F.-J., Dr.
DRK-Kinderklinik, D-Siegen

GRÄBNER, H., Frau Dr.
Klinik für Kinder- und Jugendmed., Bezirkskrankenhaus Heinrich Braun,
D-Zwickau,

GRAFENHAFER, H., Frau, Dr.,
Universitätsklinik für Innere Medizin I, A-Wien

GRAW, J., Prof. Dr.
GSF-Forschungszentrum f. Umwelt und Gesundheit GmbH,
Inst. f. Säugetiergenetik, D-Oberschleißheim

GRIENBERGER, H., Dr.
Facharzt für Kinderheilkunde, A-Salzburg

GROSS, J., Dr.
Abt. Klinische Hämostaseologie und Transfusionsmed.,
Universitätskliniken des Saarlandes, D-Homburg

GROSS, W., Prof. Dr.
Franz-von-Prümmer-Klinik, D-Bad Brückenau

GÜLDENRING, H., Dr.
Kinderklinik, Städtisches Krankenhaus Dresden-Neustadt, D-Dresden

GÜRTLER, L., Prof. Dr.
Institut für Med. Mikrobiologie, Universität Greifswald, D-Greifswald

GUTENSOHN, K., Dr.
Abt. Transfusionsmed., Transplantationsimmunologie,
Universitätskrankenhaus Eppendorf, D-Hamburg

GÜTHNER, CH., Frau Dr.
Abt. Innere Med. III, Universitätsklinik und Poliklinik, D-Ulm

HALBMAYER, M., Dr.
Zentrallaboratorium, Krankenhaus der Stadt Wien-Lainz, A-Wien

HARTL, H.K., Dr.
Inst. für Sozialmedizin der Universität Wien, A-Wien

HARTMANN, S., Frau Dr.
   Ärztin für Hämatologie und Onkologie, CH-Chur

HASAN, C., Frau Dr.
   Abt. Päd. Hämatologie/Onkologie, Zentr. f. Kinderheilkunde der Universität
   Bonn, D-Bonn

HASLER, K., Frau Prof. Dr.
   Abt. Hämatologie und Onkologie, Zentrum Innere Med. I/Klinikum
   der Albert-Ludwigs-Universität, D-Freiburg

HAUSHOFER, A., Dr.
   Zentrallabor, Krankenhaus der Stadt Wien-Lainz, A-Wien

HEIDEMANN, P., Prof. Dr.
   Klinik für Kinder und Jugendliche, Krankenhauszweckverband Augsburg,
   D-Augsburg

HEINRICHS, CH., Frau Doz. Dr.
   Abt. Klinische Hämostaseologie, Hämophilie-Zentrum, Krankenhaus im
   Friedrichshain, D-Berlin

HELLSTERN, P., Prof. Dr.
   Inst. für Transfusionsmed. und Immunhämatologie,
   Klinikum der Stadt Ludwigshafen, D-Ludwigshafen

HEMPELMANN, L., Dr.
   Kinderklinik Lindenhof, Krankenhaus Lichtenberg, D-Berlin

HERPERTZ, CH., Dr.
   Gerinnungslabor, Universitätsspital, CH-Zürich

HERRMANN, F.H., Prof. Dr. Dr.
   Inst. für Humangenetik, Med. Fakultät der Ernst-Moritz-Arndt-Universität,
   D-Greifswald

HERTWICH, CH., Frau
   Kurpfalzkrankenhaus Heidelberg und Hämophiliezentrum gGmbH,
   D-Heidelberg

HESS, L., Dr.
   Inst. für Experimentelle Hämatologie und Transfusionsmed. der Universität,
   D-Bonn

HILGENFELD, E., Frau Dr.
   D-Berlin

HOFFMANN, M., Dr.
Med. Klinik A, Klinikum der Stadt Ludwigshafen, D-Ludwigshafen

HOFFMANN-OTTENJANN, J., Dr.
Abt. Hämostaseologie, Med. Klinik Innenstadt der Ludwig-Maximilians-
Universität, D-München

HOFMANN, H., Dr.
Facharzt für Transfusionsmed., D-Töplitz

HOFMANN, KL., Dr.
Abt. Hämatologie und Onkologie, Kinderklinik, Klinikum Chemnitz gGmbH,
D-Chemnitz

HOFMANN, S., Frau Dr.
Kinderklinik, Universitätsklinikum Carl-Gustav-Carus, D-Dresden

HOLZHÜTER, H., Prof. Dr.
Hämophilie-Zentrum Nordwest, D-Bremen

HOVY, L., PD Dr.
Orthopädische Universitätsklinik, Friedrichsheim, D-Frankfurt/Main

HUBER, K., Dr.
Abt. Hämatologie, Universitätsklinik Regensburg, D-Regensburg

HUMBERT, J., Prof. Dr.
Service d'hématologie Pédiatrique, Hôpital des Enfants, CH-Genève

HUTH-KÜHNE, A., Frau Dr.
Kurpfalzkrankenhaus Heidelberg und Hämophiliezentrum gGmbH,
D-Heidelberg

IFSITZ, A., Frau
Wiener Gebietskrankenkasse, A-Wien

IMAHORN, P., P.
Kinderarzt, CH-Brig

INGERSLEV, J., Dr.
Dept. Clinical Immunology, Hemophilia Center and Coagulation Laboratory,
University Hospital, DK-Aarhus

IVASKEVICIUS, V.
Inst. für Humangenetik, Biozentrum, Universität Würzburg, D-Würzburg

JAGER, R., Frau Dr.
Vertranszfuzios Allomas, H-Szombathely

JOACHIM, D., Frau Dr.
Kinderklinik, Städt. Klinikum Görlitz GmbH, D-Görlitz

JULEN, E., Dr.
CH-Zermatt

JUNG, A., Frau Dr.
Hemofilicentret, Rigshospitalet, DK-Copenhagen

KAISER, R., Dr.
Institut für Virologie der Universität, D-Köln

KALNINS, W., Dr.
Orthopädische Abteilung, Eifelhöhenklinik, D-Marmagen

KARMANN, K., Frau
D-Ludwigshafen

KECSKÉS, M., Dr., Frau
Inst. Dept. of Int. Med., Med. University of Pécs, H-Pécs

KEIL, F., Dr.
Klinische Abt. f. Hämatologie und Hämostaseologie,
Universitätsklinik für Innere Med., A-Wien

KENTOUCHE, K., Dr.
Klinik für Kinder- und Jugendmedizin Jussuf Ibrahim,
der Friedrich-Schiller-Universität, D-Jena

KIESEWETTER, H., Prof. Dr. Dr.
Inst. für Transfusionsmed. und Immunhämatologie, Campus Charité Mitte,
D-Berlin

KJELLMAN, H.
S-Skinnskatteberg

KLAMROTH, R., Dr.
Abt. Klinische Hämostaseologie, Hämophilie-Zentrum,
Krankenhaus im Friedrichshain, D-Berlin

KLARE, M., Dr.
III. Innere Klinik, Klinikum Berlin-Buch, D-Berlin

KLOSE, H.J., PD Dr.
Arzt für Kinderheilkunde, D-München

KNÖBL, P., Prof. Dr.
Klin. Abt. für Hämatologie und Hämostaseologie,
Universitätsklinik für Innere Med., A-Wien

KNÖFLER, R., Dr.
Klinik und Poliklinik für Kinderheilkunde/Universitätsklinikum
Carl-Gustav-Carus, D-Dresden

KOBELT, R., Dr.
Arzt für Kinderheilkunde, CH-Wabern

KÖHLER-VAJTA, K., Frau Dr.
Ärztin für Kinderheilkunde, D-Grünwald

KOKSCH, M., Dr.
Klinische Hämostaseologie, Med. Klinik und Poliklinik I, Universität Leipzig,
D-Leipzig

KOMRSKA, V., Dr.
II. Detska Klinika, FN Motol, CZ-Praha

KOSCH, A., DR., Frau
Kinderklinik/Kinderonkologie der Med. Einrichtungen
der Westfälischen Wilhelms-Universität, D-Münster

KOSCIELNY, J., Dr.
Inst. für Transfusionsmed. und Immunhämatologie, Campus Charité Mitte,
D-Berlin

KÖSTENBERGER, M., Dr.
Universitäts-Kinderklinik, A-Graz

KÖSTERING, H., Prof. Dr.
Lemgo

KRALL, G., Dr.
Head Hemophilia Care Center, H-Budapest

KRAUSE, M., Frau Dr.
Zentrum der Inneren Med., Hämophilieambulanz,
Klinikum der J.-W.-Goethe-Universität, D-Frankfurt/Main

KREUZ, W., PD Dr.
Zentrum der Kinderheilkunde, Klinikum der J.-W.-Goethe-Universität,
D-Frankfurt am Main

KRISPONEIT, D., Dr.
Med. Klinik I, Zentralkrankenhaus St.-Jürgen-Str., D-Bremen

KRIZ, G., Frau
Universitätsklinik für Kinderheilkunde, A-Wien

KÜHN-WALZ, K., Frau Dr.
Inst. für Transfusionsmed. und Klinische Hämostaseologie,
St. Willibrord-Spital, D-Emmerich

KÜHNEL, G., Frau
Zentr. für Innere Med., Klinikum der Justus-Liebig-Universität, D-Gießen

KUNZE, M., Prof. Dr.
Inst. für Sozialmedizin, A-Wien

KURME, A., Dr.
Arzt für Kinderheilkunde, D-Hamburg

KURNIK, K, Dr., Frau
Kinderklinik im Dr. von Hauner'schen Kinderspital der Ludwig-Maximilians-
Universität, D-München

KURNIK, P., Dr.
Kinderinterne Abt., Allg. Österr. Landeskrankenhaus, A-Klagenfurt

KUSE, R., Prof. Dr.
Abt. Hämatologie, Allg. Krankenhaus St.Georg, D-Hamburg

KYANK, U., Frau Dr.
Universitäts-Kinderklinik, Med. Fakultät, Universität Rostock, D-Rostock,

LAGES, P., Dr.
Kurpfalzkrankenhaus Heidelberg und Hämophiliezentrum gGmbH,
D-Heidelberg

LECHLER, E., Prof. Dr.
D-Esslingen a.N.

LENK, H., PD Dr.
Klinik für Kindermed., Universität Leipzig, D-Leipzig

LESCHNIK, B., Frau
Universitätskinderklinik, A-Graz

LESTIN, H.-G., Prof. Dr.
Inst. für Labormed., Klinikum Schwerin, D-Schwerin

LEUTNER, E., Frau Dr.
Abt. Innere Med., Fachkrankenhaus Neckargemünd gGmbH, D-Neckargemünd

LEX, CH., Frau Dr.
Zentrum der Kinderheilkunde, Med. Einrichtungen der Heinrich-Heine-Universität, D-Düsseldorf

LIMBACH, H.G., Dr.
Kinderklinik, Universitätskliniken des Saarlandes, D-Homburg

LORETH, R.M., Dr.
Abt. für Klin. Hämostaseologie, Med. Klinik III, Westpfalz-Klinikum GmbH, D-Kaiserslautern

LÜHR, C., Frau
Abt. Hämophilie/Med. Poliklinik, Med. Hochschule Hannover, D-Hannover

LUTZE, G., Prof. Dr.
Inst. für Klin. Chemie und Laboratoriumsdiagnostik, Otto-von-Guericke-Universität, D-Magdeburg

MAAK, B., PD Dr.
Thüringen-Klinik Georgius Agricola Saalfeld, D-Saalfeld

MAGENS, M.
Abt. Transfusionsmed., Transplantationsimmunologie, Universitätskrankenhaus Eppendorf, D-Hamburg

MALY, J., Dr.
FN Hradec Kralove, Interne Clinic - Hematology, CZ-Hradec Kralove

MANNHALTER, CH., Frau Prof. Dr.
Klinisches Inst. für Med. und Chem. Labordiagnostik, A-Wien

MARBY, P., Frau Dr.
Kinderklinik und Ambulanz, Städtisches Klinikum Dessau, D-Dessau

MAREK, R., Dr.
Wiener Gebietskrankenkasse, A-Wien

MARSMANN, G., Dr.
Arzt für Kinderheilkunde, D-Varel

MARTINKOVÁ, I., Frau Prim. Dr.
odd. Hematologie, Fakultni nemocnice v Plzni, CZ-Plzen-Bory

MARX, G., Dr.
Gerinnungslabor, Chirurgische Klinik, Universitätskrankenhaus Eppendorf,
D-Hamburg

MÄRZ, M., Frau
Abt. Transfusionsmed., Transplantationsimmunologie,
Universitätskrankenhaus Eppendorf, D-Hamburg

MATERN, H., Dr.
D-Münster

MATYSKOVA, M., Frau Dr.
Dept. of Hematology, II. Interni Klinika, CZ-Brno

MATZDORF, A., Dr.
Abt. für Hämatologie und Onkologie, Zentrum für Innere Med./Klinikum
der Justus-Liebig-Universität, D-Gießen

MAURER, M., Prof. Dr.
D-Bernau/Chiemsee

MEDGYESSY, I., Frau Dr.
Vertranszfuzios Központ, H-Debrecen

MEILI, E.O., Frau Dr.
Gerinnungslabor, Abt. Innere Med., Universitätsspital, CH-Zürich

MIHAILOV, D., Dr., Frau
Clinica I-a Pediatrie, University of Medicine, R-Timisoara

MINGERS, A.-M., Frau Prof. Dr.
D-Würzburg/Lengfeld

MÖBIUS, D., Frau Dr.
Kinderklinik und Kinderpoliklinik, C.-Thiem-Klinikum, D-Cottbus

MOHREN, M., Dr.
Abt. Innere Med. II, Klinikum der Eberhard-Karls-Universität, D-Tübingen

MONDORF, W., Dr.
Praxis und Labor zur Diagnostik und Therapie, D-Frankfurt/Main

MORGENSCHWEIS, K., Dr.
Abt. Anästhesie, Kreiskrankenhaus Mechernich, D-Mechernich

MÖSSELER, J., Dr.
Arzt für Kinderheilkunde, D-Dillingen

MUNTEAN, E., Prof. Dr.
Universitäts-Kinderklinik, A-Graz

MUSS, N., Dr.
Facharzt für Innere Medizin, A-Salzburg

NAGY A., Dr., Frau
1st Dept. of Internal Med., Med. University of Pécs, H-Pécs

NAGY Z., Dr.
Semmelweis Kórhárz, II. Belosztály, H-Miskolc

NEIDHARDT, B., Dr.
Abt. für Transfusionsmed., Chirurgische Universitätsklinik, D-Erlangen

NIEKRENS, C., Frau Dr.
Kinderklinik, Städtische Krankenanstalten, D-Delmenhorst

NIENHAUS, K., Dr.
Chirurgische Intensivstation, Universitätskliniken des Saarlandes, D-Homburg

NIMTZ, A., Frau Dr.
Klinik für Kinder- und Jugendmed., Klinikum Frankfurt/Oder, D-Frankfurt/Oder

NOHE, N., Frau
Kinderklinik im Dr. von Hauner'schen Kinderspital
der Ludwig-Maximilians-Universität, D-München

OLDENBURG, J., Dr.
Inst. für Humangenetik, Biozentrum, Universität Würzburg, D-Würzburg

PABINGER, I., Frau Prof. Dr.
Universitätsklinik für Innere Med. I, A-Wien

PECHLANER, CH., Dr.
Gerinnungslaboratorium, Universitätsklinik für Innere Med., A-Innsbruck

PHILIPP, S., Frau Dr.
Deutsche Angestellten Krankenkasse (DAK), D-Hamburg

PILLKAHN, R., Frau Dr.
Abt. Hämatologie, Med. Klinik I, Waldklinik GmbH, D-Gera

PINDUR, G., PD Dr.
Abt. Klin. Hämostaseologie und Transfusionsmedizin,
Universitätskliniken des Saarlands, D-Homburg

PLENDL, H., Dr.
Inst. für Humangenetik, Klinikum der Christian-Albrechts-Universität, D-Kiel

POEK, KL.
Deutsche Hämophiliegesellschaft, D-Berlin

POLLMANN, H., Dr.
Abt. für Hämostaseologie, Kinderklinik Med. Einrichtungen
der Westfälischen Wilhelms-Universität, D-Münster

PROHASKA, W., Dr.
Inst. für Laboratoriums- und Transfusionsmed.,
Herzzentrum Nordrhein-Westfalen, D-Bad Oeynhausen

RAGER, K., PD Dr.
Kinderklinik, Caritas-Krankenhaus, D-Bad Mergentheim

RAMSCHAK, H., Doz. Dr.
I. Med. Universitätsklinik, A-Graz

RASCHE, H., Prof. Dr.
Med. Klinik I, Zentralkrankenhaus St-Jürgen-Str., D-Bremen

RAUCH, R., Dr.
Kinderklinik mit Poliklinik der Universität Erlangen-Nürnberg, D-Erlangen

REDDEMANN, H., Prof. Dr.
Verein zur Unterstützung krebskranker Kinder und Krebsforschung
im Kindesalter, D-Greifswald

RIES, M., PD Dr.
Kinderklinik mit Poliklinik der Universität Erlangen-Nürnberg, D-Erlangen

ROCKSTROH, J., Dr.
Med. Klinik, Med. Einrichtung der Rheinischen Friedrich-Wilhelms-
Universität, D-Bonn

ROMMEL, F., Dr.
Abt. Hämostaseologie, Med. Klinik Innenstadt der Ludwig-Maximilians-
Universität, D-München

ROSCHITZ, B., Dr., Frau
Universitäts-Kinderklinik, A-Graz

ROTTMANN, M., Dr.
Med. Klinik, Städt. Kliniken Dortmund, D-Dortmund

RUES, S., Frau
Kurpfalzkrankenhaus Heidelberg und Hämophiliezentrum gGmbH,
D-Heidelberg

SCHARRER, I., Frau Prof. Dr.
Zentrum der Inneren Medizin, Hämophilieambulanz,
Klinikum der J.-W.-Goethe-Universität, D-Frankfurt/Main

SCHEEL, H., Dr.
Klinische Hämostaseologie, Med. Klinik und Poliklinik I, Universität Leipzig,
D-Leipzig

SCHEEL-WALTER, H. Dr.
Abt. Hämatologie und Onkologie, Universitäts-Kinderklinik, D-Tübingen

SCHEIRING, H., Dr.
Tiroler Gebietskrankenkasse, A-Innsbruck

SCHELLE, G.
IGH, D-Bonn

SCHIMPF, KL., Prof. Dr.
D-Heidelberg

SCHMANDT, S., Frau Dr.
Abt. für Transfusionsmed., Med. Einrichtungen der Heinrich-Heine-Universität,
D-Düsseldorf

SCHMELTZER, B., Frau Dr.
Ärztin für Kinderheilkunde, D-Potsdam

SCHMID, L., Dr.
Inst. für klin. Chemie und Hämatologie, Kantonsspital, CH-St.Gallen

SCHMIDT, I., Dr.
Paul-Ehrlich-Institut, Bundesamt für Sera und Impfstoffe, D-Langen/Hess.

SCHMIDT, O., Dr.
Tagesklinik für Angiologie und Phlebologie, D-Magdeburg

SCHMITT, K., Prim. Dr.
Kinder- und Infektionsabteilung, Landes-Kinderkrankenhaus, A-Linz

SCHMUTZLER, R., Prof. Dr.
D-Wuppertal

SCHRAMM, K., Frau, cand. med.
D-München

SCHRAMM, W., Prof. Dr.
Abt. Hämostaseologie, Med. Klinik Innenstadt der Ludwig-Maximilians-
Universität, D-München

SCHRÖDER, J.
Inst. für Humangenetik, Biozentrum, Universität Würzburg, D-Würzburg

SCHULTE-OVERBERG, U., Frau Dr.
Kinderklinik, Campus Virchow Klinikum, D-Berlin

Schulz, M., Frau Dr.
Abt. Blutspende- und Transfusionsmed. der Ernst-Moritz-Arndt-Universität,
D-Greifswald

SCHWAAB, R., Dr.
Inst. für Exp. Hämatologie und Transfusionsmed. der Universität Bonn, D-Bonn

SCHWARZ, R., Dr.
Landeskinderklinik, A-Linz

SCHWARZ, H., Frau Dr.
Kinderklinik, Klinikum Suhl gGmbH, Südthüringen, D-Suhl

SEITZ, H., Dr.
Abt. Hämatologie und Transfusionsmed., Paul-Ehrlich-Institut, D-Langen/Hess.

SEITZ, R., Prof. Dr.
Abt. Hämatologie und Transfusionsmed. Paul-Ehrlich-Institut, D-Langen/Hess.

SERBAN, M., Frau Dr.
Clinica I-a Pediatrie, University of Medicine, R-Timisoara

SEUSER, A., Dr.
Kaiser-Karl-Klinik, Fachklinik für Orthopädie, D-Bonn

SEVERIN, TH., Dr.
Abt. Hämatologie und Hämostaseologie,
Kinderklinik/Klinikum der Albert-Ludwigs-Universität, D-Freiburg

SIEGEMUND, A., Frau Dr.
Inst. für Klin. Chemie, Gerinnungslabor Inn. Med., Universität Leipzig, D-Leipzig

SIEMENS, H.-J., Dr.
Hämatologie-Labor, Klinik für Innere Med. II, Med. Universität zu Lübeck,
D-Lübeck

SIEMENSEN, M., Frau
Abt. Transfusionsmed., Transplantationsimmunologie,
Universitätskrankenhaus Eppendorf, D-Hamburg

SILLER, M.
Berlin

SIRB, H., Dr.
Klinik für Kinder- und Jugendmed., Heinrich-Braun-Krankenhaus, D-Zwickau

STENSZKY, V., Frau Doz. Dr.
Vertransfuzios Központ, H-Debrecen

STIGENDAL, L, Dr.
Koagulationscentrum, Sahlgrensk Sjukhuset, S-Gothenburg

STREIF, W., Dr.
Universitätsklinik für Kinderheilkunde, A-Innsbruck

STOLZ, P.
D-München

SUBERT, R., Frau Dr.
Abt. für Hämatologie und Onkologie, Klinik für Innere Medizin II,
Klinikum Schwerin, D-Schwerin

SULOVSKA, I., Frau Dr.
Hämatologische Klinik, Fakultäts-Krankenhaus, CZ-Olomouc

SUTOR, A., H., Prof. Dr.
Abt. Hämatologie und Hämostaseologie, Kinderklinik,
Klinikum der Albert-Ludwigs-Universität, D-Freiburg

SYRBE, G., PD Dr.
Innere Abt., Landesfachkrankenhaus Stadtroda, D-Stadtroda

THÜRMEL, K., Dr.
Abt. Hämostaseologie, Med. Klinik Innenstadt der Ludwig-Maximilians-
Universität, D-München

TIMR, P., Dr.
Children's Dept., Nemocnice Ceske Budejovice, CZ-Ceske Budejovice

TOURANI, S., Dr.
Abt. Transfusionsmed., Transplantationsimmunologie,
Universitätskrankenhaus Eppendorf, D-Hamburg

TÜRK-KRAETZER, B., Frau Dr.
Ärztin für Kinderheilkunde, D-Oldenburg

ULSENHEIMER, K., Prof. Dr.
D-München

UNKRIG, CH., Dr.
Med. Universitäts-Poliklinik, D-Bonn

VAHLENSIECK, U., Frau Dr.
Abt. Hämatologie und Transfusionsmed., Paul-Ehrlich-Institut, D-Langen/Hess.

VAN DEN BERG, M., Frau Dr.
Van Creveld Clinic, Academisch Ziekenhuis, NL-Utrecht

VIGH, TH.
Zentrum der Inneren Medizin, Hämophilieambulanz,
Klinikum der J.-W.-Goethe-Universität, D-Frankfurt/Main

VOERKEL, W., Dr.
Gemeinschaftspraxis für Labormed., Mikrobiologie, Transfusionsmed., D-Leipzig

VOGT, B., Frau
Abt. für ambulante und soziale Pädiatrie, Universitäts-Kinderklinik Leipzig,
D-Leipzig

VON DEPKA PRONDZINSKI,
Abt. Hämophilie, Med. Poliklinik, Med. Hochschule Hannover, D-Hannover

VONDRYSKA, F., Dr.
Czech Hemophilia Society, CZ-Praha

VORLOVA, Z., Frau Dr.
Inst. für Hämatologie und Bluttransfusion, CZ-Praha

WALLNY, TH., Dr.
Orthopädische Klinik, Med. Einrichtung der Rheinischen Friedrich-Wilhelms-
Universität, D-Bonn

WANK, H., Dr.
St.-Anna-Kinderspital, A-Wien

WATZKE, H., Prof.
Universitätsklinik für Innere Med. I, A-Wien

WEILANDT, M., Frau
Abt. Transfusionsmed., Transplantationsimmunologie,
Universitätskrankenhaus Eppendorf, D-Hamburg

WEIPPERT-KRETSCHMER, M., Dr.
Abt. Transfusionsmed. und Gerinnungsphysiologie,
Klinikum der Philipps-Universität, D-Marburg

WEISSBACH, G., Prof. Dr.
Klinikum Bavaria Zscheckwitz, Rehabilitationszentrum für Kinder
und Jugendliche, D-Kreischa

WEISS, J.
Österr. Hämophiliegesellschaft, A-Wien

WELTERMANN, DR.
Universitätsklinik für Innere Med. I, A-Wien

WENDISCH, J., Dr.
Klinik und Poliklinik für Kinderheilkunde,
Universitätsklinikum Carl-Gustav-Carus, D-Dresden

WENDISCH, E., Dipl.-med., Frau
D-Dresden

WENK, S., Frau
Abt. Transfusionsmed., Transplantationsimmunologie,
Universitätskrankenhaus Eppendorf, D-Hamburg

WENZEL, E., Prof. Dr.
Abt. Klin. Hämostaseologie und Transfusionsmed.,
Universitätskliniken des Saarlandes, D-Homburg

WERMES, C., Frau Dr.
Abt. Hämophilie/Med. Poliklinik, Med. Hochschule Hannover, D-Hannover

WOLF, H.-H., Dr.
Klinik und Poliklinik für Innere Med. IV, Med. Fakultät,
Martin-Luther-Universität Halle-Wittenberg, D-Halle

WOLF, K., Dipl.-Med.
Klinik f. Innere Medizin, Krankenhaus Küchwald, Klinikum Chemnitz,
D-Chemnitz

WOLLINA, K., Frau Dr.
Klinik Inn. Med. II, Friedrich-Schiller-Universität, D-Jena

WULFF, K., Frau Dr.
Inst. für Humangenetik, Med. Fakultät der Ernst-Moritz-Arndt-Universität,
D-Greifswald

WYSS, M., Frau Prof. Dr.
Hôpital de la Tour, Service de pédiatrie, CH-Meyrin

ZEGNER, M., Frau
Hämophilieambulanz, Universitätsklinik für Innere Med. I, A-Wien

ZEITLER, P., Dr., Frau
Kinderklinik und Poliklinik der Julius-Maximilians-Universität, D-Würzburg

ZELLHOFER
Österr. Hämophiliegesellschaft, A-Wien

ZHANG, W.W., Dr.
GenStar Therapeutics/UroGen Corp., San Diego, CA, USA

ZIMMERMANN, R., Prof. Dr.
Kurpfalzkrankenhaus Heidelberg und Hämophilie-Zentrum gGmbH,
D-Heidelberg

ZÖHRER, B., Frau Dr.
Hämostaseologie, Universitäts-Kinderklinik, A-Graz

I. HIV Infection and Epidemiology in Hemophilia

Chairmen:

I. PABINGER (Vienna)
R. SEITZ (Langen)

Causes of Death and AIDS-Related Disease in Hemophilia Patients in Germany (Inquiries 1999)

W. Schramm, H. Krebs, S. Fleissner
for the GTH Hemophilia Commission

Basis of Inquiries

In 1983, Prof. Landbeck started an annual inquiry about causes of death and AIDS-related disease in the former West Germany. The questionnaires focused on the date of infection, the outbreak of AIDS, the diagnosis of AIDS-defining diseases, and the cause of death, if it occurred.

Since the year 1998, data about hepatitis, cause of death of non-HIV-infected patients with hemophilia, and information about antiretroviral therapies have also been gathered.

In future, this inquiry will be supported by data from the German Hemophilia Registry of the GTH Hemophilia Commission.

Participating Centers

From the beginning of the inquiry, the number of participating centers increased each year, especially after 1991 when hemophilia-treating centers of the former East Germany started to take part. Today these centers contribute significant data to the inquiry (see Fig. 1). Fortunately, in the year 1999, the number of reporting centers again slightly increased to 126, compared to 108 in 1998 (see Table 1). The overall number of reported patients this year has decreased from 6353 to 4507.

Table 1. Numbers of participating hemophilia centers

	1991	1992	1993	1994	1995	1996	1997	1998	1999
East	47	62	79						
West	18	18	24						
Total	65	80	103	111	119	119	104*	108*	126*

*Including 33 centers, whose patients have died.

I. Scharrer/W. Schramm (Ed.)
30th Hemophilia Symposium Hamburg 1999
© Springer-Verlag Berlin Heidelberg 2001

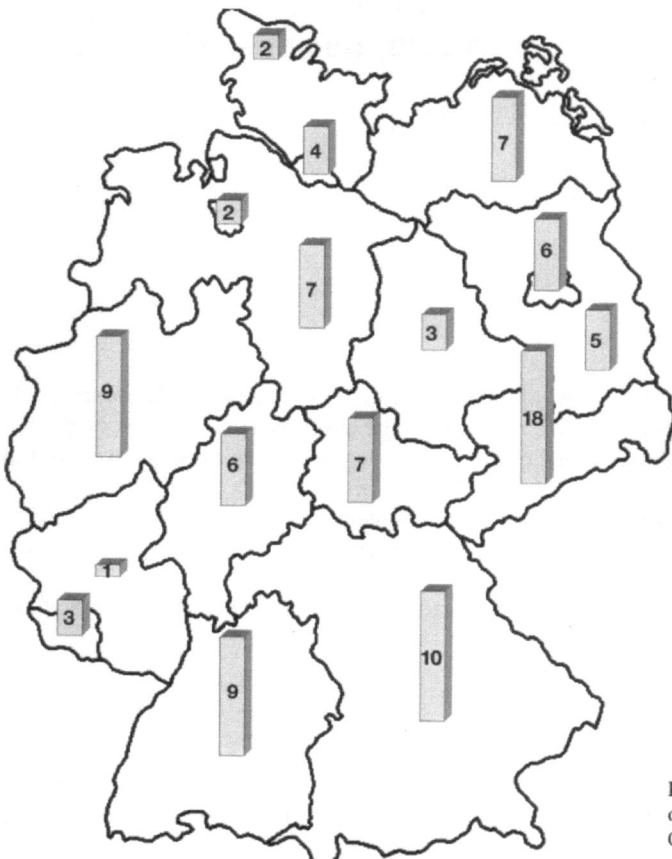

Fig. 1. Distribution
of reporting centers in
Germany

Patients

In 1999, 4507 patients with hemophilia (including possible duplicates) were reported by the participating centers (see Table 2). Of them, 1260 patients were

Table 2. Patients with hemophilia in Germany, including deceased (1999)

| | Anti-HIV-positive | | Anti-HIV-negative | | Total | |
	n	%	n	%	n	%
Alive	689	15.3	3176	70.5	3865	85.8
Died of AIDS	408	9.1	–	–	408	9.1
Died of other causes	163	3.6	71	1.6	234	5.2
Total deaths	571	12.7	71	1,6	642	14.2
Total	1260	28.0	3247	72.0	4507	100

HIV-infected, corresponding to 28.0%. A total of 642 patients died in 1999, 408 of AIDS, corresponding to 63.6%. Of all registered patients with hemophilia, 84.3% could be classified as hemophilia A, 15.7% as hemophilia B (Fig. 2). The factor activity in 54.3% of the patients was below 2%, in 35.3% of patients it was higher than 2%. Of all patients with hemophilia, 15.7% were HIV-infected, in contrast to 0.4% of the patients with vWJ syndrome (Fig. 3). To date, 8.1% of the patients with hemophilia (57) and 18.2% with vWJ syndrome (2) have fallen ill with AIDS (Table 3).

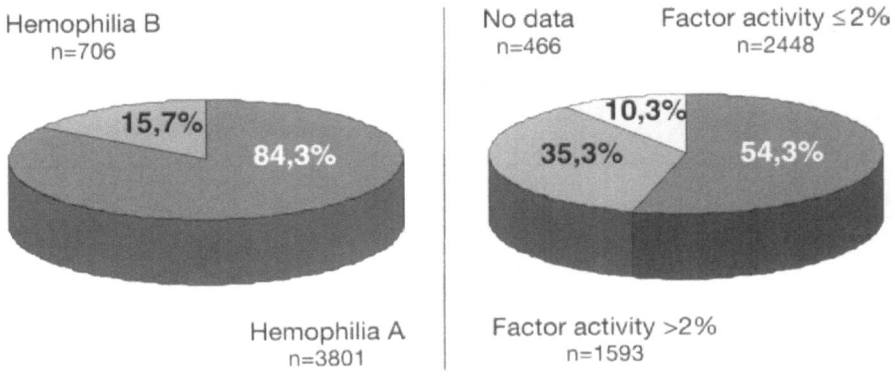

Fig. 2. Distribution and severity of illness of patients with hemophilia (*n*=4507)

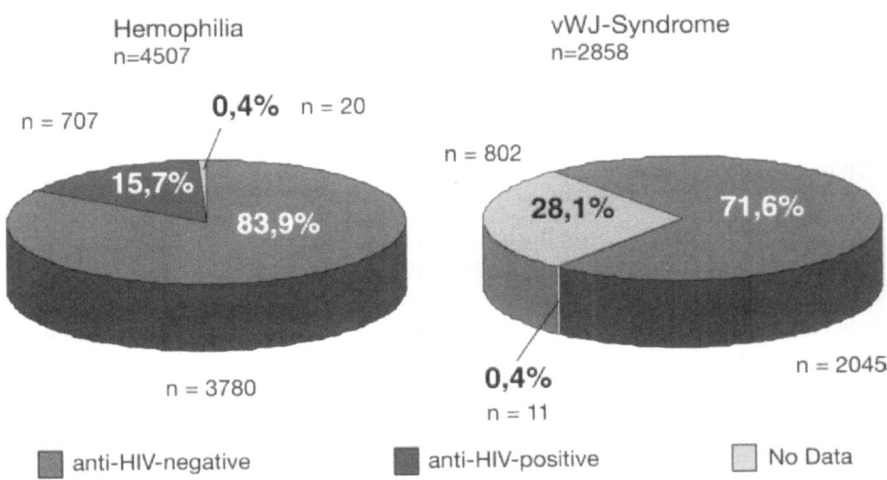

Fig. 3. HIV status of patients with hemophilia and vWJ syndrome

Table 3. 1999 aggregated data of 106 centers

	Hemophilia A		Hemophilia B		Hemophilia total		vWJ syndrome	
Total	3801		706		4507		2858	
Factor activity ≤2%	2088	54.9%	360	51.0%	2448	54.3%	739	25.9%
Factor activity >2%	1285	33.8%	308	43.6%	1593	35.3%	2009	70.3%
No data	428	11.3%	38	5.4%	466	10.3%	110	3.8%
Inhibitor low	73	1.9%	7	1.0%	80	1.8%		
Inhibitor high	109	2.9%	11	1.6%	120	2.7%		
		95.2%		97.5%	4307	95.6%		
HIV negative	3166	83.3%	614	87.0%	3780	83.9%	2045	71.6%
HIV positive total	626	16.5%	81	11.5%	707	15.7%	11	0.4%
No data	9	0.2%	11	1.6%	20	0.4%	802	28.1%
No AIDS	263	42.0%	51	63.0%	314	44.4%	7	63.6%
CD4 <200	198	31.6%	17	21.0%	215	30.4%	2	18.2%
AIDS	50	8.0%	7	8.6%	57	8.1%	2	18.2%
No data	115	18.4%	6	7.4%	121	17.1%	0	0.0%

Causes of Death

Contemplating the annual causes of death, it is striking that the formerly most frequent causes of death, such as cirrhosis and bleeding, are of only secondary importance in anti-HIV-positive patients. Up to 1995 a perpetual increase of AIDS deaths
was encountered; however, the number of patients dying of AIDS is regressing since
then. The main reason for this may be improved therapy methods. Nevertheless,
AIDS is the most frequent cause of death in the observation period. In contrast, the
number of patients dying of liver disease is evenly increasing since 1998 (Figs. 4, 6).

Comparing the causes of death of anti-HIV-positive with anti-HIV-negative
patients with hemophilia, there is, apart from AIDS, a significant difference in the
number of patients dying of liver disease. Bleeding as a cause of death is almost
equal in both groups. The lower rate of cancer in the anti-HIV-positive group is still
recognizable (Fig. 5).

GTH Hemophilia Registry

The German Society of Thrombosis and Hemostasis (GTH) intended to establish a
central register accessible to all German centers treating patients with bleeding disorders. The goal was the invention of a suitable and easy-to-use system for acqui-
ring and analyzing epidemiologic data about diseases in context with bleeding disorders. In addition, attending infections such as HIV and hepatitis had to be regarded. The register is basically made up of the annual statistics on the cause of
death in patients with bleeding disorders, and has been established in Germany
since 1983.

A unique center code, personal data, age and gender, type of illness, and auxili-
ary information about infections (HIV and hepatitis), inhibitors, and average data

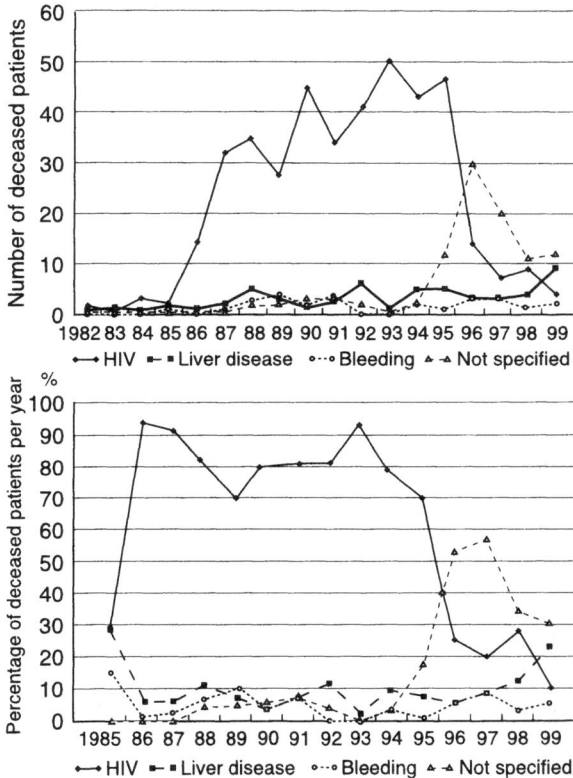

Fig. 4. Causes of death of patients with hemophilia

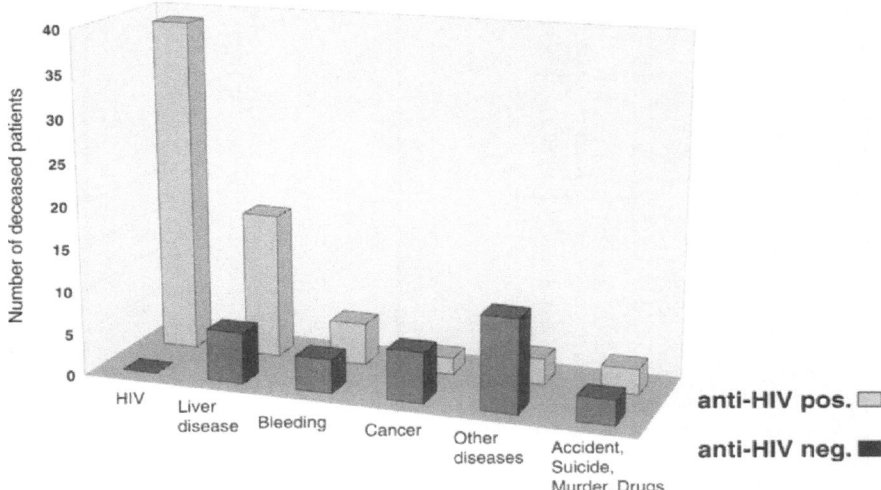

Fig. 5. Comparison of causes of death (10/1995–9/1999) of anti-HIV-positive and anti-HIV-negative patients (n=86)

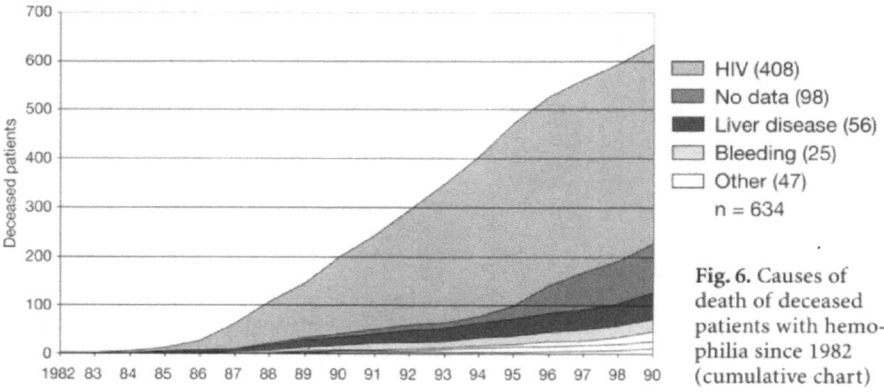

Fig. 6. Causes of death of deceased patients with hemophilia since 1982 (cumulative chart)

about consumption of blood products are entered. This information forms the basic data pool for successive studies concerning clinical, social, and economic questions. An insularity network (intranet) is used for electronic communication among the participating centers. Thereby, problems with paper-based data gathering are avoided, as are errors filling in questionnaires or transferring data into databases, which frequently occurred in former studies. Additionally, redundant efforts are eliminated by using electronic input, cutting down time consumption and therefore reducing overall costs. A modern Java-based WEB application was developed in cooperation with the Deutsches Gesundheitsnetz (D/G/N), which allows through

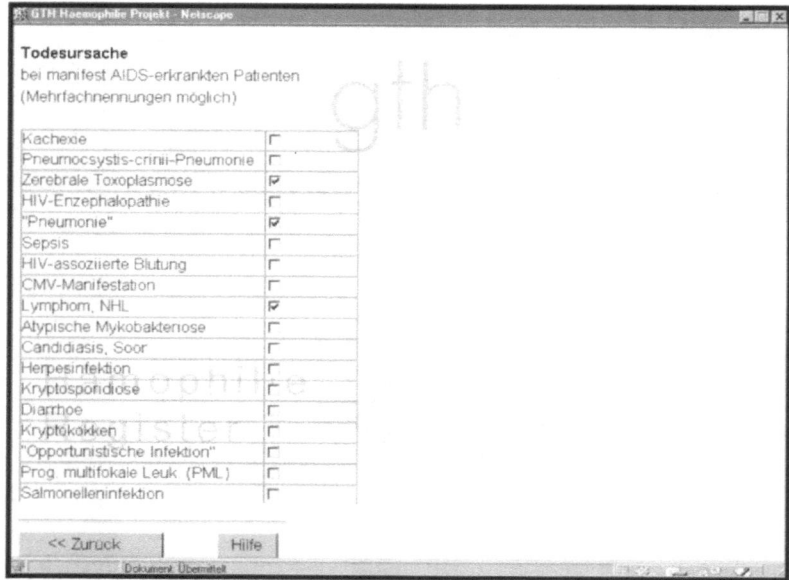

Fig. 7. Example input-mask of the GTH Hemophilia Registry

electronic data input using an usual WEB browser and proprietary cipher software (Fig. 7). The participating centers use remote data transmission to log on to a central server. Successive data entry is done online using a convenient graphical user interface (GUI). After a concluding confirmation, data are saved in a relational database. On the other hand, simple queries can be made to receive global data. A high level of data security is assured by a restricted access mechanism to the intranet using unique PINs and memory cards. Patient data are anonymized and scrambled using secure encoding. The definitive network was implemented at the beginning of 2000. Data entry began immediately thereafter, so at present, detailed data are already available on our database. Additional features, such as comfortable data im- and export are planned for subsequent versions of the software. Also, extending the system to other European countries might be possible in future. The initiators expect a distinct improvement of epidemiologic knowledge for prospective decisions regarding enhanced therapy of patients with bleeding disorders and subsequent cost cuts. By establishing this registry, we hope to reach an additional improvement of completeness and validity of data.

Acknowledgements. Peter Heidemann, Astrid Guekow, Augsburg; Schlimok, Linné, Augsburg; K. Rager, Bad Mergentheim; Lothar Hempelmann, Berlin; Günter Henze, Frau U. Schulte Overberg-Schmidt, Berlin; Christiane Beck, Dorothea Kroll, Berlin; Ch. Heinrichs, Frau Stumpe, Berlin; H. Koop, M. Klare, Berlin; H. Kiesewetter, Koscielny, Berlin; H.-H. Brackmann, Bonn; Wolfgang Eberl, Braunschweig; G. Auerswald, Bremen; Holzhüter, Bremen; H. Leithäuser, Celle; F. Fiedler, Kerstin Wolf, Chemnitz; Klaus Hofmann, Chemnitz; J. Oppermann, Elisabeth Holfeld, Dagmar Möbius, Cottbus; Johann Böhmann, Claudia Niekrens, Delmenhorst; Joachim Mößeler, Dillingen; Wolfgang Kotte, Heiner Güldenring, Dresden; Jörg Wendisch, Dresden; Heiner Trobisch, Duisburg; U. Göbel, Lex, Düsseldorf; G. Vogel, Frau Winterstein, Erfurt; Jens Klinge, M. Girisch, Erlangen; R. Eckstein, Erlangen; Christian Klinkenstein, Frankfurt (Oder); Frau I. Scharrer, Frankfurt/Main; W. Kreuz, Klarmann, Frankfurt/Main; W. Mondorf, Frankfurt/M; Antje Nimtz, Frankfurt/Oder; A.H. Sutor, Barbara Ziegler, Freiburg; R. Mertelsmann, Karola Hasler, Freiburg; Pralle, PD Bettina Kemkes-Matthes, Giessen; G. Berger, Wilke (I Med), Doris Joachim, Görlitz; Rosemarie Schobeß, Halle-Wittenberg/S; Anatol Kurme, Burkhard Pauka, D.K. Hossfeld, Barbara Eifrig, Hamburg; Rolf Kuse, Wittkowsky, Hamburg; Schneppenheim, N. Muenchow, Hamburg; L. Balleisen, Hamm; A. Ganser, M. von Depka, Hannover; K. Welte, C. Wermes, Hannover; Rainer Zimmermann, Heidelberg; E. Wenzel, Pindur, Homburg/Saar; F.C. Sitzmann, Gerd Dockter, Annegret Seider, Homburg/Saar; F. Zintl, Karim Kentouche, Jena; K. Höffken, K. Wollina, Fricke, Jena; Hirschmann, Frau B. Eggeling, Kassel; U.R. Fölsch, H.D. Bruhn, Kiel; Eckhard Lechler, Köln (Lindenthal); Mario Koksch, Leipzig; Harald Lenk, Leipzig; H. J. Siemens, Lübeck; Peter Hellstern, Ludwigshafen; R. Herbert, Lüneburg; D. Franke, Magdeburg; Uwe Mittler, von Aumann, Magdeburg; Volker Kretschmer, Monika Weippert, Marburg; K.U. Freiberger, K. Morgenschweis, Mechernich; Karin Kurnik, München; W. Schramm, Franz Rommel, München; H. Pollmann, Sr. Heike, Münster; C. G. Lipinski, J. Weisser, Neckargemünd; R. Arndt, Neubrandenburg; B. Berthold, Neubrandenburg; Jürgen Drescher, Oldenburg; Th.

Wüst, Pforzheim; M. Karl, Maria Anstadt, Plauen; R. Pasold, Potsdam; Beate Schmeltzer, Potsdam-Drewitz; Prof. Andreesen, Karl Huber, Regensburg; H. Konrad, Rostock; I. Richter; Ulrike Kyank, Rostock; M. Freund, O. Anders, Rostock; Bernhard Maak, Saalfeld; P.C. Clemens, R. Schumacher, Schwerin; Rita Subert, Schwerin; F.J. Göbel, Siegen; Osswald, Singen (Hohentwiel); Günter Syrbe, Schw. M.Stephan, Schw. H. Hädrich, Stadtroda; H. Edelmann, Heidrun Schwarz, Suhl; D. Niethammer, H. Scheel-Walter, Tübingen; L. Kanz, Jaschonek, M. Mohren, Tübingen; Debatin, W. Behnisch, Ulm; Dieter Böttcher, Wuppertal; F. Keller, U. Geisen, Würzburg; Speer, Petra Zeitler, Würzburg; Richter, Zella Mehlis; G. Schott, Ute Kreibich, Zwickau; Nentwich, Helga Gräbner, Zwickau

II. Gene Therapy in Hemophilia

Chairmen:

I. PABINGER (Vienna)
R. SEITZ (Langen)

Genotype–Phenotype Correlation in Hemophilia A

J. Graw, H.-H. Brackmann, J. Oldenburg, W. Schramm, R. Schwaab

Aim of the Study

Hemophilia is understood as a disturbance of the blood coagulation system and includes hemophilia A (factor VIII deficiency), hemophilia B (factor IX deficiency), and von Willebrand's disease (VWD). Because of limited resources, the project will concentrate on X-linked hemophilia A. The clinical phenotype of hemophilia A is highly variable, ranging from mild forms to very severe diseases including the formation of antibodies to exogenous factor VIII; substitution by exogenous factor VIII concentrates is the main form of medical treatment. In Germany, about 5800 patients are affected; the average cost for the treatment is about 100,000 DM per patient per year, totaling more than 500 million DM per year. Worldwide, only 20% of patients can be treated because of the expense of the therapy.

The aim of the study is to determine the genotype of all severe cases in Germany (about 3000 patients). Together with the present database of about 550 hemophilia A patients at the University of Bonn, new data allow the formation of an accurate hemophilia A register at the University of Munich. The study will correlate systematically the genotype of the mutation in the affected gene (*FVIII* gene) to:

1. The severity of the disease including the frequency and localization of bleeding episodes
2. The treatment regimen (on demand or prophylaxis, dosages, type of concentrate)
3. The orthopedic situation
4. The production of alloantibodies to factor VIII concentrates
5. The success rate of the immune tolerance therapy that is used to overcome the neutralizing activity of these inhibitors
6. The domains of the factor VIII molecule responsible for the antibody formation.

The data will provide the basis to define predictive parameters for inhibitor formation. This information is important for the pharmaceutical industry to improve their products with respect to an economically optimized therapy, to the formulation of less immunogenic factor VIII concentrates, and to the development of new therapeutic drugs for immune tolerance induction.

In this study, five groups at four institutes will cooperate connecting several national and international efforts in hemophilia A research in Germany. It opens the possibility for tremendous synergistic effects:

I. Scharrer/W. Schramm (Ed.)
30th Hemophilia Symposium Hamburg 1999
© Springer-Verlag Berlin Heidelberg 2001

1. The Institute of Experimental Hematology at the University of Bonn and the Medical Clinic at the University of Munich (LMU) offer their databases of long-lasting therapeutic experience in hemophilia A and combine them to the German hemophilia A register.
2. The already existing genotyping group at the Institute of Human Genetics of the University of Würzburg will be expanded.
3. A new hemophilia A genotyping unit will be established at the Institute of Mammalian Genetics of the GSF Research Center for Health and Environment (Neuherberg).
4. The Institute of Experimental Hematology at the University of Bonn uses this new technique of epitope screening of human anti-FVIII antibodies in hemophilia A patients with an actual inhibitor.

State of Research

Clinical Aspects of Hemophilia A

Hemophilia A is caused by decreased activity of blood coagulation factor VIII. The corresponding gene comprising 26 exons and 186 kb (9 kb coding sequence) is mapped at the X-chromosome (Xq28). Affected individuals develop a variable phenotype of hemorrhage into joints and muscles, easy bruising, and prolonged bleeding from wounds. The disorder is mainly caused by heterogeneous mutations in the *F8* gene (for details, see next chapter). The severity and frequency of bleeding in hemophilia A is inversely related to the amount of residual factor VIII (<2%, severe; 3–5%, moderate; and 6–30%, mild). The proportion of cases that are severe, moderate, and mild are about 50, 10, and 40%, respectively. The joints are frequently affected causing swelling, pain, decreased function, and degenerative arthritis. Similarly, muscle hemorrhage can cause necrosis, contractures, and neuropathy by entrapment. Intracranial hemorrhage, while uncommon, can occur after even mild head trauma and lead to severe complications. Additionally, mortality due to ischemic heart disease is lower in hemophilia patients than in the general male population.

The symptomatic bleeding in hemophilia A is prevented by prophylactic or on-demand treatment with factor VIII concentrates that can be of plasma or recombinant origin. However, the most important complication that affects about 25% of hemophiliacs is the development of alloantibodies to substituted factor VIII (Scharrer and Neutzling 1993). These antibodies neutralize the therapeutic effect of factor VIII concentrates. Consequently, hemophiliacs with an inhibitor are prone to recurrent bleeding episodes and progressive joint damage. The only chance for these patients is the eradication of the inhibitor by the induction of immune tolerance to substituted factor VIII by application of high doses of factor VIII (Brackmann et al. 1996). After average treatment duration of about 15 months, a successful eradication of the inhibitor is achieved in around 80% of the patients. The treatment costs amount to more than 2 million DM/patient per year. This treatment regimen has been established on an empirical basis (Brackmann and Gormsen 1977). The mechanism of immune tolerance induction is still not understood and may depend on the production of anti-idiotypic antibodies (Gilles et al. 1996). In some patients, the success of inhibitor eradication depends on the type of factor VIII concentrate used, maybe on the content of von Willebrand's factor (vWF). It is speculated that vWF competes with the epitope on the factor VIII molecule that is affected by factor VIII antibodies. Moreover, it was shown recently that several factor VIII domains contain common inhibitory epitopes (Sawamoto et al. 1998; Zhong et al. 1998). However, mass spectrometric methods, which allow identifying stretches even of large proteins located at the surface, have not yet applied to factor VIII. With respect to the exorbitant costs of the immune tolerance induction therapy, there is an absolute need for solving the open questions regarding interaction of the applied drug, factor VIII concentrate, and the eradication of the anti-factor VIII antibodies.

Mutation Analysis in Hemophilia A

The heterogeneity of mutations and the size of the *FVIII* gene have made it difficult to determine all genetic defects in hemophilia A. Of the severe hemophiliac cases, 40–45% are caused by intron 22 inversions. Within the extremely long (32 kb) intron 22 of the *FVIII* gene, two other genes are located: *gene A* has the opposite orientation to the *FVIII* gene and exhibits high homology to sequences within exon 22 of the *FVIII* gene. Two additional copies of *gene A* are 500 kb upstream of the *FVIII* gene. A second gene (*gene B*) is also located within intron 22; splicing occurs together with exons 23–26 of the *FVIII* gene. A CpG island acts as bi-directional promotor for both, *gene A* and *B*. Both genes are expressed ubiquitously; their functions are still unknown (Levinson et al. 1990; Lakich et al. 1993).

The development of screening methods such as single-stranded conformational polymorphism (SSCP), chemical mismatch cleavage (CMC), and denaturing gradient gel electrophoresis (DGGE) provided efficient tools for an analysis of large genes like *FVIII*. Up to now, in the OMIM database, 266 alleles of the *FVIII* gene have been documented. Moreover, a database of nucleotide substitutions, deletions, insertions, and rearrangements was first published a few years ago (Tuddenham et al. 1991) and is routinely updated (HAMSTeRS: http://europium.csc.mrc.ac.uk).

A recent report (Antonarakis 1998) summarizes the molecular genetics of hemophilia A. The main part of severe hemophilia A is caused by inversions affecting intron 22 and the *FVIII-A* and *FVIII-B* genes (43%). Moreover, there are 270 different single-base substitutions described, about 45% of them reflect severe cases (80% produce a single amino-acid exchange, 14% a preliminary stop codon, and 6% affect the splice sites). 5 % of the severe cases are caused by a large deletion (>100 bp) leading to a significant level of development of antibodies against factor VIII concentrates. On the other hand, about 23% of the affected patients have a small deletion (<100 bp) within the *FVIII* gene; however, only 5% of the patients in this group form antibodies. Additionally, there are a few cases of sequence insertions, mainly where a stretch of A residues occur. Interestingly, these patients with small deletions/insertions at series of adenines show an unexpected mitigation of severe hemophilia A phenotype with almost no development of factor VIII inhibitors. This particular feature is caused by a »self correction« of the mutation, which is performed by additional failures during DNA replication/RNA transcription or »ribosomal frameshifting« at poly-A stretches restoring the original open-reading frame (Young et al. 1997; Oldenburg et al. 1998).

In Germany, mutation type profiles of about 550 hemophilia A patients were established at the universities of Bonn and Würzburg for non-severe and severe hemophilia A (Schwaab et al. 1995; Becker et al. 1996). In agreement with the worldwide database, almost all mutations in non-severe hemophilia A are missense mutations. In severe hemophilia A, the expected broad range of different mutations was found (inversions 40%, point mutations 35%, deletions 15%). However, in about 10–15% of patients the mutation was not detected, which might be due to an incomplete sensitivity of the screening methods (SSCP, DGGE, CMC) or to still unknown mechanisms leading to decreased factor VIII activity. However, most of these mutations are X-linked, leading to the suggestion that they occur at regions of the *FVIII* gene, which are not yet sequenced systematically. Moreover, one of the autosomal candidate genes which has to be considered is the gene encoding von Willebrand's factor. This gene is mapped to human chromosome 12p13.3, and contains 52 exons within 178 kb.

Inhibitors in Hemophilia A Treatment

The inhibitor incidence in patients with severe molecular defects is higher than for other types of mutations. A genetic predisposition to inhibitor development was proven, since inversions, large deletions, or nonsense mutations were associated with a 7–10-times higher inhibitor risk than less severe molecular defects as missense mutations and small deletions (Schwaab et al. 1995). However, there is no clear correlation possible to the affected domains in the FVIII protein. Moreover, no data are available on the impact of the parameter *FVIII* gene mutation and factor VIII epitope to the outcome (success rate, duration) of the cost-intensive immune tolerance induction therapy. In contrast, some alleles of the MHC class II system have been shown to increase risk of inhibitor formation, while others might be protective (Oldenburg et al. 1997). Other parameters such as antenatal exposure to maternal factor VIII, type of factor VIII concentrates used, and epitope characteristic of the factor VIII molecule in inhibitor patients are still in discussion. It is obvious that there must be further, non-genetic parameters because monozygotic twins have been reported with discordant inhibitor status. However, at present no sufficient data exist to answer these open questions.

Structure-Function Relationship of Altered Factor VIII Molecules

In the case of predicted single amino-acid substitutions, two categories of phenotypes are found:
1. Cases in which plasma factor VIII antigen is reduced concomitantly to activity: it might be a result of a coagulation-normal protein being either poorly expressed

or more rapidly cleared from the circulation than the wild-type form; however, the ways in which the substitutions produce this phenotype are unknown in all cases.

2. Approximately normal circulating levels of factor VIII antigen with reduced or absent factor VIII activity.

Unfortunately, the antibody status is only reported in a minority of the single amino-acid substitutions in the database. Therefore, only a few conclusions can be drawn up to now:

1. Mutations at or after critical Arg residues at thrombin cleavage sites have been shown to render the molecule resistant to thrombin activation resulting in reduced coagulation activity.
2. Mutation of a Tyr residue at the binding site for von Willebrand's factor is a frequently reported defect resulting in low plasma factor VIII antigen levels with even lower activity.
3. Mutations in I566T and M1772T result in two predicted new N-glycosylation sites, normal circulating antigen levels with grossly reduced or absent activity (HAMSTeRS 1999).

Scientific Approach of the Consortium

A schematic overview on the entire consortium is given in Fig. 1: Blood samples will be obtained from hemophilia A patients first by the clinics involved in this study (LMU Munich, Bonn, Würzburg) as well as clinics that are regional centers for hemophilia A therapy. As chairman of the Commission of Hemophilia of the German Society for Thrombosis and Hemostasis Research (GTH), Prof. Schramm (Munich) is responsible for the collection of blood samples and evaluable clinical data from the German hemophilia centers. All cases will be documented with respect to the severity of the disease, the remaining factor VIII activity, laboratory parameter, family history, treatment protocol (factor VIII concentrates used), clinical course, joint status, and inhibitor anamnesis.

Prof. Brackmann has established a mutation database at the Bonn Hemophilia Center; the phenotypic data include the severity of the disease, laboratory parameter, clinical course, joint status, inhibitor anamnesis, and factor VIII concentrates used. This information is registered for up to 20 years in an EDV-based system (IHIS, Interaktives Hämophilie Informations-System). Altogether, the complete phenotype data from a total of 800 patients from the Hemophilia Center Bonn, including 90 patients with an inhibitor anamnesis, are available. Blood from these patients has already been collected and will be investigated for the factor VIII genotype.

Blood samples will be sent to PD Dr. Oldenburg (Würzburg), and a back-up will be stored at Munich. Mutations within the *FVIII* gene will first be screened by SSCP, CMC, and DGGE procedures, and the mutation will be finally characterized by sequencing of the corresponding fragment. The Würzburg group has a database, currently comprising 500 hemophilia A patients, that is growing by

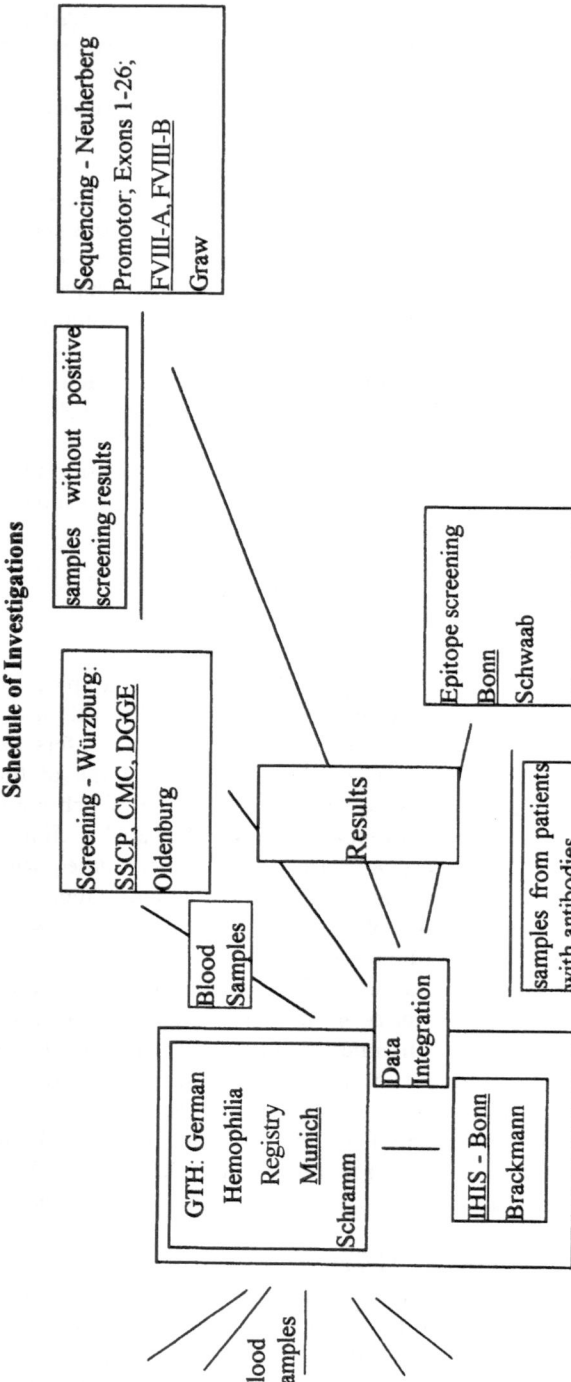

Fig. 1. The Hemophilia A Consortium within the German Human Genome Project. For details, refer to the main text

150–200 patients a year. Using the infrastructure established, the capacity of screening for mutations will be increased to 1000 patients per year.

In about 5–10% of cases, these applied methods are not sensitive enough to detect all the mutations. The corresponding samples (approximately 300 within 3 years) will be sent to Prof. Graw (Neuherberg). There, the entire *FVIII* gene including the flanking splice sites and the promoter will be amplified by PCR and sequenced. Genes *A* and *B* located within intron 22 as well as their upstream homologs will be included into the screening and sequencing program. Sequencing will be performed using a CEQ200 DNA Analysis System (Beckman) at the Genome Analysis Center within the GSF. Using the synergistic effect of the groups at Würzburg and Neuherberg, it will be possible to identify the mutations in all severely affected hemophilia A patients in Germany (about 3000 patients) within the given time period of 3 years, which allows a precise genotype–phenotype correlation. Moreover, this additional information concerning the regulation of *FVIII* gene expression, processing, or secretion is important for overcoming actual problems in the development of a somatic gene therapy of FVIII deficiency.

In parallel, samples from patients with antibodies against factor VIII concentrates will be given to PD Dr. Schwaab (Bonn) for epitope screening of human anti-factor VIII antibodies. Based upon the present data, we expect to identify about 10% of inhibitors (300 patients) within the total number of 3000 patients with severe hemophilia A. Comparison of the sequence analysis with the treatment schedules of the patients allows a correlation of the inhibitor status not only with the type of mutation (intron 22 inversion, point mutations, large deletions), but also with the domains of the protein affected by the mutation and the resulting alterations concerning the structure and stability of the FVIII protein. This information is important for the pharmaceutical industry for an optimized design of recombinant factor VIII in treatment of at least severe hemophilia A without adverse reactions. This could reduce the total amount of factor VIII and the costs for the health system.

Combined phenotypic and genotypic data of all patients investigated during this study will be centered in the German Hemophilia A Register by Prof. Schramm (Munich), and correlation between these sets of data will be calculated. A national hemophilia A register will be established combining the effort of the EDV-based system of the Bonn group and the existing database at Munich. Based upon the collected data, correlation analysis will be performed.

Perspectives and Scientific Impact of Systematic *FVIII* Mutation Analysis

There is an obvious need for a large-scale mutation analysis of *FVIII* mutations to correlate the site, size, and type of the mutation with remaining factor VIII activity, severity of disease, antibody production, and induction of immune tolerance. The expected results of the proposed study open the way for new strategies in the therapy of hemophilia A and for identifying potentially new drug targets. Moreover, new perspectives for somatic gene therapy might evolve. Furthermore, the know-how on the rapid identification of *FVIII* mutations allows application of the methods in genetic counseling. The results will be implemented into the regular updating of the HAMSTeRS database, and therefore be an important contribution to the global efforts for a systematic understanding of the molecular pathology of hemophilia A. In future, this kind of study might be extended also to other types of bleeding disorders, like hemophilia B or von Willebrand's disease.

Summary

Within the second phase of the German Human Genome Project, a series of investigations will be founded concerning a systematic genotype–phenotype correlation in hemophilia A in Germany. In particular, the hemophilia A phenotype will be correlated to the type of mutations, the affected domains in the factor VIII protein, and the production of alloantibodies. We expect to identify the genotype of all severe cases of hemophilia A in Germany within the next 3 years and to compare it with the individual treatment protocols. During this study, domains in the FVIII protein will be identified, which are mainly responsible for antibody production. The expected results of the proposed study open the way for new strategies in the therapy of hemophilia A. The project makes important contributions to our understanding of the efficacy of pharmaceutical active substances at genetically distinct targets. During the project, a large number of disease-associated alleles will be identified to avoid adverse reactions during therapy. This information is important for companies producing recombinant FVIII concentrates to allow an optimized design for novel recombinant factor VIII products.

Acknowledgements. The work is supported by the German Human Genome Project (01KW9905).

References

Antonarakis, S.E.: Molecular genetics of coagulation factor VIII gene and hemophilia A. Hemophilia 4 (1998, Suppl. 2), 1–11.
Becker, J., Schwaab, R., Möller-Taube, A., Schwaab, U., Schmidt, W., Brackmann, H.-H., Grimm, T., Olek, K., Oldenburg, J.: Characterization of the factor VIII defect in 147 patients with sporadic Hemophilia A: family studies indicate a mutation type-dependent sex ratio of mutation frequencies. Am. J. Hum. Genet. 58 (1996) 657–670.
Brackmann, H.-H., Gormsen, J.: Massive factor VIII infusion in hemophilic patients with factor VIII inhibitor. Lancet II (1977) 933.
Brackmann, H.-H., Oldenburg, J., Schwaab, R.: Immune tolerance for the treatment of factor VIII inhibitors – Twenty years »Bonn Protocol«. Vox Sang. 70 (1996, Suppl. 1) 30–35.
Fallaux, F.J., Hoeben, R.C.: Gene therapy for the hemophiliacs. Curr.Opin.Hematol. 3,1996,385–389.
Gilles, J.G., Desqueper, B., Lenk, H., Vermylen, J., Saint-Remy, J.M.: Neutralizing antiidiotypic antibodies to factor VIII inhibitors after in patients with hemophilia A. J. Clin. Invest. 97 (1996) 1382–1388.
HAMSTeRS: Review: The molecular pathology of Hemophilia A. http://europium.csc.ac.uk (last updated version: May 4, 1999).
Lakich, D., Kazazian, H.H., Antonarakis, S.E., Gitschier, J.: Inversions disrupting the factor VIII gene are a common cause of severe hemophilia A. Nat. Genet. 5 (1993) 236–241.

Levinson, B., Kenwrick, S., Lakich, D., Hammonds, G., Gitschier, J.: A transcribed gene in an intron of the human factor VIII gene. Genomics 7 (1990) 1–11.

Oldenburg, J., Picard, J.K., Schwaab, R., Brackmann, H.-H., Tuddenham, E.G.D., Simpson, E.: HLA genotype of patients with severe Hemophilia A due to intron 22 inversion with and without inhibitors of factor VIII. Thromb. Haemost. 77 (1997) 238–242.

Oldenburg, J., Schröder, J., Schmitt, C., Brackmann, H.-H., Schwaab, R.: Small deletion/insertion mutations within poly-A runs of the factor VIII gene mitigate the severe haemophilia A phenotype. Thromb. Haemost. 79 (1998) 452–453.

Sawamoto, Y., Prescott, R., Zhong, D., Saenko, E.L., Mauser-Bunschoten, E., Peerlinck, K., van den Berg, M., Scandella, D.: Dominant C2 domain epitope specificity of inhibitor antibodies elicited by a heat pasteurized product, factor VIII CPS-P, in previously treated hemophilia A patients without inhibitors. Thromb. Haemost. 79 (1998) 62–68.

Scharrer, I., Neutzling, O.: Incidence of inhibitors in hemophiliacs (Review). Blood Coag. Fibrinol. 4 (1993) 753–758.

Schwaab, R., Brackmann, H.H., Meyer, C., Seehafer, J., Kirchgesser, M., Haack, A., Olek, K., Tuddenham, E.G.D., Oldenburg, J.: Hemophilia A: mutation type determines risk of inhibitor formation. Thromb. Haemost. 74 (1995) 1402–1406.

Tuddenham, E.G.D. et mult. al.: Database of nucleotide substitutions, deletions, insertions and rearrangements of the factor VIII gene. Nucleic Acids Res. 19 (1991) 4821–4833.

Young, M., Inaba, H., Hoyer, L.W., Higuchi, M., Kazazian, H.H.jr., Antonarakis, S.E.: Partial correction of a severe molecular defect in hemophilia A, because of errors during expression of the factor VIII gene. Am. J. Hum. Genet. 60 (1997) 565–573.

Zhong, D., Saenko, E.L., Shima, M., Felch, M., Scandella, D.: Some human inhibitor antibodies interfere with factor VIII binding to factor IX. Blood 92 (1998) 136–142.

III. *Therapy of Hepatitis C*

Chairmen:

L. GÜRTLER (Greifswald)
E. LECHLER (Cologne)

Current Therapy of Hepatitis C Virus Infection

H.M. DIEPOLDER

Hepatitis C virus (HCV) was discovered 11 years ago as the principal cause of post-transfusion non-A–non-B hepatitis [2, 8]. Worldwide, about 3% or 150–200 million individuals are chronically infected with HCV. The prevalence in Europe and North America ranges from 0.5 to 3% [3]. Today, chronic hepatitis C accounts for 70% of cases of chronic hepatitis, and 20–40% of those will develop cirrhosis within 10–20 years after onset of disease [6, 14]. In cirrhotic patients the incidence of hepatocellular carcinoma is 1–4% per year [5]. In most Western countries, HCV-related liver disease is now the leading indication for liver transplantation.

Blood products were the major source of infection until efficient blood donor screening could be implemented in the early 1990s; subsequently, the risk of infection by blood products has dropped dramatically and is now estimated to be around 1:100,000 per unit of blood [15]. Nevertheless, due to the peak of new infections in the late 1980s and the typical lag period before complications arise from chronic hepatitis C, the number of new cases of HCV-related liver cirrhosis and other complications will continue to rise until 2010–2020 [4]. Available therapies may induce viral eradication in about a third of patients, and therefore it is a major public health goal to identify patients with chronic hepatitis C and to further improve current treatment strategies.

Diagnosis

Inexpensive and reliable ELISAs are available for the initial screening of patients. They may be false negative in the early phase of acute hepatitis C and in immuno-compromised and hemodialysis patients. In a low-risk population like blood donors the false positive rate may be up to 25%. In these patients, an immunoblot or Western blot should be performed. Eventually all patients testing positive for HCV antibodies or those who are suspected to be false negative should be tested qualitatively for HCV-RNA by RT-PCR. The quantitative determination of viral load as well as genotyping have no prognostic value regarding the natural course of disease but are important prognostic markers for the response to therapy. Therefore, viral load and genotype should be determined before the start of treatment [1].

I. Scharrer/W. Schramm (Ed.)
30th Hemophilia Symposium Hamburg 1999
© Springer-Verlag Berlin Heidelberg 2001

Screening

The prevalence of HCV infection in Western countries has been estimated to 1–3%. Only a minority of these patients know about their disease. Given the asymptomatic course of the disease over many years and the potential for serious complications like cirrhosis and liver cancer after several decades, identification and treatment of HCV-infected individuals is a major public health issue. Since population-wide screening is usually not feasible, the Centers of Disease Control in Atlanta have made the following recommendations for the USA [15]: screening should be offered to individuals who have ever injected illegal drugs, received clotting factor concentrates before 1990, are or were on hemodialysis, have abnormal liver function tests, or received a blood transfusion or organ transplant before 1992. Until detailed epidemiological data are available from Europe, it may be reasonable to extend these guidelines to most European countries.

Treatment

Due to a series of large multicenter studies, the interferon-α/ribavirin combination therapy has become the treatment of choice for treatment-naive patients (Fig. 1) [16, 18]. It consists of 3 MU interferon-α three times a week injected subcutaneously and 1000 mg or 1200 mg ribavirin (for body weight >75 kg) daily, given orally in two divided doses, for 6–12 months.

Major side effects of interferon-α are flu-like symptoms, depression, cytopenias, and tiredness, which are readily reversible once treatment is stopped. Persistent thyroid dysfunction, either hypo- or hyperthyroidism may occur, particularly in women with elevated pretreatment thyroid antibodies, and appropriate tests should

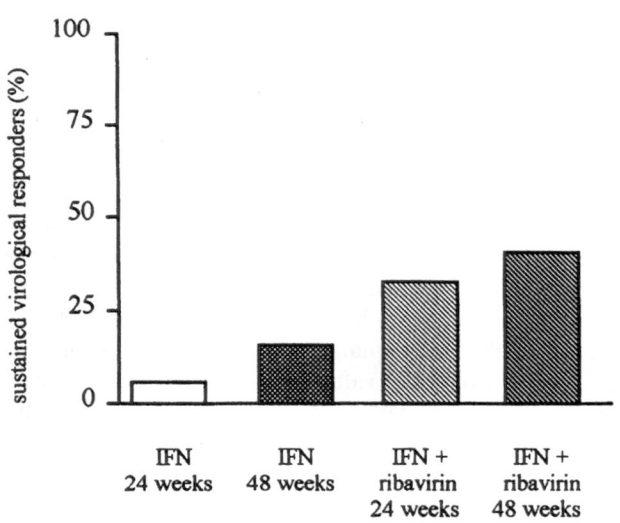

Fig. 1. Sustained virological response rates with interferon-α (*IFN*) alone for 24 or 48 weeks, or combination of IFN with ribavirin for 24 or 48 weeks. (Adapted from [18] and [16])

Table 1. Common side effects of interferon-α and ribavirin treatment

Side effect	Action
Flu-like symptoms	Paracetamol
Cardiac symptoms (chest pain, arrhythmias)	Stop medication
Depression	Psychiatric evaluation
Thyroid dysfunction	Treat appropriately
Anemia	
Hemoglobin <10 g/l	50% reduction of ribavirin dose
Hemoglobin <8.5 g/l	Stop ribavirin
With increased cardiac risk:	
hemoglobin drop >2 g/l	50% reduction of ribavirin dose
hemoglobin <12 g/l	Stop ribavirin
	Restart ribavirin after recovery at 50% of previous dose
Neutropenia	
<0.75 G/l	50% reduction of interferon-α dose
<0.5 G/l	Stop interferon-α
Thrombopenia	
<50 G/l	50% reduction of interferon-α dose
<30 G/l	Stop interferon-α

be performed during the course of treatment. Main side effects and the appropriate action are summarized in Table 1. The major side effect of ribavirin is dose-related hemolysis, which can occasionally be severe and may necessitate dose reduction or cessation of treatment (Table 1). Dangerous complications may occur in patients with preexisting heart disease, and special care should be taken with this patient group. Ribavirin is a highly teratogenic drug, and reliable contraception is mandatory during treatment and for 6 months after treatment has been completed.

Who Should Be Treated?

Chronic Hepatitis C – Treatment Naive

The decision to treat should take into account a series of variables, including age of the patient, general health, likelihood of response, and absolute or relative contraindications to interferon-α or ribavirin. In general, in the absence of contraindications (Table 2), patients who are symptomatic or young enough to have a significant risk of suffering HCV-related complications and have serological or histological evidence of hepatitis should be offered treatment. Patients with genotype 2 or 3 have a much higher rate of sustained response to treatment (60% vs 30% for genotype 1); nevertheless, the genotype should not lead to the denial of treatment.

»Healthy Carriers«

Patients for whom treatment probably offers little benefit are those with persistently normal aminotransferases. If a liver biopsy confirms the absence of inflammation

Table 2. Contraindications to interferon-α and ribavirin treatment

Interferon-α	Ribavirin
Absolute contraindications	
Present or past psychosis or severe depression	End-stage renal failure
Neutropenia or thrombopenia	Anemia
Organ transplantation except liver	Hemoglobinopathies
Symptomatic heart disease	Severe heart disease
Decompensated cirrhosis	Pregnancy
Uncontrolled seizures	No reliable method for contraception
Active alcoholism or drug abuse	
Relative contraindications	
Uncontrolled diabetes	Uncontrolled arterial hypertension
Autoimmune disorders, esp. thyroiditis	Old age

or shows only very mild inflammatory changes, these patients have a very low likelihood for disease progression. Also, the treatment response in this group is probably very low and presently only regular follow-up is recommended [21].

Relapsers and Non-Responders

Patients who have failed previous interferon monotherapy are candidates for combination therapy. The treatment response is good in patients who achieved a transient response to interferon monotherapy and relapsed after treatment was stopped. There is no clear recommendation for patients who did not respond at all to interferon monotherapy or did not achieve a sustained response after 12 months of combination therapy. Preferentially, these patients should be enrolled in clinical trials [7, 19, 20].

Acute Hepatitis C

The treatment of patients with acute hepatitis C is controversial due to the fact that a considerable number of patients who present with *symptomatic* acute hepatitis C spontaneously clear the virus (up to 50%). Before randomized studies are available, it may be a rational strategy to defer treatment for 3–4 months and treat only those patients with persistent viremia.

HIV Coinfection

The treatment of HIV-coinfected patients is problematic. HIV–HCV coinfection is frequent, and it is now clearly established that HCV infection is a more aggressive disease in patients with concomitant HIV infection. However, although treatment responses in HIV-infected patients with preserved immune function occur, the additive drug toxicities are frequently limiting.

These guidelines have recently been reviewed by a consensus panel of the European Association for the Study of the Liver (EASL) [1].

How Long Should Patients Be Treated?

Recent large multicenter trials have clearly answered this question. In patients with genotypes 2 or 3, regardless of viremia level, the duration of treatment is 6 months. In patients with genotype 1, the duration is also 6 months if the viremia level is below 2 million copies/ml. For highly viremic patients with genotype 1, treatment for 12 months is recommended [1, 16, 18].

When Should Treatment Be Stopped?

With interferon-α monotherapy, the absence of a virological response after 3 months was usually considered an indication to stop treatment. However, in combination treatment, as many as 10–15% of patients with detectable HCV-RNA at 3 months may nevertheless clear HCV-RNA after 6 months of treatment. Therefore, if side effects can be tolerated, treatment should be for 6 months before a patient is considered a non-responder [1, 6].

Monitoring During Treatment

Weekly monitoring of full blood counts including thrombocytes is recommended during the first 4 weeks. Thereafter, intervals can be extended to 4–6 weekly controls. Every 3 months, a thyroid function test should be performed. In combination treatment, HCV-RNA and liver function tests should be determined at 6 months, at the end of treatment, and 6 months after the treatment has been stopped. Interferon-α/ribavirin doses should be adjusted according to Table 1 [1, 6].

Future Therapies

Although up to 40% of patients with chronic hepatitis C can be cured with the current combination therapy, the majority cannot and the rate of response seems to be lower in those patients with the strongest indicators of disease progression, like fibrosis or early cirrhosis. New therapies are urgently required to prevent the threat of increasing HCV-related morbidity and mortality [4].

While different interferon-α subtypes or increased doses may not hold any promise for major improvement, the pegylated form of interferon-α, which has a longer half-life and requires only one injection per week, may improve the sustained response rate particularly in patients with genotype 1 [6]. The results of large multicenter trials with pegylated interferon-α will soon be published.

Antiviral approaches aiming, for example, at the viral protease are eagerly pursued. The conformational characteristics of the active site of the HCV protease, however, make the design of a high-affinity antagonist more difficult than in HIV.

A very promising approach both for the development of a preventive vaccine as well as for the development of an immunotherapy for chronically infected patients comes from the study of the antiviral immune response [10]. In acute self-limited hepatitis C, a strong and maintained HCV-specific CD4+ T cell response has consistently been linked with viral clearance [11, 17]. Very recent data on HCV-specific CD8+ T cell responses during this critical phase of disease have revealed a strong HCV-specific CD8+ T cell response during viral elimination, which, however, disappears a few months following viral clearance. Several highly conserved CD4+ T cell epitopes have been identified and characterized, and these epitopes are currently among the prime candidates for an HCV vaccine [9, 13]. New vaccine delivery systems like DNA vaccines, peptide vaccines, antigen-pulsed dendritic cells, or recombinant viruses may be able to overcome the relative immune tolerance of chronic infection and may have the potential to induce viral clearance in patients with chronic hepatitis C [12].

Summary

The combination of interferon-α and ribavirin can cure 30–40% of patients with chronic hepatitis C. These results may be even better as soon as pegylated interferons become readily available. Nevertheless, the treatment is expensive and a large number of patients will not respond to the current treatment or may not be able to tolerate the considerable side effects. Moreover, patients with the most advanced liver disease, i.e., decompensated cirrhosis, cannot be treated with interferon. New therapeutic strategies involve antiviral agents like protease inhibitors and immunological approaches, which may revolutionize the treatment of hepatitis C in the next 5–10 years.

References

1. EASL International Consensus Conference on hepatitis C. 1999. Paris, 26–27 February 1999. Consensus statement. J Hepatol. 31 Suppl 1:3–8.
2. Alter, M. J. 1997. Epidemiology of hepatitis C. Hepatology. 26:62s–65s.
3. Alter, M. J., D. Kruszon-Moran, O. V. Nainan, G. M. McQuillan, F. Gao, L. A. Moyer, R. A. Kaslow, and H. S. Margolis. 1999. The prevalence of hepatitis C virus infection in the United States, 1988 through 1994. N Engl J Med. 341:556–62.
4. Armstrong, G. L., M. J. Alter, G. M. McQuillan, and H. S. Margolis. 2000. The past incidence of hepatitis C virus infection: implications for the future burden of chronic liver disease in the United States. Hepatology. 31:777–82.
5. Bellentani, S., C. Tiribelli, G. Saccoccio, M. Sodde, N. Fratti, C. De Martin, and G. Cristianini. 1994. Prevalence of chronic liver disease in the general population of northern Italy: the Dionysos Study. Hepatology. 20:1442–9.
6. Boyer, N., and P. Marcellin. 2000. Pathogenesis, diagnosis and management of hepatitis C. J Hepatol. 32:98–112.
7. Buti, M., and R. Esteban. 1999. Retreatment of interferon relapse patients with chronic hepatitis C. J Hepatol. 31 Suppl 1:174–7.
8. Choo, Q. L., G. Kuo, A. J. Weiner, L. R. Overby, D. W. Bradley, and M. Houghton. 1989. Isolation of a cDNA clone derived from a blood-borne non-A, non-B viral hepatitis genome. Science. 244:359–362.

9. Diepolder, H. M., J. T. Gerlach, R. Zachoval, R. M. Hoffmann, M. C. Jung, E. A. Wierenga, S. Scholz, T. Santantonio, M. Houghton, S. Southwood, A. Sette, and G. R. Pape. 1997. Immunodominant CD4+ T cell epitope within nonstructural protein 3 in acute hepatitis C virus infection. J Virol. 71:6011–6019.

10. Diepolder, H. M., R. M. Hoffmann, J. T. Gerlach, R. Zachoval, M.-C. Jung, and G. R. Pape. 1998. Immunopathogenesis of HCV infection. Curr Stud Hematol Blood Transf. 62:135–151.

11. Diepolder, H. M., R. Zachoval, R. M. Hoffmann, E. A. Wierenga, T. Santantonio, M. C. Jung, D. Eichenlaub, and G. R. Pape. 1995. Possible mechanism involving T-lymphocyte response to non- structural protein 3 in viral clearance in acute hepatitis C virus infection. Lancet. 346:1006–1007.

12. Inchauspe, G. 1999. DNA vaccine strategies for hepatitis C. J Hepatol. 30:339–46.

13. Lamonaca, V., G. Missale, S. Urbani, M. Pilli, C. Boni, C. Mori, A. Sette, M. Massari, S. Southwood, R. Bertoni, A. Valli, F. Fiaccadori, and C. Ferrari. 1999. Conserved hepatitis C virus sequences are highly immunogenic for CD4(+) T cells: implications for vaccine development. Hepatology. 30:1088–98.

14. Liang, T. J., B. Rehermann, L. B. Seeff, and J. H. Hoofnagle. 2000. Pathogenesis, natural history, treatment, and prevention of hepatitis C. Ann Intern Med. 132:296–305.

15. Mast, E. E., M. J. Alter, and H. S. Margolis. 1999. Strategies to prevent and control hepatitis B and C virus infections: a global perspective. Vaccine. 17:1730–3.

16. McHutchison, J. G., S. C. Gordon, E. R. Schiff, M. L. Shiffman, W. M. Lee, V. K. Rustgi, Z. D. Goodman, M. H. Ling, S. Cort, and J. K. Albrecht. 1998. Interferon alfa-2b alone or in combination with ribavirin as initial treatment for chronic hepatitis C. Hepatitis Interventional Therapy Group [see comments]. N Engl J Med. 339:1485–92.

17. Missale, G., R. Bertoni, V. Lamonaca, A. Valli, M. Massari, C. Mori, M. G. Rumi, M. Houghton, F. Fiaccadori, and C. Ferrari. 1996. Different clinical behaviors of acute hepatitis C virus infection are associated with different vigor of the anti- viral cell-mediated immune response. J Clin Invest. 98:706–714.

18. Poynard, T., P. Marcellin, S. S. Lee, C. Niederau, G. S. Minuk, G. Ideo, V. Bain, J. Heathcote, S. Zeuzem, C. Trepo, and J. Albrecht. 1998. Randomised trial of interferon alpha2b plus ribavirin for 48 weeks or for 24 weeks versus interferon alpha2b plus placebo for 48 weeks for treatment of chronic infection with hepatitis C virus. International Hepatitis Interventional Therapy Group (IHIT) [see comments]. Lancet. 352:1426–32.

19. Poynard, T., J. Moussali, V. Ratziu, C. Regimbeau, and P. Opolon. 1999. Effects of interferon therapy in »non responder« patients with chronic hepatitis C. J Hepatol. 31 Suppl 1:178–83.

20. Schalm, S. W., J. T. Brouwer, F. C. Bekkering, and T. G. van Rossum. 1999. New treatment strategies in non-responder patients with chronic hepatitis C. J Hepatol. 31 Suppl 1:184–8.

21. Tassopoulos, N. C. 1999. Treatment of patients with chronic hepatitis C and normal ALT levels. J Hepatol. 31 Suppl 1:193–6.

Interferon Alpha-2a Treatment in Patients with Hepatitis C and Bleeding Disorders

R. Zimmermann, A. Huth-Kühne, A. Skibbe, P. Lages, T. Göser

Introduction

In 1943, Beeson observed a connection between the transfusion of blood products and the emergence of hepatitis [1]. Jaundice developed in seven patients 1–4 months after the administration of whole blood or plasma. Further reports on the development of hepatitis in hemophilia patients were published in the mid-1970s [2, 3, 4]. Today, it is generally accepted that the hepatitis C virus causes the majority of cases of post-transfusion hepatitis in the Western world. It is responsible for most chronic liver disorders observed in hemophilia patients treated with clotting factor concentrates. The hepatitis C infection can be associated with replacement therapy involving clotting factor concentrates applied in the early 1970s [2, 5, 6].

Hepatitis often follows an asymptomatic course, but at least 50% of patients infected with the virus develop chronic hepatitis and up to 30% develop cirrhosis of the liver within 10–20 years following diagnosis. Of all those infected, 10% develop a liver cell carcinoma within a further 10 years [7, 8]. Of the variants known, six more frequently occurring genotypes (types 1–6) are described, although each type can be differentiated further [9]. The six most common genotypes have varying nucleotide sequences in the 5-noncoding region (NCR).

Interferon alpha ($IFN-\alpha_{2a}$) is an effective treatment for chronic hepatitis C, but only 15–30% of patients show a sustained response after treatment. HCV-positive hemophiliacs in Europe present mostly with genotype 1a/1b, and thus may have an even more poor response rate to $IFN-\alpha_{2a}$. It has been shown that higher dosage regimens (cumulative dose) are more effective.

Patients and Methods

We treated 14 patients, 12 with hemophilia A and 2 with von Willebrand's disease, with the following dosage regimen: 6 MU s.c. daily for 4 weeks, followed by 6 MU three times per week for 22 weeks; the dose was then reduced to 3 MU three times per week for the next 6 months.

Inclusion criteria were the presence of anti-HCV antibodies, HCV-RNA (detected by nested PCR), and elevated transaminases (ALT). The clinical course, transaminases, quantitative HCV-RNA, HCV-genotype, and immunological parameters were evaluated before treatment, 2, 4, 8, 12, 38, and 52 weeks after start of treatment, and 6 months after discontinuation of therapy.

I. Scharrer/W. Schramm (Ed.)
30th Hemophilia Symposium Hamburg 1999
© Springer-Verlag Berlin Heidelberg 2001

Results

Preliminary data showed normalized ALT-levels in 10 of the 14 patients. At the end of the study, only two patients demonstrated levels in the normal range. After 12 weeks of treatment, ALT could be reduced by 40%.

HCV-RNA normalized in 6 out of 14 patients (42%) after 12 weeks of treatment. However, at the end of the treatment (52 weeks), only 2 out of 14 patients (14%) were HCV-RNA negative. A sustained response could be demonstrated only in 2 (14%) out of 14 patients 26 weeks after the end of interferon treatment. An 80% reduction of the HCV-RNA values was seen after 12 weeks of therapy.

Side Effects

Influenza-like symptoms' initially observed in most of the patients disappeared within a few weeks. In two patients the interferon dose had to be reduced because of a depression of platelets or leukocytes. Two patients reported mental depression, and two stomatitis and leukoplakia.

Discussion

Few studies have been published concerning interferon treatment of chronic hepatitis C in patients with hemophilia. In the study of Makris et al. [10] only 3 of the 18 patients showed a sustained response. Similar results were reported by Laursen and coworkers [11]. In the latter study, 47 patients were enrolled and received 3 MU interferon thrice weekly for 3 months. In 26 non-responders the dose was increased to 6 MU thrice weekly for additional 3 months. Only 16% of the patients could be treated successfully, with a sustained response documented 26 weeks after discontinuation of therapy.

The high-dose interferon regimen applied in our study with an initial dose of 6 MU daily within the first 4 weeks was not able to induce a higher response rate. Out of the 14 patients, 11 displayed genotypes 1a or 1b (79%); 3 patients presented with genotype 1a (1), genotype 2a (1), and genotype 3a (1). The high incidence of genotype 1 may explain the poor response rate to the high interferon regimen.

The 80% reduction of HCV-RNA in all patients demonstrates the great potency of the high-dosage regimen. Perhaps a prolonged high initial dosage or a combination therapy may have a more pronounced effect and better long-term results.

Summary

Our preliminary data of the high-dosage treatment with interferon show that the virus load of HCV-RNA could be reduced in all patients by 80%. HCV-RNA disappeared transiently in 6 out of 14 patients during 12 weeks, but a high recurrence has to be considered in most of the patients. A sustained response could be observed in 2 (14%) of our patients. Influenza-like symptoms could be observed in nearly all patients but disappeared in most of them within a few weeks. Depression of platelets or leukocytes necessitated a dose reduction of interferon in 2 patients. One reason for the lower response rate may be the predominant genotype 1a and 1b (79%) in our patient group. Therefore, we have initiated a new prospective study including the same IFN-α_{2a} dosage regimen in combination with ribavirin and amantadine, which seems to be very promising.

References

1. Beeson PB. Jaundice occurring one to four months after transfusion of blood or plasma: report of seven cases. J Am Med Assoc 1943; 121: 1332–4.
2. Hasiba UW, Spero JA, Lewis JH. Chronic liver dysfunction in multitransfused haemophiliacs. Transfusion 1977; 17: 490.
3. Kasper CK, Kipnis SA. Hepatitis and clotting-factor concentrates. JAMA 1972; 221: 510.
4. Laursen AL, Scheibel E, Ingerslev J, Clausen NC, Wantzin P, Oestergaard L, Schou G, Black FT, Krogsgaard K. Alpha interferon therapy in Danish hemophiliac patients with chronic hepatitis C: results of a randomized controlled open label study comparing two different maintenance regimens following standard interferon-alpha-2b treatment. Haemophilia 1998; 4:25–32.
5. Makris M, Preston FE, Triger DR, Underwood JCE, Westlake L, Adelman MI. A randomized controlled trial of recombinant interferon-α in chronic hepatitis C in hemophiliacs. Blood 1991; 78:1672–7.
6. Makris M, Preston FE, Triger DR, Underwood JC. The natural history of chronic liver disease in haemophilia: more rapid progression relates to age and mild disease (abstract). Br J Haematol 1992; 81 (Suppl. 1): 72
7. Mannucci PM, Capitanio A, del Nino E, Colombo M, Pareti F, Ruggeri ZM. A symptomatic liver disease in haemophiliacs. J Clin Path 1975; 28: 620–4.
8. Preston FE, Jarvis LM, Makris M, Philp L, Underwood JCE, Ludlam CA, Simmonds P. Heterogeneity of hepatitis C virus genotypes in haemophilia: relationship with chronic liver disease. Blood 1995; 85: 1259–62.
9. Schimpf K, Zimmermann R. Hepatitishäufigkeit, serologische Befunde und Leberhistologie nach Therapie schwerer hämorrhagischer Diathesen mit Gerinnungsfaktorenkonzentraten. In: Fibrinogen, Fibrin and Fibrin Glue. Side effects of therapy with clotting factor concentrates. Schimpf K Ed, Schattauer Verlag 1980; 299–308
10. Simmonds P, Holmes EC, Cha TA, Chan SW, McOmish F, Irvine B, Beall E, Yap PL, Kolberg J, Urdea MS. Classification of hepatitis C virus into six major genotypes and a series of subtypes by phylogenetic analysis of the NS-5 region. J Gen Virol 1993; 74: 2391.
11. Zeuzem S, Roth WK, Herrmann G. Virushepatitis C. Z Gastroenterol 1995; 33: 117–32.

Report on Experience in the Treatment of Hepatitis C in HIV-Coinfected Hemophiliacs

J.K. ROCKSTROH

Introduction

Hepatitis C and HIV represent global health problems. To date, over 35 million people have become infected with HIV. The hepatitis C virus is found generally in 1–3% of the population with an assumed worldwide number of between 60 and 180 million infected persons. Coinfection with hepatitis C virus and HIV frequently occurs because of the same route of transmission via blood and blood products. This applies especially to drug addicts and hemophiliacs. In Germany it is estimated that there are about 5600 HIV/HCV-coinfected patients. In view of the rapid progress of hepatitis C in the presence of HIV infection, especially in advanced immunodeficiency, treatment of hepatitis C in the presence of HIV coinfection is becoming increasingly important. Up to now, however, the poor therapeutic success and considerable side effects of the current forms of treatment (especially interferon-α monotherapy) have been limiting factors. The following paper deals with the data so far collected on the therapeutic possibilities for hepatitis C in HIV-infected hemophiliacs.

Interferon Monotherapy

Patients with hepatitis C without HIV infection exhibit a sustained response, which is defined as normalization of transaminases and negativation of HCV-RNA 6 months after completing interferon treatment, in only up to 20% of cases treated with interferon-α. Evaluation of the combined results of studies on the treatment of hepatitis C in HIV-infected patients with interferon-α monotherapy essentially showed even poorer treatment results. Table 1 summarizes the data obtained from controlled studies on the treatment of chronic hepatitis C in patients coinfected with HIV with interferon-α monotherapy.

Briefly, it can be said that the response rates for interferon-α monotherapy vary markedly between the different studies given. Thus the response rates range from 0 to 28% after 6–12 months of interferon-α treatment. Reasons for the different results of treatment may be partly due to the different degrees of immunodeficiency at the start of the studies, but also to the different dosages and lengths of treatment. It was found that patients with longer duration of treatment and higher interferon dosages tended to show an overall better response to treatment. In addition, patients

I. Scharrer/W. Schramm (Ed.)
30th Hemophilia Symposium Hamburg 1999
© Springer-Verlag Berlin Heidelberg 2001

Table 1. Review of controlled studies on the treatment of chronic hepatitis C in HIV-coinfected patients with interferon-α

Reference	Year	Patients with HIV/HCV coinfection (n)	Patients with HCV alone (n)	CD4 cell count at baseline for HIV-positive patients	Study design	Dose of IFN-α 3x a week	Duration of treatment (weeks)	Primary response rate %	Sustained response rate % 6 months	Sustained response rate % 12 months
DeSanctis et al.	1993	20	20	NA	Prospective comparative	3	78	–	–	25%
Marcellin et al.	1994	20	20	350/µl	Prospective comparative	3	6	30 vs 75%	3 months 15 vs 30%	–
Pol S. et al.	1994	16	12	–	Prospective comparative	3	24	18.8 vs 64.5%	0 vs 40.3%	–
Soriano et al.	1996	90	29	>200/µl	Prospective Comparative	5 (3 months) 3 (9 months)	54	32.5 vs 37%	–	22.5 vs 25.9%
Piliero et al.	1997	Group A 14 Group B 14	0 0	A: Mean 573 B: Mean 392	Prospective Comparative	5 (Group A) 3 (Group B)	24	A: 11% B: 25%	0%	
Mauss et al.	1998	17	0	Median 400/µl (range 0–160/µl)	Prospective	5	54	46%	28%	–

with a helper cell count of more than 500 absolute/µl at the start of treatment showed the best response rates, which again clearly underlines the importance of a good immune function before starting therapy as a prognostic factor. In view of the poor treatment results, especially with the advanced loss of helper cells, a study was set up by the Klinische Arbeitsgemeinschaft AIDS Deutschland (KAAD; Clinical Working Party on AIDS Germany) which investigated higher dosages of interferon-α in HIV/HCV-coinfected patients who still had helper cell counts in an immunologically well-compensated range of more than 350/µl, and had a RNA replication rate of less than 5000 copies/ml either in the spontaneous course or under highly potent antiretroviral therapy. Nine patients were enrolled in this investigation. None of the patients showed any success of treatment, which was defined as negativation of the HCV-RNA and normalization of the transaminases 6 months after withdrawal of interferon therapy. After publication of the more favorable data on treatment of hepatitis C with interferon and ribavirin as a combined therapy, this KAAD study was closed. Overall, it should be noted that, in view of the poorer treatment success with interferon-α monotherapy in HIV/HCV coinfection, it is currently generally no longer indicated. Instead, more promising combined therapies or new interferon forms should be used, and these are reported on below.

Interferon/Ribavirin Combined Therapy

Investigations on the treatment of hepatitis C with interferon and ribavirin as combined therapy showed a clearly improved response in patients with HCV alone without simultaneous HIV infection [9]. In the meantime, interferon/ribavirin combined treatment has become standard therapy for hepatitis C. In the past, ribavirin could be used in the presence of HIV; however, there were still several unanswered questions. For example, ribavirin exhibits an antagonistic action to the inhibitory effects of various nucleoside analogues, such as azidothymidine, on HIV-1 replication in vitro. It must therefore be postulated that the use of ribavirin simultaneously with antiretroviral therapy may lead to an abolition of the antiviral action of the nucleoside analogues used. To date, however, no resistant phenotypes have been induced by ribavirin therapy. In addition, ribavirin exhibits an intrinsic activity against HIV-1. Initial investigations and pilot projects on the use of ribavirin and interferons therefore investigated especially the effects on the course of HIV-RNA and the safety of this combination used in HIV/HCV-coinfected patients. Initial data are available from Zylberberg et al. [12], who investigated the clinical relevance of the in vitro interaction between antiretroviral therapy and ribavirin. In this study, 10 HCV/HIV-infected patients, of whom 7 had manifest liver cirrhosis, and who were undergoing antiretroviral treatment with either azidothymidine (AZT; $n=5$) or stavudine (D4T; $n=5$) as a component of triple therapy with inclusion of a protease inhibitor, were treated with 1000 mg/day ribavirin and 3 million units interferon 3 times a week. The HIV viral load and helper cells were determined before treatment and then every 3 months (mean follow-up 5±1 months). Analysis showed the five patients with nondetectable HIV viremia before ribavirin/interferon therapy continued to be below the limit of detection. The five patients who exhibited persistent virus replication before treatment did not show any significant difference in their viral load before and after ribavirin/interferon combined treatment. The helper cell count did not change significantly in the course of the study. Under the combined treatment with ribavirin and interferon, four of the treated patients became negative for HCV-RNA. The authors concluded that the interaction between the nucleoside analogues and ribavirin demonstrated in vitro did not lead to any significant variation in the HIV replication in HIV/HCV-coinfected patients. In parallel, however, there was an improved response of hepatitis C viral load during the combination treatment.

Similar results were obtained in a further study which investigated the effects of treatment with interferon-α and ribavirin on HCV and HIV viral load in comparison with an interferon-α monotherapy in HIV/HCV-coinfected patients. Altogether, 23 patients were randomized to either interferon-α alone ($n=10$) or to the combination of interferon-α and ribavirin ($n=11$). After 4 months, the patients who were randomized to the interferon-α monotherapy were offered the possibility of switching to the combination treatment if their HCV viral load had not become negative at this time. The dosages of the study medications were 3 million units interferon-α 3 times a week in combination with 1000–1200 mg/day ribavirin. Table 2 shows the baseline characteristics of the enrolled study population. The results at 3 months in this ongoing study are summarized in Table 3.

In this study, therefore, there was no significant change in HIV-RNA in the combination arm compared with the administration of interferon-α alone. There was, nevertheless, in parallel a clearly greater reduction of the HCV-RNA in the combination arm. A striking finding, however, was a clear reduction in the helper cell count in the interferon-α/ribavirin combination arm. A final assessment is only

Table 2. Patient characteristics

Percentage men	90.5
Age in years (median)	40.0
Percentage of patients that received antiretroviral treatment	90.5
Hemoglobin before treatment (median, g/dl)	13.2
Fibrosis score before treatment	2.0

Table 3. Results

	Interferon-α	Interferon-α/Ribavirin
Month 0:		
HCV-RNA copies/ml	5,000,000	325,000
HIV-RNA copies/ml	1,500	<400
CD4/ml	211	529
Month 3:		
HCV-RNA copies/ml	4,350,000	850,000
HIV-RNA copies/ml	<400	<400
CD4/ml	276	277

possible to a limited degree in this ongoing study. With respect to side effects, it should be noted that 45% of the patients treated with the interferon/ribavirin developed anemia (Hb <10 g/dl) compared with only 10% of patients undergoing interferon-α monotherapy. An adequate increase in Hb was observed on substitution treatment with subcutaneous erythropoietin. The frequency of the constitutional side effects (fever, joint pains, etc.) was comparable in the two groups. The dropout rate was about 20%.

In summary, the data so far available from pilot projects on the use of ribavirin and interferon for the treatment of hepatitis C in the presence of coinfection with HIV have not shown any indications of significant changes in the HIV-RNA level as a result of interactions between ribavirin and the nucleoside analogues that were used. There is also a tendency for better response in the treatment of hepatitis C with a combination treatment in comparison with interferon-α monotherapy. In this respect, however, the analyses of further studies must be awaited.

Course of Hepatitis C Viremia During Antiretroviral Therapy

The increase in deaths due to liver failure in HIV/HCV-coinfected patients has been correlated with significantly increasing HCV-RNA levels with advancing immunodeficiency [4]. This raises the question whether, with an increase in helper cells and subsequent immune reconstitution under potent antiretroviral therapy including protease inhibitors, there is the possibility of achieving a reduction of the HCV-RNA levels. In a prospective investigation on the course of HCV-RNA levels in

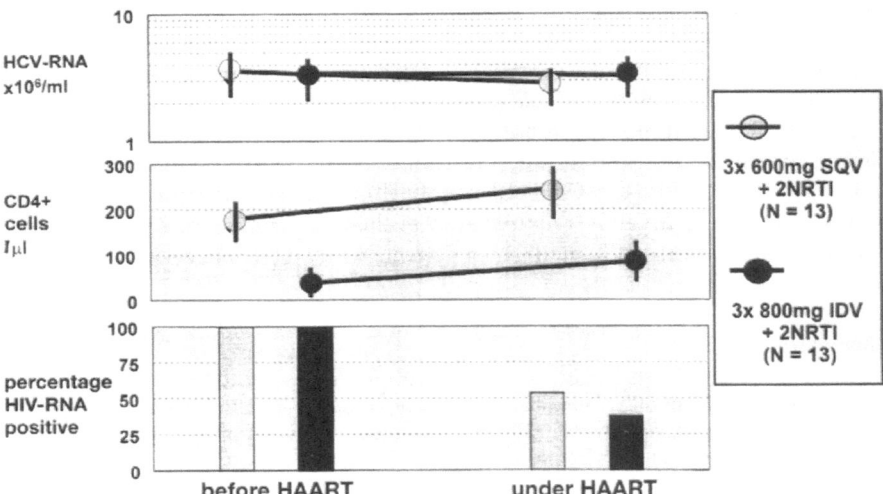

Fig. 1. Course of hepatitis C viral load during highly active antiretroviral therapy (HAART) including a protease inhibitor (SQV, saquinavir; IDV, indinavir) for 3 months

HIV/HCV-coinfected hemophiliacs undergoing antiviral triple therapy there was, however, no significant reduction of the hepatitis C viremia in spite of a significant increase in helper cells and falling HIV-RNA, either with two nucleoside analogues and saquinavir or two nucleoside analogues and indinavir (Fig. 1) [10]. It is, nevertheless, interesting to note that in the meantime data are available from the USA which show that patients with HIV/HCV coinfection who fail on their anti-retroviral combination therapy and exhibit a marked renewed rise in HIV-RNA also simultaneously show a significant rise in the HCV-RNA, so that in the context of partial immune reconstitution under HAART at least stability of the level of HCV-RNA may be achievable [2]. In this connection, attention should also be drawn to a recently published paper in which 2 out of 10 patients with HIV/HCV coinfection who were treated with a protease inhibitor and 2 nucleoside analogues developed negativation of the HCV-PCR in months 6 and 9 respectively. Thus, the question again arises whether complete clearance of hepatitis C viremia can take place through partial immune reconstitution. A study from France presented at the European AIDS Conference in Lisbon caused a great sensation. It investigated whether highly active antiretroviral therapy had an influence on the progression of fibrosis in patients with HIV/HCV coinfection [1]. In this study, liver biopsies were obtained from 162 patients with HIV/HCV coinfection. The fibrosis progression rate was defined as the rate between the fibrosis stage (METAVIR scoring system) and duration of the HCV infection. The mean duration of HCV infection was 14.4 ± 0.4 years, the helper cell count $327 \pm 18/\mu l$, and the HIV-RNA $17,283 \pm 7212$ copies/ml at the time of liver biopsy. Forty-two patients had an increased alcohol consumption of more than 50 g/day. Forty-nine patients received a highly active antiretroviral therapy including a protease inhibitor (duration 12 ± 1 month). Patients with an increased fibrosis rate were significantly older at HCV infection, more often exhibited an increased alcohol consumption, and had lower helper cell counts and underwent HAART treatment more frequently than patients with lower fibrosis rates. Regression analysis found two independent risk factors for increased fibrosis progression rates: CD4 cell counts of less than $200/\mu l$ and no treatment with a protease inhibitor. From this it may be deduced that the effect of protease inhibitors in antiviral therapy is associated with a significantly lower fibrosis progression rate and this cannot be explained by any other cofactors such as, for example, the CD4 cell count. This means that further longitudinal investigations are urgently required to reevaluate the influence of antiretroviral therapy on the course of hepatitis C in patients with HIV coinfection.

References

1. Bochet M, Benhamon Y, Colombat G, et al: Anti–protease inhibitor therapy decreases the liver fibrosis progression rate in HIV–HCV coinfected patients. In: Program and Abstracts of the 7th European Conference on Clinical Aspects and Treatment of HIV–Infection, Lisbon, 1999; 33:248
2. Busch C, Nagabhairu L, Markowitz M, et al: Changes in HCV viral load in HIV patients during HAART therapy and after therapy failure. In: Program and Abstracts of the 6th Conference on Retroviruses and Opportunistic Infections, Chicago, 1999; 192

3. DeSanctis GM, Errera G, Barbacini G, et al: Long–term outcome of chronic hepatitis infection in HIV± subjects treated with interferon. In: Program and Abstracts of the 9th International Conference on AIDS, Berlin, Germany, 1993:B19
4. Eyster ME, Fried MB, Di Bisceglie AM, et al: Increasing hepatitis C virus RNA levels in hemophiliacs: Relationship to human immunodeficiency virus infection and liver disease. Blood 1994; 84:1020–1023
5. Marcellin P, Boyer N, Areias J, et al: Comparison of efficacy of α-interferon in former intravenous drug addicts with chronic hepatitis with or without HIV–infection. Gastroenterology 1994; 106:A938
6. Mariott E, Navas S, del Romero I et al: Treatment with combinant α-interferon of chronic hepatitis C in anti–HIV–positive patients. J Med Virol 1993; 40:107–111
7. Mauss S, Klinker H, Ulmer A, Willers R, Weißbrich B, Albrecht H, Häussinger D, Jablonowski H: Response to treatment of chronic hepatitis C with interferon α in patients infected with HIV-1 is associated with higher CD4- cell count. Infection 1998; 26:16–19
8. Piliero PJ, Szebenyi S, Bartholomew C, et al: Recombinant interferon therapy for chronic hepatitis C in patients with HIV. In: Program and Abstracts of the 4th Conference on Retroviruses and Opportunistic Infections, Washington, 1997:673
9. Reichard O, Norkrans G, Fryden A, et al: Randomized double–blind placebo–controlled trial of interferon-α 2b with and without ribavirin for chronic hepatitis C. Lancet 1998; 351:83–87
10. Rockstroh JK, Theisen A, Kaiser R et al: Antiretroviral triple therapy decreases HIV-viral load but does not alter hepatitis C virus serum levels in HIV/HCV–coinfected hemophiliacs. AIDS 1998; 12:829–830
11. Soriano V, Garcia-Samaniego J, Bravo R, et al: Interferon-α for the treatment of chronic hepatitis C in patients infected with human immunodeficiency virus. Clin Infect Dis 1996; 23:585–591
12. Zylberberg H, Landau A, Chai XML, et al: Ribavirin does not modify HIV–replication in HCV/HIV–coinfected subjects under antiretroviral regimen. Hepatology 1998; 28:479a

IV. *Inhibitors in Hemophilia*

Chairman:

R. Burger (Berlin)

A New Therapeutic Option for Inhibitor Elimination in Patients with Acquired Hemophilia

A. Huth-Kühne, P. Lages, R. Zimmermann

Introduction

Antibodies to factor VIII:C (FVIII:C) and factor IX may arise in response to replacement therapy in patients with congenital hemophilia (alloantibodies), or in patients with previously normal FVIII:C activity in association with a diverse variety of clinical settings (autoantibodies).

Autoantibodies to FVIII:C constitute the most common spontaneous inhibitor to any coagulation factor. Inhibitor formation is rare with an incidence of 0.2–1 per 1 million persons per year [5]. Conditions associated with spontaneous inhibitor formation include autoimmune diseases, such as rheumatoid arthritis, bronchial asthma, myasthenia gravis, and systemic lupus erythematosus, as well as the postpartum period and malignancies [6, 16]. However, in approximately 50% of cases no underlying disease is found [5, 12].

Factor VIII:C antibodies are characterized as non-complement-fixing, heterogeneous, non-precipitating immunoglobulins of the IgG class, predominantly of the IgG4 heavy-chain subclass, and rarely IgA or IgM class [10]. Such antibodies are directed against functional epitopes of FVIII:C in a time- and temperature-dependent manner.

The clinical course of patients with acquired hemophilia is characterized by progressive and dramatic hemorrhages and presents a different bleeding pattern from patients with congenital hemophilia and inhibitors. Severe soft tissue bleeds, major life-threatening abdominal and retroperitoneal hemorrhages, as well as extensive muscle bleeding predominate and may lead to a fatal outcome in up to 22% of cases [5, 12].

Treatment goals consist of two objectives: management of the acute bleed and permanent inhibitor elimination. New therapeutic options are the management of acute bleeds with recombinant factor VIIa (rFVIIa) [8, 9] and permanent inhibitor elimination with a modified Malmö protocol.

The reminder of this article will refer to the management of permanent inhibitor elimination. There are a number of immune-tolerance protocols including the Malmö protocol introduced by Nilsson et al. [14, 2], which have been successfully applied to patients with congenital hemophilia and inhibitors. To date, none of these protocols have been applied to patients with acquired hemophilia. The Malmö protocol consists of high-dose FVIII administered several times a day as bolus injections with an initial dose of intravenous immunoglobulin (IVIG) (2.5–5 g);

I. Scharrer/W. Schramm (Ed.)
30th Hemophilia Symposium Hamburg 1999
© Springer-Verlag Berlin Heidelberg 2001

cyclophosphamide for 8–10 days, first intravenously for 2 days then orally; as well as 0.4 g/kg IVIG for 5 days beginning on day 4 of treatment. If the initial inhibitor level exceeds 10 BU, treatment is preceded by Immunoadsorption (IA) to protein A to remove the antibodies.

A modification of this protocol was introduced in 1997 for the treatment of patients with acquired hemophilia, and promising preliminary data have recently been reported [11, 18]. It comprises combined treatment with IA, high-dose FVIII, IVIG, and immunosuppressive therapy. Major modifications include the mode of application of IA, which represents a substantial part of the modified protocol and is regarded as an immunomodulatory strategy, and the introduction of a new extra-corporal adsorption technique (Ig-Therasorb) based on the selective IA of specific proteins to polyclonal sheep antibodies immobilized on sepharose columns. This antibody–antigen reaction currently represents the most selective approach to extract plasma components and eliminates all four subclasses of IgG, as well as IgM, IgA, and circulating immunocomplexes. This adsorption technique, introduced by Knöbl et al. [13], has been successfully applied to auto- and alloantibodies to FVIII:C.

The current report describes the successful, permanent inhibitor elimination in five patients with acquired hemophilia who were referred to the modified Malmö regimen.

Methods and Patients

The modified Malmö treatment protocol includes:
1. IA (Therasorb) on 2–5 consecutive days each week. Length of treatment was based on a Monday-to-Friday schedule and was therefore determined by the day of patient admission.
2. IVIG (0.3 g/kg) (Polyglobin, Bayer) on 3 consecutive days (Friday to Sunday) in between adsorption cycles, starting on the day of the last IA.
3. High-dose rFVIII (Kogenate, Bayer) starting after the first IA.
4. Immunosuppressive therapy until remission, beginning at the same time as IA and including 2 mg/kg per day cyclophosphamide and 1 mg/kg per day prednisolone to avoid autoantibody rebound.

For dosing with rFVIII, we administered a bolus of 200 IU/kg rFVIII followed by 200 IU/kg per day as continuous infusion starting after the first IA. As soon as plasma FVIII:C levels increased to normal (>60%), the rFVIII dose was gradually reduced in steps of 50 IU/kg. The treatment cycles were continued until patients reached normal FVIII:C levels without replacement therapy. Following remission, immunosuppressive therapy was continued for 2–4 weeks and IVIG twice a week for 4 weeks. To treat acute bleeds, all patients received rFVIIa applied as continuous infusion (0.75–1 KIU/kg per hour) following one or two initial bolus injections (4.5–6.0 KIU/kg). When FVIII:C levels increased to more than 30% under this specific therapy, treatment with rFVIIa was discontinued.

Results

Between October 1997 and May 1998, five patients with acquired antibodies to FVIII:C were referred to this modified Malmö protocol. All patients were transferred to our hospital because of severe bleeding complications. The median age of patients was 73 years (range 60–82) with a gender distribution of 3 males and 2 females. Three of the five patients showed an associated underlying medical condition (Table 1). The effect of the immunomodulatory treatment on inhibitor titers and FVIII:C activity in two patients is shown in Figs. 1 and 2. After a mean of 4.8 adsorptions, patients' FVIII:C levels were more than 30%, while the presence of inhibitor in plasma was no longer detectable. Remission in all patients required continuous rFVIII replacement for a mean of 19 days and 17 adsorptions (Table 2).

Therapy was well tolerated by all patients without severe side effects. To date, after follow-up periods of 26 months (2 patients), 25 months (1 patient), 20 months (1 patient), and 18 months (1 patient), all patients continue to be in remission.

Table 1. Patient characteristics

Case	Age	Sex	Underlying medical condition	Type or site of bleeding	Previous treatment
1	60	M	Bronchial asthma	Hematuria Retroperitoneal hematoma Soft tissue bleeds Intramuscular bleeds	Corticosteroids
2	77	F	None	Hematuria Hemarthrosis Subcutaneous hematoma Muscle bleeding Corticosteroids	Cyclophosphamide
3	82	M	None	Intra-abdominal bleeding Muscle bleeding and compartment syndrome	None
4	72	F	Rheumatoid arthritis	Subcutaneous hematoma Hematuria Hemarthrosis	Corticosteroids
5	74	M	Insulin-dependent diabetes mellitus Chronic obstructive lung disease	Hematuria Extensive hemorrhage following transurethral resection of the prostate	None

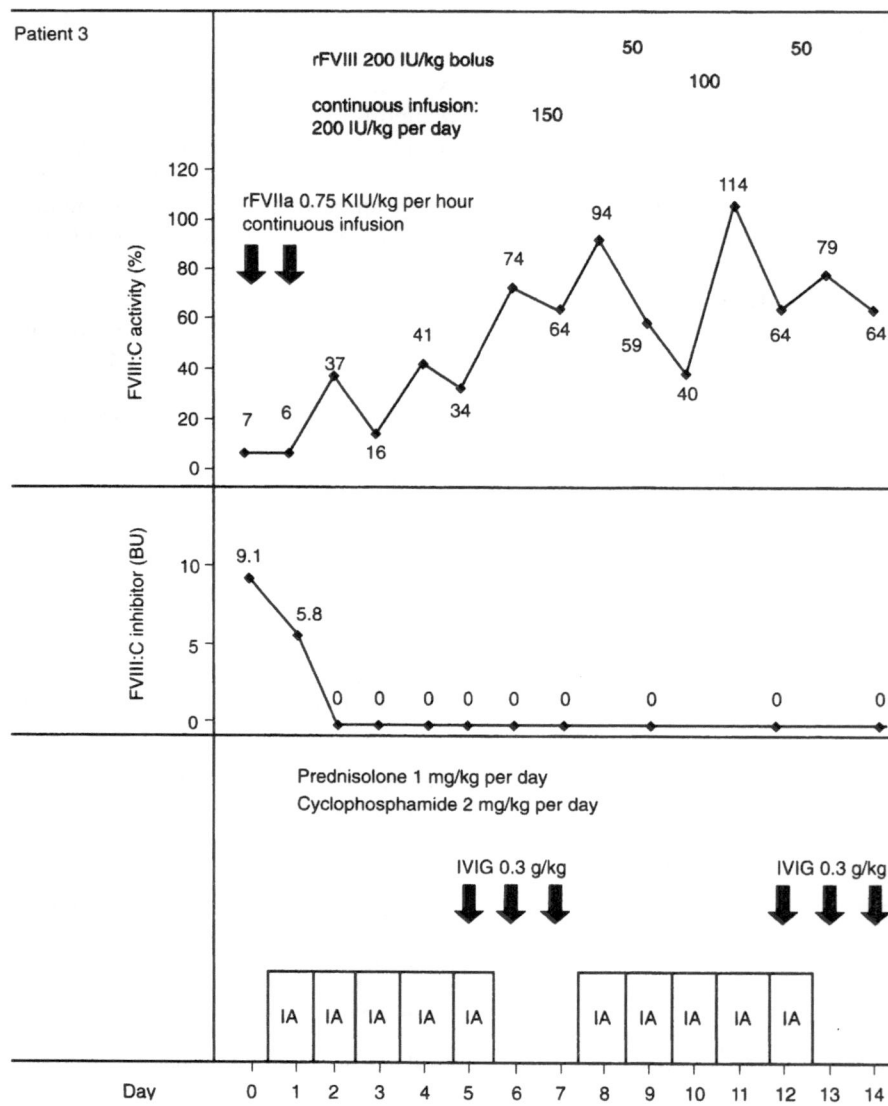

Fig. 1. Dosing schedules for rFVIII, rFVIIa, prednisolone, cyclophosphamide, IVIG, and application of immunoadsorption (*IA*), for the first 14 days of therapy in patient 3. FVIII:C activity is expressed as percentage of activity in normal plasma. FVIII:C inhibitor titer is expressed in Bethesda units (*BU*)

Discussion

Treatment of patients with FVIII:C or FIX autoantibodies still represents a major challenge. In most cases, immediate therapeutic intervention to control the acute bleeding is necessary and any choice of therapeutic modality should be based on an

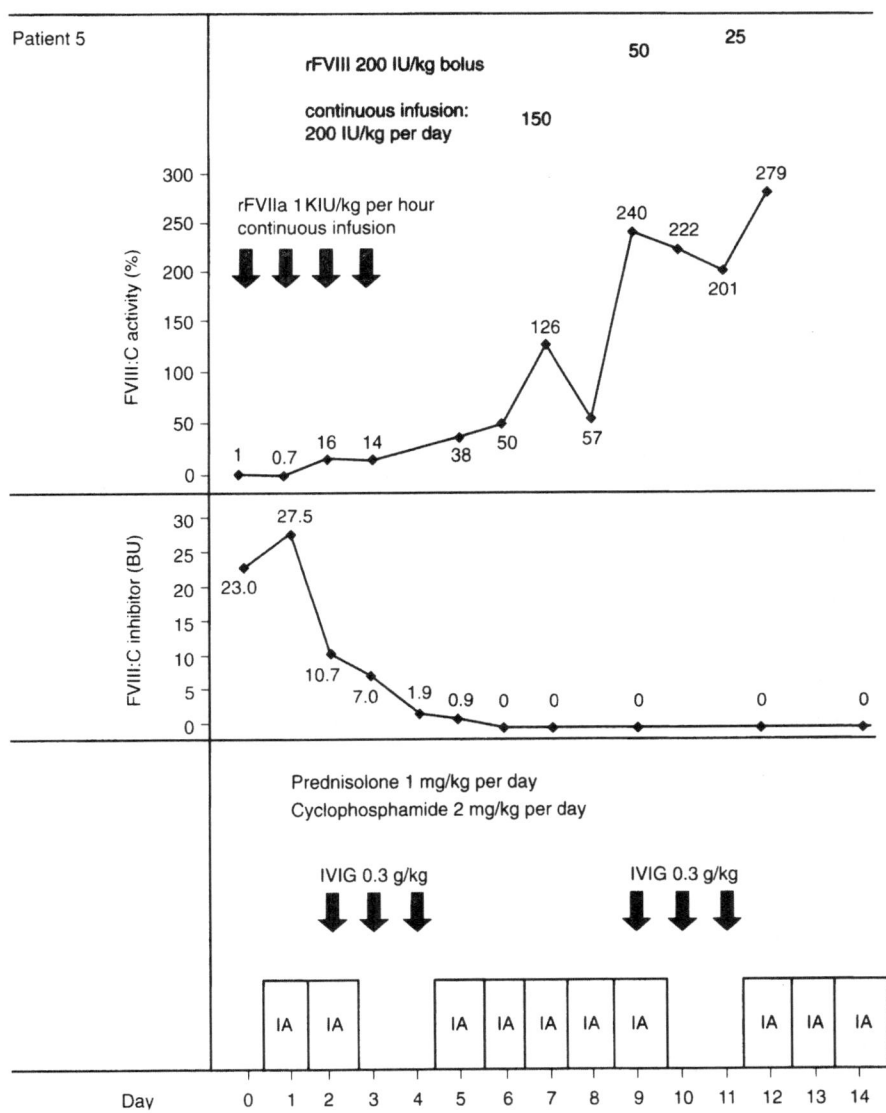

Fig. 2. Dosing schedules for rFVIII, rFVIIa, prednisolone, cyclophosphamide, IVIG, and application of immunoadsorption (*IA*), for the first 14 days of therapy in patient 5. FVIII:C activity is expressed as percentage of activity in normal plasma. FVIII:C inhibitor titer is expressed in Bethesda units (*BU*)

algorithm which considers age, inhibitor titer, residual FVIII:C activity, as well as the underlying medical condition.

We referred five patients to the modified Malmö protocol, where IA is considered an immunomodulatory strategy and applied as long-term treatment. Inhibitor elimination was achieved in all patients and, after a period of

Table 2. Details of treatment and outcome

Case	Number of IAs until FVIII >30%	Total number of IAs	Duration of FVIII replacement (days)	Outcome
1	5	20	23	Resolved
2	2	7	12	Resolved
3	4	17	16	Resolved
4	10	31	32	Resolved
5	3	10	12	Resolved
Mean	4.8	17.0	19.0	

IA, immunoadsorption

18–26 months, all patients continue to be in remission. Therapy was well tolerated without any serious side effects. For the management of acute bleeding, all but one patient received rFVIIa as first-line therapy and bleeding was successfully controlled in all patients. In contrast to the treatment protocol as applied by Zeitler and Brackmann in Bonn (bolus injections of rFVIII 100–200 IU/kg q.i.d.), we applied a modified factor VIII regimen so that a single bolus of 200 IU/kg was followed by 200 IU/kg per 24 h as continuous infusion. This mode of application was as effective as the original, despite a 50% reduction in dose, and yielded additional cost benefits.

Immunosuppressive therapy, IVIG, high-dose FVIII, and extracorporal IA comprise the modified Malmö protocol [11, 18]. Because each of these immunomodulatory strategies, described below, target a different aspect of the immune system and work, in part, synergistically, we believe this treatment protocol to be very promising.

Immunosuppressive and Cytotoxic Agents

Corticosteroids suppress immune responses mediated by B and T lymphocytes. By inhibiting interleukin-2, they prevent B cells from responding to T-helper lymphocytes, thus reducing immunoglobulin production [1].

Cytotoxic agents kill actively proliferating cells, acting preferentially on cancer cells and cells of the immune system.

Immunoglobulins

IVIG exerts its effect by complex formation with the circulating antibody mediated via anti-idiotype antibodies present in the normal antibody population and represented in the pooled plasma that comprises IVIG [3, 15]. The fact that the binding of Fab2 fragments from the immunoglobulin preparation to the autoantibody was responsible for the suppression of the autoantibody provided the first convincing evidence for the manipulation of the immune system by anti-idiotypic antibodies [17].

Re-Induction of Immune Tolerance with High-Dose FVIII

Mechanisms by which high doses of FVIII reduce the anti-FVIII:C antibodies are not clearly understood. They can induce anti-idiotypic antibodies, which bind to the variable region of the anti-FVIII:C antibodies and neutralize them [4]. Alternatively, high-dose FVIII may stimulate the pathological cell clone responsible for antibody synthesis via antigen presentation and render it more susceptible to immunosuppressive and cytotoxic agents [7]. High-dose continuous FVIII infusion, applied in our protocol as an alternative to bolus injections, seems to be an alternative approach to presenting sufficient antigen at a constant level.

Extracorporal IA (Ig-Therasorb)

This new adsorption technique was introduced for the treatment of acquired hemophilia by Knöbl and coworkers [13]. It leads to an extensive reduction of immunoglobulins from intravascular space and changes the distribution of antibodies and immune complexes between intra- and extravascular compartments leading to mobilization of antibodies from interstitial sites, especially when applied as long-term treatment.

In summary, combination of the four different immunomodulatory strategies described above proved successful in all five patients. Considering the side effects of immunosuppressive therapy, which should be part of any regimen for inhibitor elimination, a major advantage of our protocol is the relatively short time-course of immunosuppressive therapy. We achieved inhibitor elimination in less than 3 weeks (mean) and all patients continue to be in remission.

The modified Malmö protocol for the treatment of patients with acquired inhibitors to FVIII:C represents an alternative therapeutic strategy requiring further evaluation.

References

1. Dwyer JM. Manipulating the immune system with immune globulin. N Engl J Med 1992; 326: 107–16.
2. Freiburghaus C, Berntorp E, Ekman M, Gunnarsson M, Kjellberg B-M, Nilsson IM. Tolerance induction using the Malmö treatment model 1982–1995. Haemophilia 1999; 5: 32–9.
3. Gilles JG, Saint-Remy JM. Healthy subjects produce both anti-factor VIII and specific anti-idiotypic antibodies. J Clin Invest 1994; 94: 1496–505.
4. Gilles JG, Desqueper B, Lenk H, Vermylen J, Saint-Remy JM. Neutralizing antiidiotypic antibodies to FVIII inhibitors after desensitization in patients with haemophilia A. J Clin Invest 1996; 97: 1382–8.
5. Green D, Lechner K. A survey of 215 non-hemophilic patients with inhibitors to factor VIII. Thromb Haemost 1981; 45: 200–3.
6. Green D. The management of factor VIII inhibitors in non-hemophilic patients. Prog Clin Biol Res 1984; 150: 337–52.
7. Green D. Suppression of an antibody to factor VIII by combination of factor VIII and cyclophosphamides. Blood 1971; 37: 381–7

8. Hay CRM, Negrier C, Ludlam A. The treatment of bleeding in acquired haemophilia with recombinant factor VIIa: A multicentre study. Thromb Haemost 1997; 78: 1463-7.

9. Hedner U, Glazer S, Falch J. Recombinant activated factor VII in the treatment of bleeding episodes in patients with inherited and acquired bleeding disorders. Transfus Med Rev 1993; 7: 78-83.

10. Hoyer LW, Scandella D. Factor VIII inhibitors: structure and function in autoantibody and hemophilia A patients. Semin Hematol 1994; 31(Suppl. 4): 1-5

11. Huth-Kühne A, Lages P, Hampel H, Zimmermann R. Long-Term Ig-Immunoadsorption, High-Dose Factor VIII, Immunoglobulins And Immunosuppressive Therapy In Acquired Hemophilia – A Modified Malmö – Protocol. Thromb Haemost 1999; (Suppl.): 277 (abstr)

12. Kessler CM, Ludlam CA. The treatment of acquired factor VIII inhibitors: worldwide experience with porcine factor VIII concentrate. Semin Hematol 1993; 30: 22-7.

13. Knöbl P, Derfler K, Korninger L, Kapiotis S, Jäger U, Maier-Dobersberger T, Hörl W, Lechner K, Pabinger I. Elimination of acquired factor VIII antibodies by extracorporal antibody-based IA (Ig-Therasorb®). Thromb Haemost 1995; 74: 1035-8.

14. Nilsson IM, Berntorp E, Zettervall O. Induction of immune tolerance in patients with hemophilia and antibody to factor VIII by combined treatment with intravenous IgG, cyclophosphamide, and factor VIII. N Engl J Med 1988; 318: 947-50.

15. Rossi F, Sultan Y, Kazatchkine MD. Antiidiotypes against auto-antibodies and allo-antibodies to VIII:C (antihemophilic factor) are present in therapeutic polyspecific normal immunoglobulins Clin Exp Immunol 1988; 74: 311-6.

16. Shapiro SS, Hultin M. Acquired inhibitors to the blood coagulation factors. Semin Thromb Hemost 1975; 1: 336-85.

17. Sultan Y, Kazatchkine MD, Maisonneuve P, Nydegger VE. Antiidiotypic suppression of autoantibodies to factor VIII (antihaemophilic factor) by high-dose intravenous gamma-globulin. Lancet 1984; 2: 765-8.

18. Zeitler H, Unkrig C, Brackmann H-H, Effenberger C, Hanfland D, Stier S, Ko Y, Vetter H. An immunomodulatory treatment of acquired hemophilia A with long-term IgG IA, immuno-suppression, and antigen substitution – a modified Bonn protocol inducing immuno-tolerance. Blood 1997; 90 (Suppl. 1): 36 A (abstr)

V. Long-Term Results After Joint Replacement

Chairmen:

H.H. BRACKMANN (Bonn)
L. HOVY (Frankfurt/Main)

Long-Term Results After Total Knee and Total Hip Replacement in Hemophilic Arthropathy

L. Hovy, S. Müller, I. Scharrer

Severe hemorrhagic diatheses are complicated by spontaneous joint bleedings. The joint cartilage is damaged through the free intra-articular blood, probably caused by the formation of reactive oxygen metabolites which are catalyzed by iron [18]. Parallel inflammatory reactions occur in the synovial membrane and may lead to a secondary catabolic destruction of the cartilage [7, 12, 18]. This hemophilic arthropathy results in severe secondary arthrosis within a few years. The end stages of hemophilic arthropathy are characterized by severe cartilage destructions, deformities, and fibrous contractures. Especially in the lower extremities, this results in an early handicap. Therefore, timely diagnosis is necessary in cases with clinical and radiological progressive joint destructions.

Indication for Total Joint Replacement

The synovial membrane is cicatrized in the end stages of hemophilic arthropathy, and hemorrhages only occur seldom [7, 12]. Mechanical impulse, bone and cartilage desquamation, and cell detritus provoke severe inflammations with opaque joint effusions. These resultant inflammations should be classified as an activated arthrosis. The acute or chronic synovitis mentioned above must be differentiated [7]. Joint-space narrowing, sclerosis, subchondral cysts, and axial malalignment can be detected radiologically.

We see the indication for a total replacement of the knee or hip joint in patients presenting at least two of the following criteria:

1. Arthropathy in stage III–V [1].
2. Progressive joint destruction (X-ray: Pettersson score more than 6 points [15]).
3. Flexion contracture more than 15° (assessment by WFH joint score [4]).
4. Knee: axial malalignment more than 15° valgus or more than 5° varus.
5. Pain refractory to conservative treatment.
6. Recurrent joint effusions with or without hemarthrosis.

I. Scharrer/W. Schramm (Ed.)
30th Hemophilia Symposium Hamburg 1999
© Springer-Verlag Berlin Heidelberg 2001

Methods

Total Knee Arthroplasty

A total of 31 total knee arthroplasties (TKAs) were implanted in 22 patients (18 hemophilia A, 2 vWS, 2 complex clotting disorder) between 1981 and 1999. The patients' age ranged from 26 to 66 years (mean: 46.3 years). Six full-constrained TKAs with axis (Blauth type) were inserted using bone cement containing gentamycine. Twenty-three joints were replaced with non-constrained bicondylar TKA (16 PFC, 5 LCS) using bone cement, and two TKAs (1 LCS, 1 Miller-Galante) were implanted without bone cement. Two more patients received a primary mono-condylar prosthesis (Tönnis type).

Total Hip Arthroplasty

We implanted 15 primary total hip arthroplasties (THAs) in 13 patients (11 hemophilia A, 2 vWS) from 1972 to 1999. The average age at the time of operation was 47.6 years (range 32–67 years). A cemented fixation of the cup and stem (2 Müller-Charnley, 2 Müller straight stem, 1 Euroform) was performed in five patients using bone cement with gentamycine. Seven more patients received hybrid THA with cement-free threaded cups (2 Zweymüller, 5 Hofer) and cemented stems (2 Müller straight stem, 5 Euroform). In three patients the THA was performed using cement-less implants (2 Zweymüller cup, 1 Hofer cup, 2 Spotorno stem, 1 Egoform stem).

Results

Total Knee Arthroplasty

Results are based on the clinical and radiological follow-up of 17 patients with 25 TKAs and a mean follow-up interval of 48.3 months (minimum 12 up to 145 months) postoperatively. The evaluation is based on the HSS score according to Ranawat and Shine [17]. Full-constrained, non-constrained bicondylar and mono-condylar TKAs were assessed separately (Isonorm 7201/1).

Using either type of TKA, the average extension improved from 14.3° preoperatively to 5° postoperatively. A similar improvement from 69.5° to 77.5° on average was noted for active knee flexion. The patients with non-constrained bicondylar TKA (PFC, LCS, and Miller Galante type) achieved a lesser extension deficit combined with a better overall result (8 excellent, 6 good, 2 fair, 1 bad) in comparison to the full-constrained TKA. Constrained prostheses with an axis (Blauth type) were rated good (6), fair (2), and bad (2) in the HSS score (see Table 1). However, these patients presented severe preoperative flexion contractures from 10° to 40° and valgus malalignments up to 35°. The bad overall result in one patient with two full-constrained TKAs resulted from the coincident septic complication on both operated hips.

Table 1. Results of TKA in hemophilic arthropathy (HSS score, *n*=23)

	Excellent	Good	Fair	Bad
Bicondylar TKA (*n*=17)	8	6	2	1
Full-constrained TKA (*n*=6)		2	2	2

The tibial component subsided and loosened causing progressive instability in a 62-year-old woman suffering from severe vWS and rheumatoid arthritis, 36 months after implantation of a medial monocondylar prosthesis. The exchange to a full-constrained TKA yielded a good result 106 months postoperatively. In another 41-year-old hemophiliac with monocondylar replacement, subsidence of the tibial plateau occurred 139 months postoperatively without radiological loosening of the components. Simultaneously, the arthropathy progressed in the other compartments to stage III. After exchange to a bicondylar TKA (PFC), the end result could be rated as good. A bicondylar TKA (LCS type), implanted cement-free on the contralateral side in the same patient, developed a radiolucent line of 1–2 mm and subsidence of the tibial plateau 55 months after implantation without loosening. Unfortunately, the patient died 2 years later of a brain tumor. Two more patients died of AIDS, 2 and 7 years postoperatively.

A 44-year-old hemophiliac with bicondylar TKA on both knees developed a complete loosening of both components on the left side following a minor trauma 10 months postoperatively. Therefore, the overall result had to be rated bad. Revision operation verified a complete aseptic loosening, so that exchange to a full-constrained TKA (Blauth type) was performed. The overall result could be rated as fair.

Early or late infections did not occur. Neither were any peri- or postoperative complications registered. Two joints required manipulation 2–3 weeks postoperatively.

Total Hip Arthroplasty

All patients could be followed up clinically and radiologically. However, this study is based on the data of 10 patients including 12 THAs and a follow-up of 12–325 months (mean 98.3 months). The evaluation was carried out using the score according to Charnley [2] (see Table 2). The mean total range of movement (ROM) in three dimensions improved in all patients from 90° preoperatively to 189° postoperatively, correlating with an increase from 2.9 to 4.6 points (Charnley score). In particular, the subjective rating of pain (maximum 6 points) improved from 2.0 to 5.4 points. Walking ability improved from 2.0 to 4.6 points, likewise.

Our first patient receiving a THA in 1972 developed an aseptic loosening of the cemented cup 14 years later. The sequela of a fall on the right hip was another aseptic loosening of the threaded cup 5 years later. Follow-up 8 years after the exchange

Table 2. Results of THA in hemophilic arthropathy (Charnley score, $n=12$)

	Preoperative	Follow-up
Total ROM	90°	189°
Mobility (maximum 6 points)	2.9	4.6
Function (maximum 6 points)	2	4.6
Pain (maximum 6 points)	2	5.4

revealed no signs of loosening of the cup or stem. All other THAs also showed no signs of radiologic loosening.

An HIV-positive hemophiliac developed septic loosening of his left hip co-incident with an abscess on the right side replaced with THA. After exchange on the left side and contralateral drainage, both THAs remained stable for 7 years till the patient's death due to AIDS. Another HIV-positive patient developed simultaneously a hematogeneous fungal abscess on both operated hips 5 respectively 10 months post-THA without loosening. The patient died 5 years after local revision due to AIDS with both THAs in situ. Besides these late infections in HIV-positive patients, no other peri- or postoperative complications occurred.

Discussion

End stages of hemophilic arthropathy are complicated by recurrent painful effusions due to the secondary arthrosis combined with contractures and axial malalignment [1, 11]. The synovial membrane is cicatrized [7, 12] so that acute hemarthrosis seldom occurs. Furthermore, these patients are handicapped because of other joints. Endoprosthetic replacement of the knee and hip joint is indicated in stages III–V [1, 3, 6, 8–11, 14].

Hemophilic arthropathy is more common in the knee. Four patients had to be operated on their hip and knee joints.

Six full-constrained TKAs with axis (Blauth type) were inserted in five patients aged 41–65 years. These cases revealed severe flexion contractures up to 40° combined with axial malalignment up to 35° and ligamentous instabilities. At follow-up, four cases had a good or fair result in the HSS score [17] and only two cases had a bad result (see Table 1). The two bad results with insufficient ROM and function in one HIV-positive patient were related to the septic complication on both total hip replacements. The other 17 patients achieved significantly better overall results 48.3 months postoperatively (8 excellent, 6 good, 2 fair, 1 bad; see Table 1). These patients had lesser limitations of movement and muscular atrophies preoperatively. All patients remained without pain and were able to walk without a cane. Perioperative complications did not occur; two joints required manipulation. Two patients died of AIDS, 2 and 7 years postoperatively without any joint infection.

A radiolucent line combined with subsidence of the tibial plateau could be detected only in one case 55 months after cement-free TKA. This patient also developed subsidence of a monocondylar prosthesis without definite loosening on the contralateral side 139 months post-implantation. The involved joint has undergone revision. Another monocondylar prosthesis had to be changed to a full-constrained TKA after 36 months. Moreover, we registered one aseptic loosening 10 months after bicondylar TKA affording a revision. All other TKAs remained radiologically uneventful up to 145 months.

Several authors report excellent or good results using different bicondylar TKAs [3, 5, 9–11, 19]. However, Figgie [3] noticed postoperative complications in 10 of 19 cases with TKA (6 bleeding, 3 nerve palsy, 1 infection, 6 skin necrosis) as well as radiolucent lines beneath the polyethylene tibia plateau in 13 TKAs combined with subsidence in 3 cases. Radiolucent lines on the tibial side were also reported by Lachiewicz [10] in 8 of 24 total condylar prostheses. Manipulation was necessary in 14 cases. In the series of Luck [11], complications occurred in 8 of 46 TKAs, including 2 infections and 3 early aseptic loosenings. Significant lower perioperative complication rates were reported by Kjaersgaard-Anderson [9] from Denmark and by Heeg [5] from the Netherlands. Heeg only had one aseptic loosening 6.9 years after implantation. The rate of radiolucent lines was 76% in the Danish series [9] 43 months postoperatively. HIV infection obviously does not have an influence on the infection rate in TKA [16,19].

In our series, 12 total hip arthroplasties in 10 patients achieved very good long-term results according to the Charnley score [2] with a mean follow-up of 98 months (12–325) (see Table 2). All patients remained without pain and are able to walk. Perioperative complications did not occur.

Only two HIV-positive patients developed late complications in the form of hematogeneous infections with bacterial or fungal abscesses on both operated hips 5–14 months postoperatively. This progressed to a septic loosening of the THA in the first patient, which remained uneventful after revision for 6 years. Two of three HIV-positive patients died 5 and 9.5 years after THA due to AIDS. Moreover, only one aseptic loosening of the cup occurred 14 years after THA. The cemented stem is radiologically still stable 27 years postoperatively in this patient. Radiological loosening was not detected in any other case.

However, in the literature high complication and revision rates are reported reaching 60% in a 20-year period [11]. Kelley [8] recently reported in a multicenter study revision rates of 23% for the acetabulum and of 21% for the stem in a total of 34 THAs. Only 3 of 23 cemented cups were radiologically stable, whereas all 6 cementless THAs remained uneventful. In Great Britain, Nelson [14] registered a rate of 36.4% for aseptic loosening 7.6 years postoperatively affecting the stem predominantly.

Conclusion

Very good long-term results with a low rate of complications could be achieved in this series using total knee and total hip arthroplasty in hemophiliacs. A cemented fixation of the endoprosthetic components is recommended especially for TKA due to frequent periarticular osteoporosis. TKA should be indicated early, i.e., before the development of severe contractures. Progressive arthrofibrosis and muscular atrophy in the late stages of hemophilic arthropathy counteract satisfactory function of total knee arthroplasty.

Summary

The end stages of hemophilic arthropathy are characterized by severe destructions, deformities, and fibrous contractures. Total joint replacement can prevent progressive handicap. We report about the indication and long-term results of 25 total knee arthroplasties and 12 total hip arthroplasties with a mean follow-up of 48.3 and 98.3 months, respectively.

The best overall result was achieved using cemented bicondylar TKA before the development of severe contractures. No perioperative complications or infections occurred. One aseptic loosening 10 months postoperatively afforded revision. All other TKAs remained clinically and radiologically uneventful up to 145 months.

In THA, only one aseptic loosening of the acetabular cup occurred 14 years postoperatively. Two late septic complications in HIV-positive patients required revision operations. Besides these, no perioperative complications or infections occurred. The overall results up to 27 years could be rated good to excellent.

References

1. Arnold WD, Hilgartner MW (1977) Hemophilic arthropathy. J Bone Joint Surg 59:287–305
2. Charnley J (1972) The long-term results of low-friction arthroplasty of the hip performed as a primary intervention. J Bone Joint Surg 54-B: 61–76
3. Figgie MP, Goldberg VM, Figgie HE, Heiple KG, Sobel M (1989) Total knee arthroplasty for the treatment of chronic hemophilic arthropathy. Clin Orthop 248: 98–107
4. Gilbert MS (1993) Prophylaxis: Musculoskeletal Evaluation. Sem Hematology 30 (Suppl 2): 3–6
5. Heeg M, Meyer K, Smid WM, Van Horn JR, van der Meer J (1998) Total knee and hip arthroplasty in haemophilic patients. Haemophilia 4: 747–751
6. Hovy L (1997): Indikation zu Gelenkersatz bei Hämophilie – Langzeitergebnisse. In: Scharrer I, Schramm W (Hrsg.) 26. Hämophilie-Symposium Hamburg 1995. Springer, Berlin, Heidelberg, New York. pp 75–80
7 Hovy L (1999) Diagnostik und Behandlung der Synovitis bei Hämophilen. In: Scharrer I, Schramm W (Hrsg.): 29. Hämophilie-Symposion 1998. Springer Verlag Berlin, Heidelberg pp 25–30
8. Kelley SS, Lachiewicz PF, Gilbert MS, Bolander ME, Jankiewicz JJ (1995) Hip Arthroplasty in Hemophilic Arthropathy. J Bone Joint Surg 77: 828–834
9. Kjaersgaard-Anderson P, Christiansen SE, Ingerslev J, Sneppen O (1990) Total knee arthroplasty in classic hemophilia. Clin Orthop 256:137–146
10. Lachiewicz PF, Inglis AE, Insall JN, Sculco TP, Hilgartner MW, Bussel JB (1985) Total knee Arthroplasty in Hemophilia. J. Bone Joint Surg Vol. 67-A, 9: 1361–1366
11. Luck JV, Kasper CK (1989) Surgical management of advanced hemophilic arthropathy. Clin Orthop 242: 60–82
12. Mohr W (1993): Pathogenese der Arthropathie. In: Scharrer I, Schramm W (Hrsg.): 23. Hämophilie-Symposion Hamburg 1992. Springer, Berlin, Heidelberg, New York: pp 83–94
13. Montane I, McCollough NC, Lian EC-J (1986) Synovectomy of the knee for hemophilic arthropathy. J Bone Joint Surg 68: 210–216

14. Nelson IW, Sivamurugan S, Latham PD, Mathews J, Bulstrode CJK (1992) Total Hip Arthroplasty for Hemophilic Arthropathy. Clin Orthop 276: 210–213
15. Pettersson H, Ahlberg A, Nilsson IM (1980) A radiologic classification of hemophilic arthropathy. Clin Orthop 149: 153–159
16. Philips AM, Sabin CA, Ribbans WJ, Lee CA (1997) Orthopaedic surgery in hemophilic patients with human immunodeficiency virus. Clin Orthop. 343: 81–87
17. Ranawat CS, Shine JJ (1973) Duocondylar total knee arthroplasty. Clin Orthop 94: 185–195
18. Roosendaal G, van den Berg HM, Lafeber FPJ, Bijlsma J (1999): Pathologie der Synovitis und hämophilen Arthropathie. Orthopäde 28: 323–328
19. Unger S, Kessler CM, Lewis RJ (1995) Total knee arthroplasty in human immunodeficiency virus-infected hemophiliacs. J of Arthroplasty Vol. 10 No 4: 448–452

Total Knee Prosthesis in Hemophiliacs with Multilocular Hemophilic Arthropathy – The Zurich Experience

E.O. Meili, M. Rodriguez

From 1985 to 1999, 31 total knee replacements were performed in 23 hemophilic patients at the Orthopedic University Hospital Zurich. Mean postoperative observation time was 5 4/12 years (range 4 months–13 years). In all patients surgery was performed by the same orthopedic surgeon (M.R.); perioperative hemostaseologic management and stand-by at the operation were carried out by the same hemostaseologist (E.O.M.).

Patients

Mean patient age at the time of surgery was 44 years (23–68 years). Of the patients, 18 had severe hemophilia A, 2 moderate hemophilia A, 2 severe hemophilia B, and 1 patient had combined factor V/VIII deficiency. Two hemophiliacs with three prostheses were HIV-infected, asymptomatic, with a postoperative observation time of 10, 6, and 4/12 years. One of these two patients underwent splenectomy because of thrombocytopenia in 1992, 1 year prior to orthopedic surgery. Both HIV-infected patients are well at present, still with asymptomatic HIV-infection and with a good function of the prostheses. Three hemophiliacs have died since the time of surgery; death was unrelated to surgery and arthropathy.

Indication for Total Knee Prosthesis

The indication was an anatomically and functionally severely altered, disabling knee with pain in all patients, flexion contracture in most patients (≥20° in 19 cases), and frequent hemorrhages in several patients (>12 per year in 9 cases). There was a striking sudden type of hemorrhage, probably due to bleeding from bone cysts communicating with the joint cavity.

Surgery

Surgery was done under routine antibiotic prophylaxis. PCA or Duracon prostheses were implanted, most cementless despite osteopenia. In single cases cementation was necessary in one compartment. Bone cysts were filled with spongiosa from the resected bone. A synovectomy as total as possible was performed.

I. Scharrer/W. Schramm (Ed.)
30th Hemophilia Symposium Hamburg 1999
© Springer-Verlag Berlin Heidelberg 2001

Replacement Therapy

Within 2 weeks before the operation, a thorough coagulation examination with inhibitor exclusion as the main point was done, including a differential blood count and platelet function analysis. A pharmacokinetic study was not carried out. Apart from cost considerations, this test does not seem to be useful enough due to the altered pharmacokinetics during the initial postoperative period. Immediately before surgery, prior to spinal or general anesthesia, an i.v. bolus injection of 50 IU kg^{-1} body weight of a factor VIII concentrate is administered in hemophilia A patients, and 80 IU kg^{-1} of a factor IX concentrate in hemophilia B patients. During surgery, blood loss is compensated with 500 IU factor VIII or IX per 500 ml measurable blood loss. In three cases, 1 g of tranexamic acid was given i.v. immediately before tourniquet withdrawal. With the last eight cases, postoperative replacement therapy was administered by continuous infusion, starting immediately postoperatively with 3 IU kg^{-1} hr^{-1}, with the aim of a factor VIII or IX level of 80–120 IU/dl. No thromboembolic prophylaxis was done, since all patients had severe coagulopathies. NSAIDs were only administered topically (Flector Tissugel); perhaps with selective Cox 2 inhibitors this attitude will change. The last four patients had a mean coagulation factor requirement of 61250 IU during the 3-week hospital stay (56000–69000, body weight 70–92 kg): two with a plasma-derived concentrate, two with a recombinant concentrate. Further replacement therapy was adapted to the intensity of rehabilitation measures and continued usually for a total of 6–10 weeks.

Postoperative Rehabilitation

Continuous passive motion started on the day following surgery, active assisted physiotherapy on day 3, walking on day 3–5. Patients walked on crutches for 6–12 weeks. With the postoperatively altered position of their knee joint, they had to learn a new gait until they felt safe with it. They had to be aware of the flexion tendency of the knee and to resist to it. Most patients continued with physiotherapy after the 3-week hospital stay; half of the patients had physiotherapy longer than 3 months. Intensive physiotherapy is essential to prevent more than the usual postoperative loss in range of motion of about one third, compared with the one which is reached during surgery.

Complications

As an early complication, ten postoperative hemorrhages occurred in the operated knee, most frequently during day 8–10. One hemorrhage required an arthroscopic evacuation, one an open revision. A further early complication was the fibrosis of the suprapatellar recessus, which was observed in 14 cases. An open arthrolysis in one case was unsuccessful. There were no late complications, especially no loosing of the prosthesis and no infections. All patients had a radiologic control within the last 14 months. Up to now, no replacement of prosthesis was necessary. The course of the three HIV-infected cases was as favorable as in the non-infected patients.

Results

At present, 26 patients are pain-free in the operated knee. The remaining five patients have mild pain, without the need of analgesics, without impairment of activity. Twenty-nine patients are free of hemorrhage. The remaining two have less than three hemorrhages per year. Seventeen patients have full extension, the remaining have extension deficits of ≤15°; 20 patients have flexion of ≥90°. In 16 cases flexion increased, in seven it decreased. Range of motion as a whole augmented in most patients. Walking distance remained decreased in 12 patients, due to the other impaired joints. None of the patients is dependent on a cane or crutch. Going upstairs is without problems in 20 patients, going downstairs in 12. Seven patients regularly use a bike.

Conclusion

Surgery for total knee prosthesis in hemophiliacs is a very demanding treatment for the patient, the doctors, the physiotherapists, the nurses, and the cost provider. Surgery must take place in a hospital setting, where a 3-week hospital stay is possible. If total knee replacement is done in close interdisciplinary cooperation at a center with experience in hemophilia treatment, the risk is nearly the same as in hemostatically normal patients. Patients will be free from pain and hemorrhage, and will have a stable leg with a good extension. All in all, there will be a marked increase in quality of life, in spite of severe arthropathy in other joints.

Corrective Osteotomy of the Lower Extremity in Hemophilic Arthropathy of the Knee and Hip Joint

T. WALLNY, H.H. BRACKMANN, L. HESS, H. REICH, A. SEUSER

A physiologic leg axis depends upon a correct anatomic axis, a stable cartilage situation, and intact interrelation of muscle agonists and antagonists. Hemophilic arthropathy of the lower extremity disturbs muscle action and changes the anatomic axis, resulting in axis deviation mainly affecting the hip and knee [12]. The axis deviation is secondarily reinforced by cartilage insufficiency. Abnormal weight-bearing enhances the bleeding tendency in hemophiliacs and accelerates joint destruction as a result. By the same token, axis correction lowers the bleeding tendency [12, 26].

In view of the extensive joint abnormalities present, joint replacement at an early stage is commonly advocated. However, joint replacement is not the ideal solution in a young patient population as the artificial joints have a limited service life. Axis correction is intended to avoid or at least defer implantation of an artificial joint. The two methods should not be looked upon as fundamental competitors. Either method may be indicated in a given situation [8]. The criteria for deciding in favor of corrective osteotomy or joint replacement are similar in osteoarthrosis and hemophilic arthropathy, and include:

1. Patient's biological age and life expectancy
2. Capacity to bear at least some weight
3. Cartilage instability
4. Patient's body weight
5. Bone quality sufficient to maintain stable osteosynthesis
6. Extent of preoperative mobility
7. Patient's occupation and subjective preference [2, 8, 13, 19]
8. Degree of axis deviation: deviation in excess of 25 may give rise to surgical and neurogenic complications [6]

Hemophilic patients' fairly young age should be given particular consideration when weighing up a decision in favor of joint replacement. In this paper, we present corrective osteotomy as an alternative joint-conserving measure. Long-term outcomes are provided.

Patients and Methods

From 1974 to 1984, 52 knee osteotomies and 9 hip osteotomies were performed in hemophilic patients at Bonn Orthopedic University Hospital. Since then, 41 patients

I. Scharrer/W. Schramm (Ed.)
30th Hemophilia Symposium Hamburg 1999
© Springer-Verlag Berlin Heidelberg 2001

have died or are lost to follow-up. The remaining 14 patients operated about the knee and 7 operated about the hip were followed up on average 19.4 and 18.3 years after surgery, respectively. The patients' mean age at the time of surgery was 27 and 25.4 years, respectively. All patients had type A hemophilia with less than 1% residual factor activity.

The deformity requiring correction was genu varum in seven patients, genu valgum in six, and coxa valga in seven. Extension osteotomy to correct an extension deficit was performed in four patients undergoing supracondylar osteotomy. The angle of correction ranged from 10 to 30 .

Tibial head osteotomy was performed using Blount clamps in nine cases. Supracondylar osteotomy and intertrochanteric osteotomy with an AO condyle angle plate was performed in four and seven cases, respectively. Coventry's technique [3] was used in tibial head procedures and the AO technique [21] was used in supracondylar and intercondylar procedures [21]. The Advisory Committee of the World Federation of Hemophilia Score was applied and the Petterson score [22] was used for radiologic evaluation.

Tibial head osteotomy patients wore a plaster tutor for 6 weeks postoperatively. During this period, the patients practiced weight-bearing by applying their foot to the floor. The plaster cast was removed after a follow-up X-ray and physiotherapeutic aftercare was initiated. Most patients were able to bear their full weight 12 weeks postoperatively.

Patients equipped with the AO angle plate had an osteosynthesis stable enough for practice and were fit for early mobilization and heel-to-toe weight-bearing. They progressed to partial weight-bearing after 6 weeks and were able to bear their full weight 12 weeks postoperatively.

The mean preoperative WFH score was 6.2 points for the involved knee joint and 4 for the hip. The mean Petterson score was 7.1 points for the knee and 6.8 for the hip.

Results

The mean WFH score at postoperative follow-up improved to 5.7 (knee) and 3.7 points (hip). Nine (4) patients improved and three (2) saw their condition deteriorate. One (1) patient's condition remained unchanged (figures in brackets: patients operated at the hip).

The Petterson score increased to an average of 8.7 (knee) and 8.3 points (hip). Ten of the knee patients were worse at follow-up, one patient had improved and two were just the same. Five of the hip patients had deteriorated and two had improved (Fig. 1).

Breakdown of the WFH score showed that in the »pain« category, pain had improved in six patients, worsened in three, and remained at the preoperative level in four cases. The pain situation improved in four of the hip patients and stayed the same in three.

In the »mobility« category, seven of the patients operated about the knee were as mobile as before after an average of 19.4 years, and six were less mobile. In the

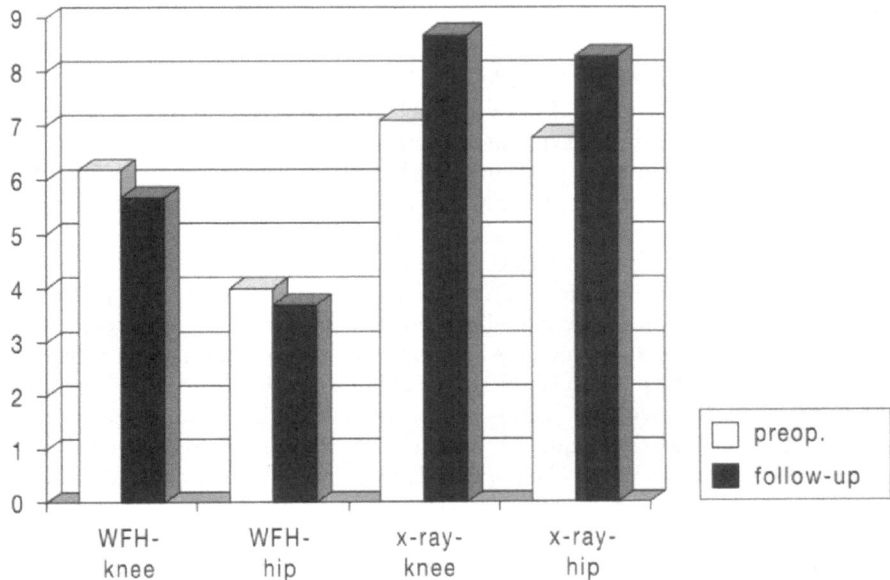

Fig. 1. Overview of clinical scores (*WFH*) and Petterson scores (X-ray) at the knee and hip preoperatively and at follow-up. Note that a clinical improvement (lower number of points) contrasts with a radiologic deterioration (higher number of points)

hip patients, mobility status was unchanged in five, improved in one, and reduced in another.

One patient required knee joint replacement 13 years post-osteotomy in one leg and 8 years post-osteotomy in the other leg. The remaining patients derived a sustained benefit according to their subjective estimation.

Of the 41 patients who were deceased or had dropped out, 38 had undergone osteotomy about the knee and three had undergone intertrochanteric osteotomy. We have data from these patients for an average follow-up period of 10.5 years (standard deviation 5.3 years) and 12.3 years (SD 2.4 years). None of these patients required joint replacement during this period.

Complications

Wound infection requiring surgical revision occurred in one case after infracondylar osteotomy. All tibial head osteotomy patients immobilized in a plaster cast required intensive physiotherapy to restore mobility. One knee joint patient had to be mobilized under anesthesia.

Discussion

Corrective osteotomy of the lower leg can bring about sustained improvement in symptoms even in advanced – but unicompartmental – cases of hemarthropathic lesions and associated axis deviations. This is due to two mechanisms.

Axis correction improves joint congruence and firms up the cartilage apparatus [11]. Movement becomes more harmonious as a result and the weight-bearing pressure on the joint is reduced.

Another explanatory approach centers on joint biology [25]. Perception of pain is mediated both through the joint capsule and the medullary space [30]. Microcirculatory congestion in the medullary sinuses, such as is seen in arthrosis [7], results in bone conversion processes [28] and causes compression of nerve fibers in the bone, which is believed to be the source of bone pain in arthrosis. Osteotomy of the bone opens the medullary spaces, lowers the elevated intravenous pressure, and improves the venous circulation. These mechanisms probably apply to non-hemophilic arthroses as well as to hemophilic joints, although joint damage in hemophiliacs is usually more severe than in »normal« arthrotic joints.

Although many authors recommend slight overcorrection in infracondylar osteotomies as a means of avoiding repeat varus osteotomy [14], it is important to avoid overcorrection in the contralateral compartment of the hemophilic knee, which frequently displays concomitant mild damage. Mild to moderate arthrotic lesions in the femoropatellar synovial bursa do not contraindicate osteotomy about the knee [1, 3, 10, 15, 16]. Our results show that moderately severe cartilage degeneration in the contralateral and femoropatellar compartment is tolerable upon restoration of the weight-bearing axis. Adjustment of the »better« cartilage in hemophilic arthropathy of the hip is a more difficult case. Apart from correction to a normal CCD angle range, the surgeon must attempt to derotate a less worn area of cartilage into the main weight-bearing zone. The difficulty in treating hemophilic joint degeneration, which is often polyarticular, is evident when the (equally affected) neighboring joints are taken into consideration: correction of bow legs results in compensatory coxa valga in the hip joint. Any flexion contracture of the hip needs to be rectified before correcting a genu valgum, as otherwise a functional shortening of the leg and downward displacement of the pelvis are likely. Ankle deformity with the typical medial inclination of the talus should be attempted conservatively or surgically after correction of the knee joint. Alternatively, corrective osteotomy in conjunction with supracondylar extension osteotomy or arthroscopic joint toilet for treatment of an extension deficit at the knee joint can normalize the gait length and bring the hip joint out of its flexion [25]. This indirectly relieves pressure on the neighboring joint.

The joint biology and biomechanical factors described above are highly complex and prohibit a reliable long-term prognosis. Owing to a possible individual or hemophilic particularity, our patients benefited for decades, admittedly in the presence of a reduced level of activity. Correction cannot bring about full restoration, although osteotomy is followed by major repair and regeneration processes in the joint. There is evidence in favor of structural recovery of the joint surfaces by cartilage repair and regeneration and also by radiologically documented spongiosis of the subchondral sclerotic zone following osteotomy [9, 25, 29].

The rate of good long-term responses in osteotomized non-hemophilic patients ranges from 45% to 80% [1, 4, 8, 14, 19, 23, 24, 27, 29]. It is clear, however, that good outcomes become increasingly rare as the follow-up period progresses. It is also important to note that the evaluation criteria are not uniform and therefore not comparable. There are no published data showing long-term outcomes in osteotomized hemophilic joints. Merchan and Galindo identified improvement after a mean 6.5 years of follow-up in 11 out of 14 patients who had undergone osteotomy about the knee [20].

To sum up, corrective osteotomy of the lower leg can be recommended even in advanced – primarily unicompartmental – hemarthropathic lesions and associated axis deviations. Axis correction is, however, only one prerequisite for a muscle coating, which should be trained as much as possible on the basis of the improved biomechanical situation.

Against this background, joint replacement operations must show long-term whether early intervention improves quality of life in hemophilic patients. It is important to remember that progressively worsening mobility improves only marginally when an artificial joint is implanted. Surgery should not be delayed too long in such cases. The physician should explore the options with the young patient and weigh up the goals that can be achieved in each case.

References

1. Augstburger F, Knüsel HP, Aebersold P (1990) Langzeitresultate nach valgisierender Tibiakopfosteotomie bei Varusgonarthrose. Orthop Prax 2: 122–123
2. Brocklehurst R (1984) The composition of normal and osteoarthritic articular cartilage from human knee joints. J Bone Joint Surg [Am] 66: 95–106
3. Coventry MB (1973) Osteotomy about the knee for degenerative and rheumatoid arthritis. Indications, operative technique, and results. J Bone Joint Surg [Am] 55: 23–48
4. Coventry MB (1979) Upper tibial osteotomy for gonarthrosis. The evolution of the operation in the last 18 years and long term results. Orthop Clin North Am 10: 191–210
5. Dolanc B, Weidmann D (1980) Die hohe Tibiaosteotomie in der Behandlung der Gonarthrose bei Betagten. Aktuel Gerontol 10: 497–499
6. Eickhoff HH, Klein C, Koch W, Seuser A, Oldenburg J, Brackmann HH (1992) Langzeitergebnisse der kniegelenknahen Umstellungsosteotomie bei der Behandlung der hämophilen Arthropathie. In: Scharrer I, Schramm W (Ed.) 23. Hämophilie-Symposium Hamburg 1992. Springer, Berlin Heidelberg New York
7. Ficat P, Arlet J (1975) Arthrosis: new diagnostic procedures. Acta Orthop Scand 46: 329–337
8. Fuchs S (1999) Bedeutung der Tibiakopfumstellungsosteotomie im Zeitalter von Endoprothesen. Z Orthop 137: 253–258
9. Fujisawa Y et al (1979) The effect of high tibial osteotomy on osteoarthritis of the knee. An arthroscopic study of fifty-four knee joints. Orthop Clin North Am 10: 585–608
10. Goutallier D, Delepine G, Debeyre J (1979) L'articulation femoro-patellaire dans le genou varum arthrosique. Rev Chir Orthop 65: 25–31
11. Hachenbroch, MH (1982) Degenerative Gelenkerkrankungen. In: Handbuch der Orthopädie, Band IV. Allgemeine Orthopädie. Thieme, Stuttgart
12. Hofmann, P, Rössler, H, Brackmann, HH (1977) Orthopädische Probleme bei der Hämophilie. Z Orthop 115, 342–355.
13. Holden, DL, James SL, Larson RL, Slocum DB (1988) Proximal tibial osteotomy in patients who are fifty years old or less. J Bone Jt Surg 70 A; 977–982

14. Jenny K, Jenny H, Morscher E (1985) Indikation, Operationstechnik und Resultate der transkondylären Tibiaosteotomie bei Gonarthrose. Orthopäde 14:161–171
15. Kettelkamp DB, Wenger DR, Chao EYS, Thompson C (1976) Results of proximal tibial osteotomy. J Bone Joint Surg [Am] 58:952–960
16. Koshino T (1982) The treatment of spontaneous osteonecrosis of the knee by high tibial osteotomy with and without bonegrafting or drilling of the lesion. J Bone Joint Surg [Am] 64: 47–58
17. Kozinn, SC, Scott, RD (1989) Unicondylar knee arthroplasty. J Bone Joint Surg 71 A; 145–150
18. Kummer B (1977) Biomechanische Grundlagen »beanspruchungsändernder« Osteotomien im Bereich des Kniegelenks. Z Orthop 19: 923–928
19. Legal H (1987) Die kniegelenksnahen Osteotomien in der Behandlung der Gonarthrose. Indikation und Ergebnisse. Orthop Prax 1: 53–62
20. Merchan ECR, Merchan ECR, Galindo E (1992) Proximal tibial valgus osteotomy for hemophilic arthropathy of the knee. Orthop Rev 21:204.
21. Müller ME, Allgöwer M, Schneider R, Willenegger H (1996) Manual der Osteosynthese. 3rd edition. Springer, Berlin
22. Petterson H, Ahlberg A, Nilsson IM (1980) A radiologic classification of hemophilic arthropathy. Clin Orthop 149:153–159
23. Schmitt O, Schmitt E, Mittelmeier H (1987) Die Behandlung der halbseitigen Kniegelenkarthrose durch kniegelenksnahe Umstellungsosteotomie mit der Autokompressions-Plattenosteosynthese. Orthop Prax 2: 84–89
24. Schmitt E, Schmitt O, Mittelmeier H (1987) Suprakondyläre Umstellungsosteotomien im Kniegelenksbereich. In: Küsswetter, WJ, Krais J von (Ed.) Kniegelenksnahe Osteotomien. Thieme, Stuttgart New York
25. Schultz, W (1999) Kniegelenknahe Osteotomien. Arthroskopie 12:22–28
26. Smith, MA, Urquhart, DR, Savidge, GF (1981) The surgical management of varus deformity in haemophilic arthropathy of the knee. J Bone Joint Surg 63 B: 2, 261–165
27. Träger D, Braukmann R, Dybowski W (1989) Kniegelenknahe Osteotomien Spätergebnisse. Orthop Praxis 9: 585–590
28. Trueta JM, Harrison HM (1953) The normal vascular anatomy of the femoral head in adult man. J Bone Joint Surg 35 [Br]:442–461
29. Wagner H, Zeiler G, Baur W (1985) Indikation, Technik und Ergebnisse der supra- und infracondylären Korrekturosteotomie bei der Kniegelenksarthrose. Orthopäde 14: 172–192
30. Willert H, Otte P (1979) Der Gelenkschmerz – Differenzierung arthrogener und osteogener Schmerzkomponenten. Orthop Prax 4;56–64

VI. Pediatric Hemostasiology

Chairmen:

W. KREUZ (Frankfurt/Main)
H. POLLMANN (Münster)

Anticoagulant Action of Activated Protein C is Diminished by Alpha$_2$-Macroglobulin in Newborn Plasma

G. Cvirn, S. Gallistl, J. Kutschera, W. Muntean

Introduction

The risk of thromboembolic complications is considerably less for newborns and children than adults for any given insult, due to lower plasma concentrations of vitamin K-dependent coagulation factors, i.e., prothrombin, and contact factors [1, 2]. The capacity of newborn plasma to generate thrombin is decreased to 30–50% of adult values [3, 4]. In addition, alpha$_2$-macroglobulin (α_2-M) has been suggested as a major anticoagulant protein in infancy and has been demonstrated to complex up to 49% of generated alpha thrombin in newborn plasma [5, 6]. On the other hand, α_2-M has been shown to bind activated protein C (APC) [7], one of the most important anticoagulant proteins. In addition, increased complex formation between α_2-M and APC has been demonstrated to be associated with an unfavorable outcome in patients suffering from disseminated intravascular coagulation (DIC) [8], suggesting that α_2-M might abrogate the anticoagulant action of APC. Previously, we have demonstrated a dose-dependent anticoagulant effect of APC in newborn and adult plasma using the determination of thrombin generation (thrombin potential, TP) [9]. TP has been shown to be a reliable parameter to assess the combined effects of all factors that may influence thrombin generation in a given sample [10–14]. Therefore, we investigated the effect of α_2-M on the anticoagulant action of APC by using the determination of TP. In addition, since TP does not exactly reflect the amount of prothrombin activated, we determined the generation of prothrombin fragments 1+2 (F1+2) in the presence of different concentrations of α_2-M.

Methods

Collection and Preparation of Plasma

Cord blood was obtained immediately following the delivery of 12 full-term infants (38–42 weeks gestational age). It was collected into 0.1 M citrate using a two-syringe technique, centrifuged at room temperature for 15 min at 2800 xg, pooled and stored at −70°C in propylene tubes until assayed. Clotting factors, AT, protein C, protein S, and α_2-M in the pooled cord plasma were in the normal range for neonates. In the same way, plasma from ten healthy adults was collected, prepared, and checked.

I. Scharrer/W. Schramm (Ed.)
30th Hemophilia Symposium Hamburg 1999
© Springer-Verlag Berlin Heidelberg 2001

Preparation of Plasma with Different α_2-M Concentration

The α_2-M activity of the pooled neonatal or adult plasma was decreased by supplementation of proteinase A, a metalloenzyme that forms a complex with α_2-M at a molar ratio of 1:1. Different amounts (0–20 µl) of proteinase A were added to 1 ml of plasma, resulting in α_2-M activities from 1.8 to 3.6 µM for newborn plasma and from 1.1 to 2.0 µM for adult plasma. To increase the α_2-M concentration, different amounts (0–80 µl) of purified α_2-M concentrate were added to 1 ml of plasma, resulting in α_2-M concentrations from 3.6 to 5.9 µM in newborn plasma and from 2.0 to 4.6 µM in adult plasma.

Determination of the α_2-M Concentration

Determination of the α_2-M concentration of pooled newborn and adult plasma was performed using the standard test kit Unitest Assay for α_2-macroglobulin determination in human plasma from CoaChrom Diagnostics, Vienna, Austria.

Activation of Plasma

200 µl plasma with different α_2-M concentrations were incubated with 10 µl of buffer A (containing different amounts of APC) for 1 min at 37°C. After subsequent incubation with 20 µl buffer A containing 1.0 mg/ml H-Gly-Pro-Arg-Pro-OH (GPRP, Pefabloc FG) for 1 min at 37°C to inhibit fibrin polymerization, the plasma samples were activated by addition of 200 µl Thromborel S and the clotting time was recorded on a Behring Fibrintimer from Behring Diagnostics GmbH, Marburg, Germany.

Determination of Thrombin Generation

We used a subsampling method derived from a recently described technique [10, 13]. Plasmas were prepared and activated as described above. At timed intervals, 10 µl aliquots were withdrawn from the activated plasma and subsampled into 490 µl buffer B containing 255 µM S-2238. The reagents were prewarmed to 37°C. Amidolysis of S-2238 was stopped after 6 min by addition of 250 µl 50% acetic acid. The amount of thrombin generated was quantitated by measuring the absorbance by double wavelength (405–690 nm) in the Anthos microplate reader 2001, from Anthos Labtec Instruments GmbH, Salzburg, Austria. The total amidolytic activity measured is caused by the simultaneous activity of free thrombin and α_2-M/thrombin complex [10]. The amount of free thrombin was determined by two different methods. (a) At timed intervals, aliquots of the extrinsically activated plasma were subsampled into buffer B containing heparin (20 U/ml) and AT (3.4 U/ml) to rapidly and completely inactivate free thrombin in the sample. The residual amidolytic activity was then determined as described above for the total amidolytic activity.

The amidolytic activity of the α_2-M/thrombin complex was subtracted from the total amidolytic activity [3]. (b) Free thrombin generation curves were calculated by mathematical treatment of total amidolytic activity curves using a method developed by Hemker et al. [11].

Determination of Prothrombin Fragment 1+2

Plasmas were prepared and activated as described above. At timed intervals, 5 µl aliquots were withdrawn from the plasma and subsampled into 495 µl stopping solution. After subsequent 1:10-dilution in stopping solution, the amount of F1+2 generated was quantitated using a standard enzymatic test kit.

Statistical Analysis

The results shown are expressed as means ($n=3$). Data were statistically analyzed for significance using the Kruskal-Wallis non-parametric analysis of variance taking $P<0.05$ to indicate a significant difference or by means of Pearson's correlation.

Results

Effect of APC Administration to Plasma with Different α_2-M Content on Thrombin Generation

The time-course of free thrombin generation (TP) was determined as described in Methods. A typical experiment performed in newborn plasma is shown in Fig. 1A: In the absence of APC, same amounts of free thrombin (291 nM/min) were generated in plasma containing 4.3, 3.6, and 2.0 µM α_2-M. Addition of 21 nM APC (final) to plasma containing 3.6 µM α_2-M (physiologic concentration in newborn plasma) resulted in a significantly decreased thrombin generation compared to plasma with the same α_2-M content in the absence of APC. The calculated area under the TGC decreased from 291 nM/min to 236 nM/min ($P<0.05$). Addition of 21 nM APC (final) to newborn plasma containing 2.0 µM α_2-M also resulted in a significant decrease of thrombin generation compared to the corresponding plasma in the absence of APC. The calculated area under the TGC decreased from 291 nM/min to 150 nM/min ($P<0.05$). Addition of the same amount of APC to newborn plasma containing 4.3 µM α_2-M resulted in no significant decrease of thrombin generation compared to the corresponding plasma without APC supplementation. In newborn plasma with α_2-M concentrations from 1.8 to 4.3 µM, APC supplementation to final concentrations of 21 and 42 nM resulted in a dose-dependent alteration of thrombin generation, following the equations $y=-18x+84.5$, $P<0.01$, and $y=-26.9x+124.1$, $P<0.01$, respectively. At α_2-M concentrations exceeding 4.3 µM, APC supplementation of 21 or 42 nM had no significant effect on thrombin generation (Fig. 1B). Essentially the same results were obtained in adult plasma. A typical experiment is

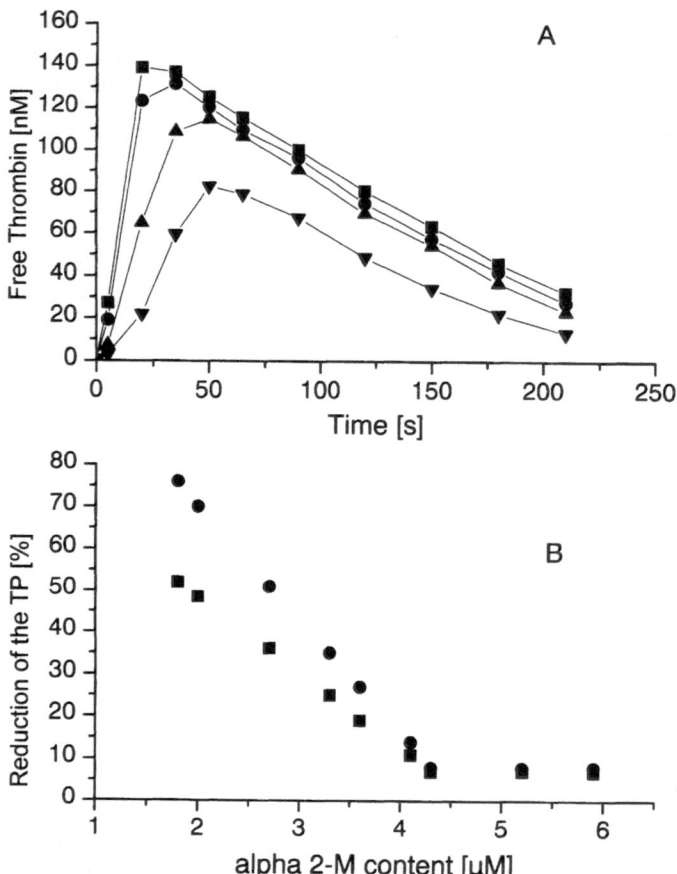

Fig. 1. A Free thrombin generation in newborn plasma containing 2.0, 3.6, or 4.3 μM α_2-M in the absence of APC (■). Effects of supplementation of 21 nM APC to plasma with different α_2-M concentrations (▼, 2.0 μM; ▲, 3.6 μM; ●, 4.3 μM) on free thrombin generation. **B** Reduction of the thrombin potential (TP) by addition of 21 nM (■) or 42 nM (●) APC to plasma containing 1.8–5.9 μM α_2-M related to corresponding plasma in the absence of APC. Results are expressed as means (n=3). SEM is not shown for clarity of graph reading, but represented less than 10% of the mean

shown in Fig. 2A: In the absence of APC in plasma containing 3.2, 2.0, and 1.4 μM α_2-M, same amounts of free thrombin (627 nM/min) were generated. Addition of 42 nM APC (final) to plasma containing 2.0 μM α_2-M resulted in a significantly decreased thrombin generation compared to the corresponding plasma without APC supplementation. The calculated area under the TGC decreased from 627 to 428 nM/min (P<0.05). Addition of 42 nM APC (final) to adult plasma containing 1.4 μM α_2-M also resulted in a significant decrease of thrombin generation compared to plasma with the same α_2-M content in the absence of APC. The calculated area under the TGC decreased from 627 to 277 nM/min (P<0.05). Addition of the same amount of APC

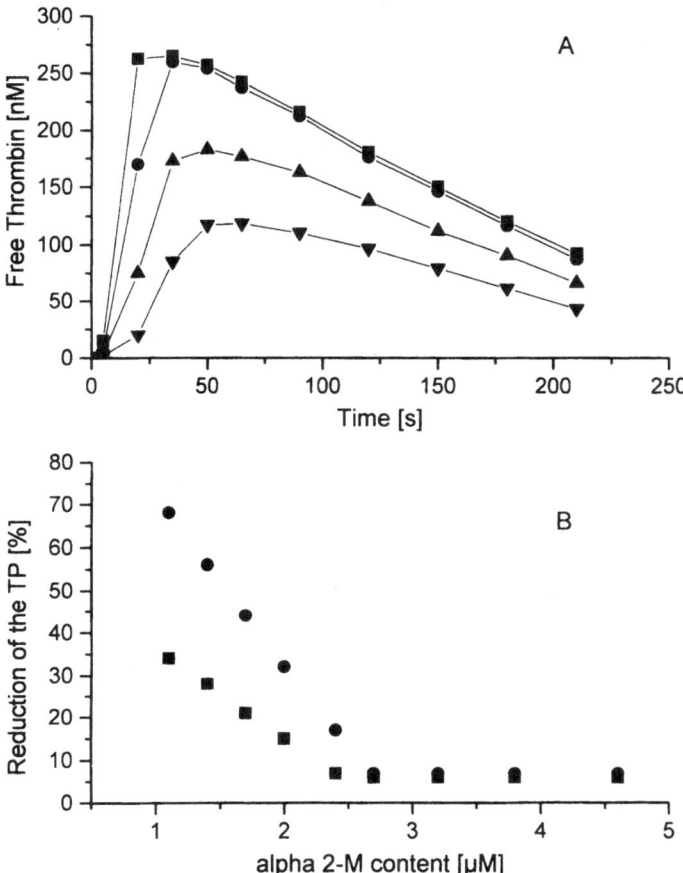

Fig. 2. A Free thrombin generation in adult plasma containing 1.4, 2.0, or 3.2 μM α$_2$-M in the absence of APC (■). Effects of supplementation of 42 nM APC to plasma with different α$_2$-M concentrations (▼,1.4 μM; ▲, 2.0 μM; ●, 3.2 μM) on free thrombin generation. **B** Reduction of the TP by addition of 21 nM (■) or 42 nM (●) APC to plasma containing 1.1–4.6 μM α$_2$-M related to corresponding plasma in the absence of APC. Results are expressed as means (n=3). SEM is not shown for clarity of graph reading, but represented less than 10% of the mean

(final) to adult plasma containing 3.2 μM α$_2$-M resulted in no significant decrease of thrombin generation compared to the corresponding plasma without APC supplementation. In adult plasma containing 1.1–2.7 μM α$_2$-M, APC supplementation to final concentrations of 21 and 42 nM resulted in a dose-dependent alteration of thrombin generation, following the equations $y=-20.9x+56.9$, $P<0.01$, and $y=-39.3x+111.1$, $P<0.01$, respectively. At α$_2$-M concentrations exceeding 2.7 μM, APC supplementation of 21 or 42 nM had no significant effect on thrombin generation (Fig. 2B).

Effect of APC Administration to Plasma with Different α_2-M Content on Prothrombin Activation

To determine prothrombin activation we recorded the time-course of prothrombin fragment 1+2 (F1+2) generation as described in Methods. A typical experiment is shown in Fig. 3A: In the absence of APC, same amounts of F1+2 (0.6 µM) were generated in newborn plasma containing 4.1 and 2.7 µM α_2-M. Addition of 21 nM APC (final) to plasma containing 4.1 µM α_2-M resulted in a significantly suppressed prothrombin activation. The end level of the F1+2 generation curve decreased from 0.60 to 0.54 µM ($P<0.05$). Addition of the same amount of APC to newborn plasma

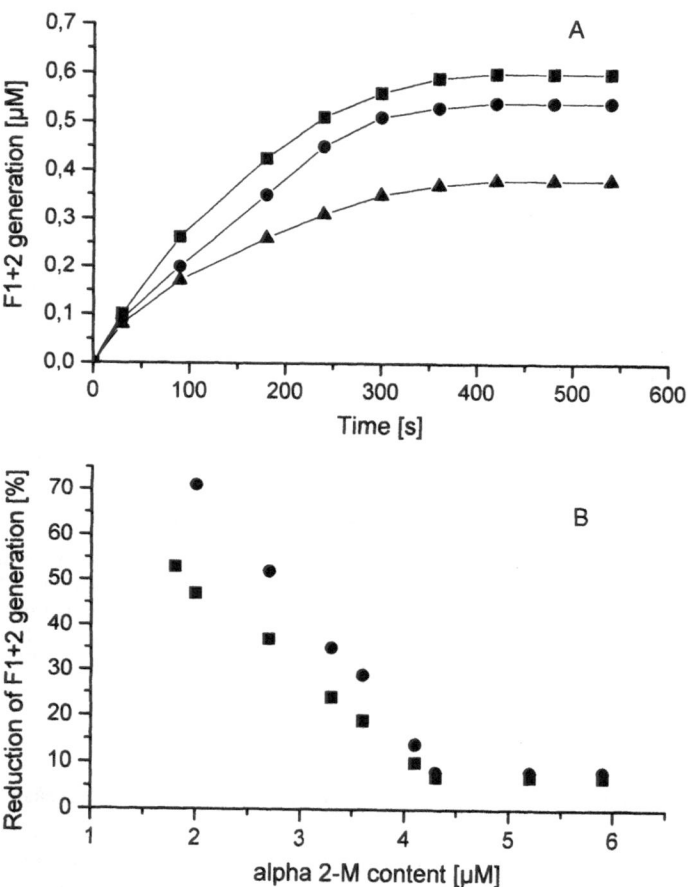

Fig. 3. A Prothrombin fragment 1+2 (*F1+2*) activation in newborn plasma containing 2.7 or 4.1 µM α_2-M in the absence of APC (■). Effects of supplementation of 21 nM APC to plasma with 2.7 µM (▲) or 4.1 µM (●) α_2-M on F1+2 generation. B Reduction of *F1+2* generation by addition of 21 nM (■) or 42 nM (●) APC to plasma containing 1.8–5.9 µM α_2-M related to corresponding plasma in the absence of APC. Results are expressed as means (*n*=3). SEM is not shown for clarity of graph reading, but represented less than 10% of the mean

containing 2.7 μM α_2-M also resulted in a significantly suppressed prothrombin activation. The end level of the F1+2 generation curve decreased from 0.60 to 0.38 μM ($P<0.05$). In newborn plasma with α_2-M concentrations from 1.8 to 4.3 μM, APC supplementation to final concentrations of 21 and 42 nM APC resulted in a dose-dependent alteration of prothrombin activation compared to corresponding plasma in the absence of APC, following the equations $y=-18.4x+85.3$, $P<0.01$, and $y=-27.1x+125.5$, $P<0.01$, respectively (Fig. 3B). At α_2-M concentrations exceeding 4.3 μM, APC supplementation of 21 or 42 nM showed no significant effect on prothrombin activation (Fig. 3B). Essentially the same results were obtained in adult plasma. A typical experiment is shown in Fig. 4A: In the absence of APC, same

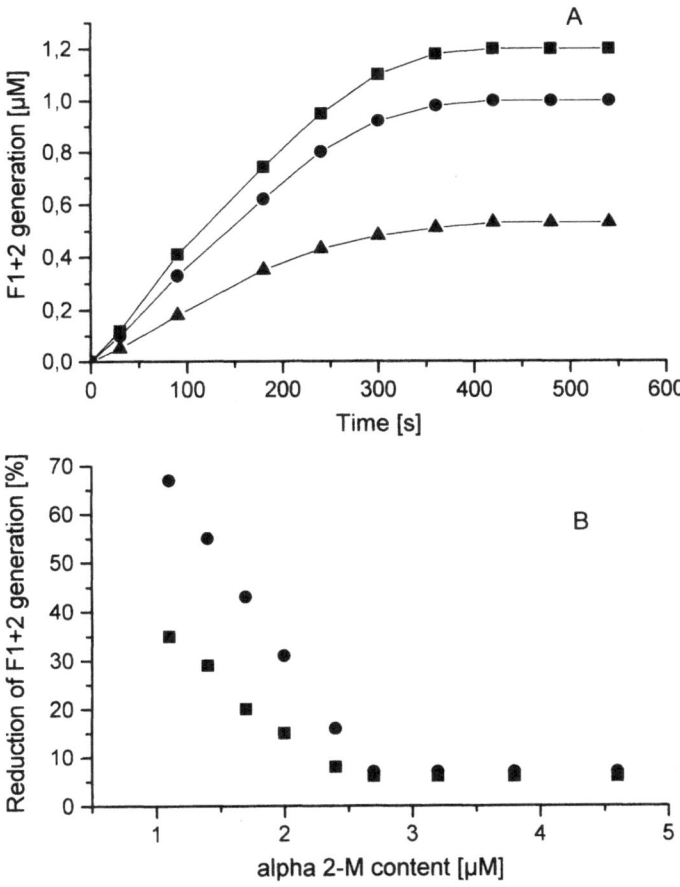

Fig. 4. A F1+2 activation in adult plasma containing 1.4 or 2.4 μM α_2-M without APC administration (■). Effects of supplementation of 42 nM APC to plasma with 1.4 μM (▲) or 2.4 μM (●) a_2-M on F1+2 generation. B Reduction of F1+2 generation by addition of 21 nM (■) or 42 nM (●) APC plasma containing 1.1–4.6 μM α_2-M related to corresponding plasma in the absence of APC. Results are expressed as means ($n=3$). SEM is not shown for clarity of graph reading, but represented less than 10% of the mean

amounts of F_{1+2} (1.2 µM) were generated in adult plasma containing 2.4 and 1.4 µM α_2-M. Addition of 42 nM APC (final) to plasma containing 2.4 µM α_2-M resulted in a significantly suppressed prothrombin activation. The end level of the F_{1+2} generation curve decreased from 1.2 to 1.0 µM ($P<0.05$). Addition of the same amount of APC to adult plasma containing 1.4 µM α_2-M also resulted in a significantly suppressed prothrombin activation. The end level of the F_{1+2}-generation curve decreased from 1.20 to 0.53 µM ($P<0.05$). In adult plasma with α_2-M concentrations from 1.1 to 2.7 µM, APC supplementation to final concentrations of 21 and 42 nM APC resulted in a dose-dependent alteration of prothrombin activation compared to corresponding plasma in the absence of APC, following the equations $y=-21.1x+57.8$, $P<0.01$, and $y=-39.3x+111$, $P<0.01$, respectively (Fig. 4B). At α_2-M concentrations exceeding 2.7 µM, APC supplementation of 21 or 42 nM showed no significant effect on prothrombin activation (Fig. 4B).

Effect of APC Administration to Plasma with Different α_2-M Content on Clotting Time

APC was added to plasma to final concentrations of 21 and 42 nM and incubated for 1 min at 37°C. Subsequently, the plasma was extrinsically activated, clotting time was recorded as described in Methods and related to clotting times of plasma with corresponding α_2-M content in the absence of APC. Administration of 21 nM APC (final) to newborn plasma (1.8–4.3 µM α_2-M) resulted in a dose-dependent alteration of clotting time, following the equation $y=-17.1x+83.7$, $P<0.01$ (Fig. 5A). Addition of 42 nM APC also resulted in a dose-dependent alteration of clotting time, following the equation $y=-22.6x+114.7$, $P<0.01$ (Fig. 5A). At α_2-M concentrations exceeding 4.3 µM, APC supplementation of 21 or 42 nM had no significant effect on clotting time. Again, the same results were obtained in pooled adult plasma. In between a concentration range of 1.1–2.7 µM α_2-M, APC supplementation to final concentrations of 21 and 42 nM resulted in a dose-dependent alteration of clotting time, following the equations $y=-17.5x+51.6$, $P<0.01$, and $y=-30.7+91.9$, $P<0.01$, respectively (Fig. 5B). At α_2-M concentrations exceeding 2.7 µM, APC supplementation of 21 or 42 nM had no significant effect on clotting time (Fig. 5).

Effect of a High-Dose Application of APC on Plasma at Physiologic and Elevated α_2-M Level

Addition of 56 nM APC (final) to newborn plasma containing 3.6 µM α_2-M (physiologic concentration in newborn plasma) resulted in a significant decrease of thrombin generation compared to plasma with physiologic concentration of α_2-M in the absence of APC. The calculated area under the thrombin generation curve decreased from 291 to 157 nM/min ($P<0.05$; Fig. 6A). Administration of the same amount of APC to newborn plasma containing 5.9 µM α_2-M resulted in no significant effect on thrombin generation compared to plasma with the same α_2-M content in the absence of APC (Fig. 6B). Comparable results were obtained in adult

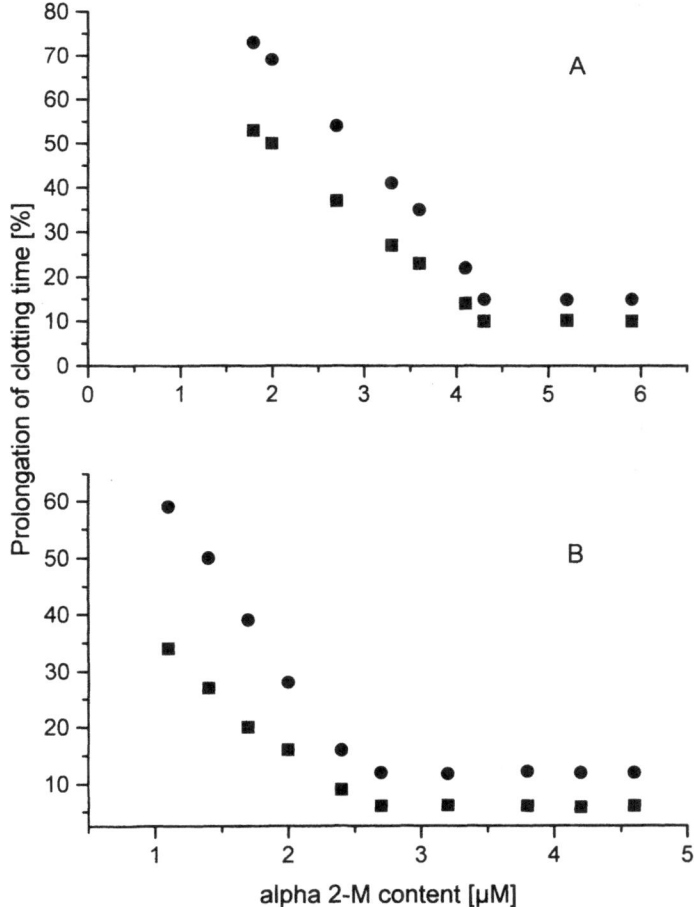

Fig. 5. A Prolongation of clotting time by addition of 21 nM (■) or 42 nM (●) APC to newborn plasma containing 1.8–5.9 μM α₂-M related to corresponding plasma in the absence of APC. **B** Prolongation of clotting time by addition of 21 nM (■) or 42 nM (●) APC to adult plasma containing 1.1–4.6 μM α₂-M related to corresponding plasma in the absence of APC. Results are expressed as means ($n=3$). SEM is not shown for clarity of graph reading, but represented less than 10% of the mean

plasma. Addition of 81 nM APC (final) to plasma containing 2.0 μM α₂-M (physiologic concentration in adult plasma) resulted in a significant decrease of thrombin generation compared to plasma with physiologic α₂-M concentration in the absence of APC. The calculated area under the thrombin generation curve decreased from 627 to 241 nM/min ($P<0.05$; Fig. 7A). Addition of the same amount of APC to adult plasma at an elevated α₂-M level (3.8 μM) resulted in no significant decrease of thrombin generation compared to plasma with the same α₂-M content in the absence of APC (Fig. 7B). Correspondingly, prothrombin activation and prolongation

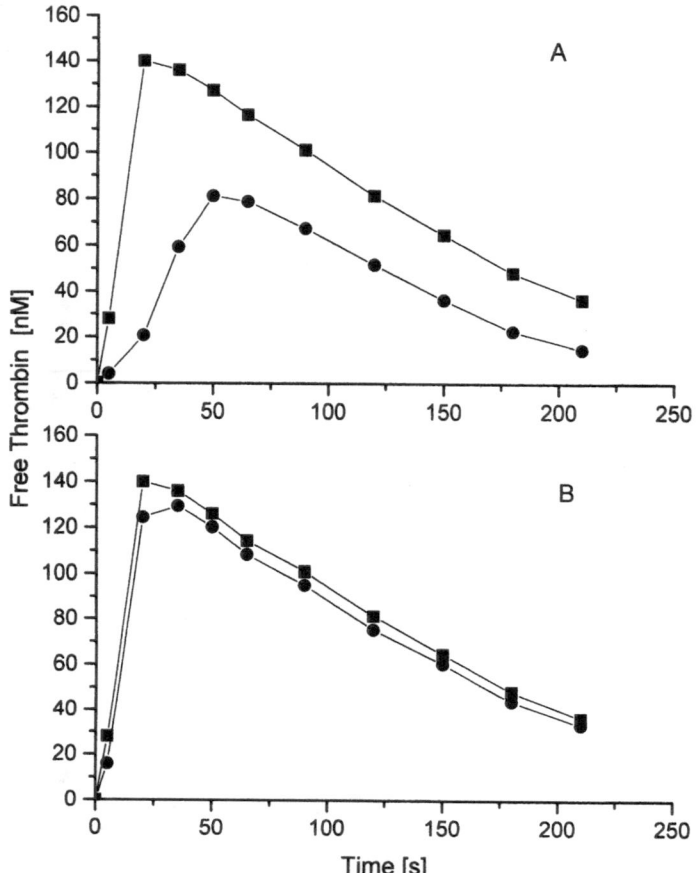

Fig. 6. A Effect of supplementation of o nM (■) or 56 nM (●) APC to newborn plasma containing 3.6 μM α_2-M on generation of free thrombin. **B** Effect of supplementation of o nM (■) or 56 nM (●) APC to newborn plasma containing 5.9 μM α_2-M on free thrombin generation. Results are expressed as means ($n=3$). SEM is not shown for clarity of graph reading, but represented less than 10% of the mean

of clotting time in both newborn and adult plasma were suppressed more effectively in plasma at an elevated α_2-M level than in plasma at a physiologic α_2-M concentration for a high-dose application of APC (data not shown).

Discussion

We have described previously a dose-dependent anticoagulant effect of APC using the determination of thrombin generation after intrinsic activation [9]. In cord and adult plasma Protac [15], induced APC reduced the amount and prolonged the lag

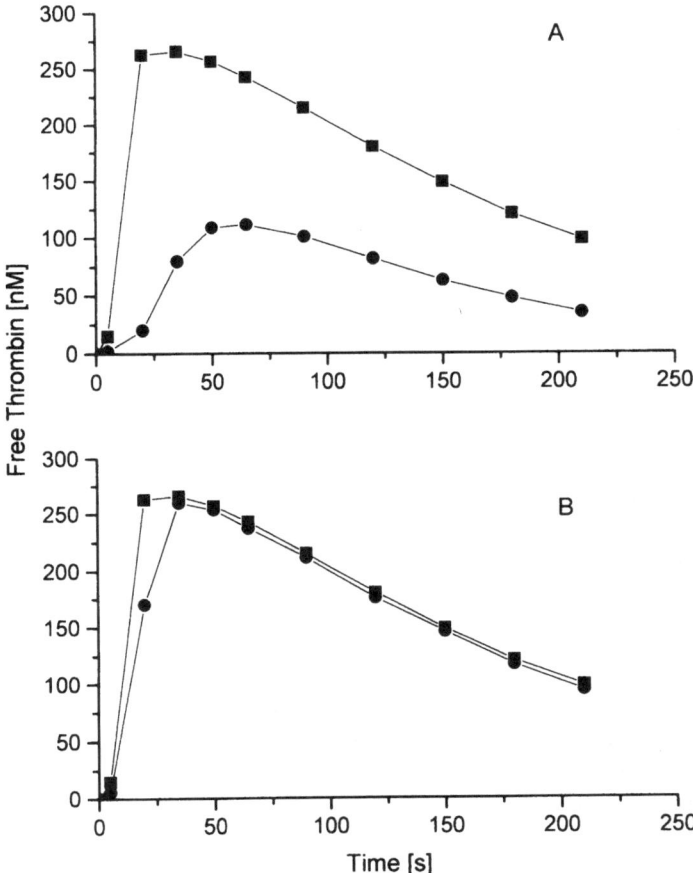

Fig. 7. A Effect of supplementation of o nM (■) or 81 nM (●) APC to adult plasma containing 2.0 μM α$_2$-M on generation of free thrombin. **B** Effect of supplementation of o nM (■) or 81 nM (●) APC to adult plasma containing 3.8 μM α$_2$-M on free thrombin generation. Results are expressed as means (n=3). SEM is not shown for clarity of graph reading, but represented less than 10% of the mean

times until the onset of free thrombin generation. These results were reproduced in the present study after addition of already activated protein C. After addition of α$_2$-M, the anticoagulant effect of APC was diminished, suggesting that α$_2$-M abrogates the anticoagulant properties of APC. In addition, the anticoagulant effect of APC was enhanced when α$_2$-M was inhibited by proteinase A [16] in both newborn (Fig. 1) and adult plasma (Fig. 2). In accordance with the effect on free thrombin generation, α$_2$-M abrogated the inhibiting effect of APC on prothrombinase activity assessed by determination of prothrombin fragment 1+2 in both newborn (Fig. 3) and adult plasma (Fig. 4). The observation that α$_2$-M abrogates the effect of APC on feedback activation of prothrombinase is intriguing since it has been shown that α$_2$-M accounts for a large amount of thrombin inhibition, especially in newborn plasma [5]. Studies dealing with thrombin inhibition by α_2-M determined thrombin/α_2-M complex formation after a certain period of plasma incubation and did not assess the time course of thrombin generation and inhibition [17, 18]. The action between α_2-M and thrombin might not be fast enough to prevent thrombin from feedback activation of factors V and VIII [19], thereby inducing prothrombinase formation. Our results suggest that the procoagulant properties of α_2-M might even surpass its anticoagulant activity. This suggestion is in contrast to the assumption that α_2-M might protect children with low antithrombin (AT) from thrombotic events, and that α_2-M is as important an inhibitor of thrombin as AT in fetal plasma [17]. Children might be protected from thromboembolic complications due to their decreased ability to generate thrombin compared to adults. This assumption is supported by the fact that free thrombin generation is increased in patients suffering from venous thromboembolic events and decreases during anticoagulant therapy [18].

Scully et al. investigated the activation of protein C and its distribution between its inhibitors in patients with DIC, and suggested that α_2-M and α_1-A appeared to assume greater roles in inhibition of APC in two fatal cases [8]. α_2-M increases during the initial phase of sepsis and subsequently decreases due to multiple complex formation with proteinases. Since availability of APC seems to be predictive of the outcome of critically ill patients and application of APC results in favorable outcome [20, 21], our data suggest that α_2-M might contribute to unfavorable loss of anticoagulant property due to inhibition of APC. In accordance with this assumption is the observation that venous thromboembolic complications in children mostly occur accompanied by associated conditions (e.g., cancer, trauma, infection) [22, 23], where APC might be consumed, probably partly due to increased concentrations of α_2-M. In our study we have shown that at elevated α_2-M levels the anticoagulant effect of even a high-dose application of APC decreases in both newborn (Fig. 6) and adult plasma (Fig. 7).

In conclusion, our study demonstrates that at elevated levels α_2-M abrogates the anticoagulant effect of APC and argues against the assumption that α_2-M protects children from thrombotic events. In addition, elevated α_2-M concentrations might even add to an unfavorable prothrombotic state in both newborn and adult plasma.

References

1. Andrew M, Paes B, Milner R, Johnston M, Mitchell L, Tollefsen DM, Powers P. Development of the human coagulation system in the fullterm infant. Blood 1987; 70: 165–170.
2. Andrew M. Developmental hemostasis: relevance to thromboembolic complications in pediatric patients. Thromb Haemost 1995; 74: 415–25.
3. Andrew M, Schmidt B, Mitchell L, Paes B, Ofosu F. Thrombin generation in newborn plasma is critically dependent on the concentration of prothrombin. Thromb Haemost 1990; 63: 27–30.
4. Andrew M, Vegh P, Johnston M, Bowker J, Ofosu F, Mitchell L. Maturation of the hemostatic system during childhood. Blood 1992; 8: 1998–2005.
5. Ling X, Delorme M, Berry L, Ofosu F, Mitchell L, Paes B, Andrew M. Alpha2-macroglobulin remains as important as antithrombin III for thrombin regulation in cord plasma in the presence of endothelial cell surfaces. Pediatr Res 1995; 37: 373–8.

6. Andrew M, Mitchell L, Vegh P, Ofosu F. Thrombin regulation in children differs from adults in the absence and presence of heparin. Thromb Haemost 1994; 72: 836–42.
7. Hoogendoorn H, Toh CH, Nesheim ME, Giles AR. Alpha 2-macroglobulin binds and inhibits activated protein C. Blood 1991; 78: 2283–90.
8. Scully MF, Toh CH, Hoogendoorn H, Manuel RP, Nesheim ME, Solymoss S, Giles AR. Activation of protein C and its distribution between its inhibitors protein C inhibitor, alpha1-antitrypsin and alpha2-macroglobulin, in patients with disseminated intravascular coagulation. Thromb Haemost 1993; 69: 448–53.
9. Cvirn G, Gallistl S, Muntean W. Effects of antithrombin and protein C on thrombin generation in newborn and adult plasma. Thromb Res 1999; 93: 183–90.
10. Hemker HC, Willems GM, Beguin S. A computer assisted method to obtain the prothrombin activation velocity in whole plasma independent of thrombin decay processes. Thromb Haemost 1986; 56: 9–17.
11. Hemker HC, Wielders S, Kessels H, Beguin S. Continuous registration of thrombin generation in plasma, its use for the determination of the thrombin potential. Thromb Haemost 1993; 70: 617–24.
12. Hemker HC, Beguin S. Thrombin generation in plasma: its assessment via the endogenous thrombin potential. Thromb Hemost 1995; 74: 134–8.
13. Gallistl S, Muntean W, Leis HJ. Effects of heparin and hirudin on thrombin generation and platelet aggregation after intrinsic activation of platelet rich plasma. Thromb Haemost 1995; 74: 1163–8.
14. Wielders S, Mukherjee M, Michiels J, Rijkers DTS, Cambus JP, Knebel RWC, Kakkar V, Hemker HC. The routine determination of the endogenous thrombin potential, first results in different forms of hyper and hypocoagulability. Thromb Haemost 1997; 77: 629–36.
15. Kisiel W, Kondo S, Smith KJ, McMullen BA, Smith LF. Characterization of a protein C activator from *Agkistrodon contortrix contortrix* venom. J Biol Chem 1987; 262: 12607–13.
16. Svoboda P, Meier J, Freyvogel TA. Purification and characterization of three α_2-antiplasmin and α_2-macroglobulin inactivating enzymes from the venom of the Mexican coast rattlesnake (crotalus basiliscus). Toxicon 1995; 33: 1331–46.
17. Mitchell L, Piovella F, Ofosu F, Andrew M. Alpha2-macroglobulin may provide protection from thromboembolic events in antithrombin III-deficient children. Blood 1991; 78: 2299–304.
18. Massicote P, Leaker M, Marzinotto V, Adams M, Freedom R, Williams W, Vegh P, Berry L, Shah B, Andrew M. Enhanced thrombin regulation during warfarin therapy in children compared to adults. Thromb Haemost 1998; 80: 570–4.
19. Jolyon J. The kinetics of inhibition of α-thrombin in human plasma. J Biol Chem 1986; 261: 10313–8.
20. Dreyfus M, Magny JF, Bridey F, Schwarz HP, Planché C, Dehan M, Tchernia G. Treatment of homozygous protein C deficiency and neonatal purpura fulminans with a purified protein C concentrate. N Engl J Med 1991; 325: 1565–8.
21. Rivard GE, David M, Farrell C, Schwarz HP. Treatment of purpura fulminans in meningococcemia with protein C concentrate. J Ped 1995; 126: 646–52.
22. David M, Andrew M. Venous thromboembolic complications in children. J Pediatr 1993; 123: 337–46.
23. Andrew M, David M, Adams M, Ali K, Anderson R, Barnard D, Bernstein M, Brisson L, Cairney B, DeSai D, Grant R, Israels S, Jardine L, Luke B, Massicote P, Silva M. Venous thromboembolic complications (VTE) in children: first analyses of the Canadian registry of VTE. Blood 1994; 83: 1251–7.

Functional Consequences of Differences in Carbohydrate Sequences of Fetal and Adult Plasminogen and Fibrinogen

M. Ries, R. Easton, M. Zenker, C. Longstaff, A. Dell, P.J. Gaffney

Introduction

The fibrinolytic system is involved in a wide variety of biological phenomena such as dissolution of fibrin blood clots, tissue remodeling, metastasis, angiogenesis, wound healing, embryogenesis, and embryo implantation [1]. The absolute and relative concentrations of various components of the fibrinolytic system in neonates differ from adults, and they are dependent on both the gestational age and postnatal age [for review see 2]. In addition, the functional behavior of fetal plasminogen and fetal fibrinogen differ from the adult forms, although electrophoretic molecular weight analyses, as well as amino-acid composition and partial amino-acid sequencing, revealed no differences between fibrinogen and the plasminogen forms 1 and 2 of neonates and adults [3–12]. Therefore, variations in functional behavior have been related to differences in carbohydrate composition [5]. Oligosaccharides linked to proteins may contribute to receptor-mediated interactions, protein stability, clearance from the circulation, and physiological function [13, 14].

Like adult plasminogen, fetal plasminogen exists in two major glycoforms: plasminogen 1 and plasminogen 2. Both contain an O-glycosylation site at Thr[345] while type 1 plasminogen contains an additional N-glycosylation site at Asn[288]. The fetal glycoforms have significantly more sialic acid than the adult forms [5]. This difference in glycosylation is possibly responsible for the lower overall activation rates of the two fetal glycoforms when t-PA is used as an activator and CNBr-fibrinogen fragments as an effector [5]. However, despite low plasminogen levels of ~50% of adult values and slower activation kinetics in the fetal plasma, the overall fibrinolytic activity measured by gross functional assays is quite similar to that of adult plasma [15–18].

Plasmin, a serine protease, is generated from its zymogen plasminogen by cleavage of the Arg[561]–Val[562] bond. This results in formation of the two-chain, disulfide-bonded plasmin with a heavy chain which contains kringles 1–5 and the lysine-binding sites (LBS) and a light chain which contains the catalytic serine protease site [19]. The reaction between α_2-antiplasmin and plasmin proceeds in a two-stage mechanism [20–25]: a very fast reaction with a loose complex (EI*), followed by a tightly bound, stable complex (EI), in which enzyme and inhibitor remain largely unchanged (Eq. 1). There is still controversy about the reversibility of the second step of the reaction.

I. Scharrer/W. Schramm (Ed.)
30th Hemophilia Symposium Hamburg 1999
© Springer-Verlag Berlin Heidelberg 2001

$$E+I \xrightleftharpoons[k_{-1}]{k_1} EI^* \xrightleftharpoons[k_{-2}]{k_2} EI$$

(Eq. 1) (E = enzyme, I = inhibitor)

The aim of our study was to look at the influence of glycosylation on plasmin activity by determining the reaction kinetics of both adult and fetal plasmin (types 1 and 2) with adult as well as fetal α_2-antiplasmin, and to investigate the stimulating effect of fetal fibrin on t-PA-mediated plasminogen activation. In addition, we performed the sequencing of carbohydrate structures of fetal plasminogen types 1 and 2 and fetal fibrinogen in comparison to the respective adult types.

Methods

All kinetic experiments were performed in a 0.01-M Hepes buffer, 0.15 M NaCl, pH 7.4, containing 0.01% Tween 20 at 37°C. After obtaining informed consent, blood samples were taken from the placenta of 45 newborn babies by atraumatic puncture of the umbilical vein immediately after the cord was clamped, but before separation of the placenta. Prior to further analyses, hereditary thrombophilia was excluded by laboratory analyses. Plasmas from healthy adults were taken as controls.

The blood was anticoagulated with 0.11 mol/l sodium citrate (1:9, v/v, anticoagulant/blood) and centrifuged at 1500 g for 15 min to obtain the plasma. Platelet-poor plasma was quickly frozen and stored at –40°C.

Purification of Plasminogen

Glu-plasminogen was isolated from plasma in the presence of aprotinin by affinity chromatography on lysine-Sepharose [26], and glycoforms 1 and 2 were separated by EACA-gradient elution as described elsewhere [27]. The plasminogen concentration was measured spectrophotometrically at 280 nm with $E^{1\%}_{1cm}$=16.8 and M_r=92,000 [28].

Preparation of Plasmin

Plasminogen was activated to plasmin by use of urokinase-Sepharose. Plasmin concentrations were determined by active site titration, essentially as described [29]. K_m and k_{cat} values for each plasmin preparation with the chromogenic substrate S-2251 were calculated from the Michaelis-Menten equation using nonlinear regression analysis (Grafit 4).

Purification of α_2-Antiplasmin

α_2-Antiplasmin was purified by affinity chromatography on LBSI followed by a gel filtration essentially as described [30]. After purification, α_2-antiplasmin was dialyzed against distilled H_2O and lyophilized. Its concentration was determined by titration against plasmin of known concentration.

Fibrinogen Purification

Human fibrinogen was prepared by β-alanine precipitation from human plasminogen-depleted plasma as described [31]. The concentration of fibrinogen was measured spectrophotometrically at 280 nm, with $E^{1\%}_{1cm} = 15.1$ and $M_r = 340,000$ [32].

Purification of Polypeptide Chains of Fibrinogen

Polypeptide chains (Aα-, Bβ-, and γ-chains) were prepared according to Raut et al. [33] with some modifications. We used guanidine-hydrochloride and DL-dithiothreitol instead of urea and β-mercaptoethanol for reduction of fibrinogen as well as a 0.05-M Tris-HCl buffer, pH 7.4, instead of 1 M Tris-HCl buffer, pH 8.6. After reduction, the samples were directly injected into an HPLC column (POROS 20-R2) and eluted with a linear gradient of 20–60% acetonitrile in 0.1% trifluoroacetic acid (TFA) (v/v).

Preparation of Soluble Fibrin and CNBr-Fibrinogen Fragments

Fibrin I monomers (des-AA fibrin monomers) were prepared by incubating fibrinogen (concentration 20 mg/ml) with batroxobin (0.3 BU/ml) in the presence of Gly-Pro-Arg-Pro (3 mg/ml) for 3 h. CNBr-fibrinogen fragments were prepared as described by Blombäck et al. [34].

Inhibition Studies

The mode of the plasmin-α_2-antiplasmin interaction was investigated by slow-binding kinetics methods according to Longstaff and Gaffney [24]. To determine inhibition constants, the onset of inhibition was monitored by adding plasmin at a final concentration of 0.5 nM to a mixture of 1 mM S-2251 and α_2-antiplasmin at concentrations from 3 to 11 nM. The final volume of each mixture was 250 μl and was overlaid by 50 μl mineral oil to prevent desiccation during the reaction period. Reactions were monitored at 8-s intervals for 40 min, followed by measurements at 55-s intervals for 5 h in order to establish good estimates of initial reaction rates as well as final steady-state rates.

Plasminogen Activation Kinetics

Plasminogen activation reactions were carried out in microtiter plates at 37°C for 4 h in reaction volumes of 100 µl. Reaction mixtures contained t-PA at a final concentration of 100 pM, Glu-plasminogen and chromogenic substrate S-2251 (final concentration 0.3 mM). Activation mixtures could also contain varying concentrations of SF, CNBr-fibrinogen fragments, Aα-, Bβ-, or γ-chains to study the stimulating effect on the activation kinetics. When plasmin formation by t-PA-catalyzed plasminogen activation in the presence of SF or CNBr-fibrinogen fragments is monitored continuously from the beginning of the reaction, maximal increase in plasmin formation is seen only after a delay period, the so-called lag phase [35, 36]. Measurement of plasmin generation used for calculation of $K_{m\ app}$ and $k_{cat\ app}$ was performed after the transition from the lag phase to maximal and constant plasminogen activation by S-2251 hydrolysis at 405 nm using a scale range of 0.1 OD. $K_{m\ app}$ and $k_{cat\ app}$ values for plasminogen activation were calculated from the Michaelis-Menten equation using nonlinear regression analysis (Grafit 4).

Carbohydrate Studies

N-glycans were isolated from adult and fetal plasminogen types 1 and 2, adult and fetal α_2-antiplasmin, as well as from adult and fetal fibrinogen Bβ- and γ-chains, and permethylated as described [37]. Briefly, after enzymic release with PNGase F, both N- and O-glycans were separated by Sep-Pak fractionization. This was followed by reductive elimination of O-glycans and by permethylation of the obtained oligosaccharides, which could then be analyzed by FAB-MS.

Results

Catalytic Constants of Fetal and Adult Plasmin Types 1 and 2 with Chromogenic Substrate S-2251

Values for K_m and k_{cat} of both fetal plasmin isoforms with S-2251 were lower than the values for the respective adult types with more abundant differences in k_{cat} than in K_m (Table 1). Whereas these catalytic constants were only slightly lower in fetal plasmin type 2 than adult plasmin type 2, marked differences could be obtained for k_{cat} of fetal plasmin type 1 compared to adult plasmin type 1.

Kinetics of Fetal and Adult Plasmin Inhibition by Fetal and Adult α_2-Antiplasmin

The data obtained for the reactions of α_2-antiplasmin with all plasmin types fitted well to the integrated rate equation for slow-binding inhibition by nonlinear regression analysis, indicating reversible slow-binding inhibition to give an initial loose

Table 1. Catalytic constants k_{cat}, K_m, and the catalytic efficiency k_{cat}/K_m of plasmin with the chromogenic substrate S-2251

Plasmin type	K_m (mM)	k_{cat} (s^{-1})	k_{cat}/K_m (M^{-1}s^{-1})
Adult type 1	0.173±0.018	21.8±0.8	12.6±1.4
Adult type 2	0.180±0.015	17.6±0.5	9.8±0.9
Fetal type 1	0.155±0.019	10.5±0.4	6.8±0.9
Fetal type 2	0.169±0.017	13.5±0.6	8.0±0.9

complex followed by a tight complex. This confirms that fetal plasmin types 1 and 2 react with α_2-antiplasmin in a two-step procedure as has been described for adult plasmin types.

However, both fetal plasmin types were significantly less inhibited by adult α_2-antiplasmin compared to the respective adult types. Detailed analyses revealed that these variations were solely due to differences in the first step of the reaction as can be seen in the higher values for the initial dissociation constant $K_{i\ initial}$ (Table 2).

No differences could be seen when fetal α_2-antiplasmin was used instead of adult α_2-antiplasmin (data not shown).

Table 2. Values for the rate constants of plasmin-α_2-antiplasmin-reaction

Plasmin type	$K_{i\ initial}$ (nM)	$K_{i\ final}$ (pM)	k_{-2} (*10^{-6} s^{-1})	k_2 (*10^{-3} s^{-1})
Adult type 1	0.34±0.06	3.59±0.47	7.41±0.66	0.69±0.07
Adult type 2	0.66±0.18	5.24±0.88	7.70±0.71	0.96±0.32
Fetal type 1	1.49±0.26	9.58±1.97	6.39±0.88	0.99±0.30
Fetal type 2	1.57±0.31	10.81±1.84	7.13±0.41	1.03±0.37

Catalytic Efficiency for t-PA-Catalyzed Glu-Plasminogen Activation in the Absence of an Effector

In the absence of an effector, adult as well as fetal Glu-plasminogen were activated to plasmin with similar kinetics (Table 3).

Effect of Fetal and Adult SF and Adult CNBr-Digested Fibrinogen Fragments on t-PA-Catalyzed Glu-Plasminogen Activation

The relative ability of each plasminogen glycoform to interact with the activation effectors SF and CNBr-fibrinogen fragments was tested at various effector concentrations ranging from 0.004 to 1.0 µM for SF and 0.195 to 50 µg/ml for CNBr-fibrinogen fragments.

Table 3. Catalytic efficiency k_{cat}/K_m for the t-PA-catalyzed activation of adult and fetal Glu-plasminogens types 1 and 2

Plasminogen type	k_{cat}/K_m (μM^{-1} min^{-1})
Adult Glu-plasminogen type 1	0.032 ± 0.004
Adult Glu-plasminogen type 2	0.041 ± 0.005
Fetal Glu-plasminogen type 1	0.027 ± 0.005
Fetal Glu-plasminogen type 2	0.033 ± 0.007

At the lowest concentration of SF tested, $K_{m\ app}$ values ranged from 0.064 to 0.089 μM for the various plasminogen molecules (Fig. 1). These values were between 0.033 and 0.043 μM when CNBr-fibrinogen fragments were used as an effector (Fig. 3). Increasing the effector concentrations resulted in a continuous increase of $k_{cat\ app}$ with only small changes in $K_{m\ app}$, until a maximum value for $k_{cat\ app}$ was reached at 0.25 μM SF and 12.5 $\mu g/ml$ CNBr-fibrinogen fragments for all plasminogen types (Figs. 1–4). Further increase of effector resulted in a decrease of $k_{cat\ app}$ and an increase of $K_{m\ app}$ (Figs. 1–4). Both fetal plasminogen types revealed lower values for $k_{cat\ app}$ with higher differences between fetal and adult plasminogen types 1 than between fetal and adult plasminogen types 2.

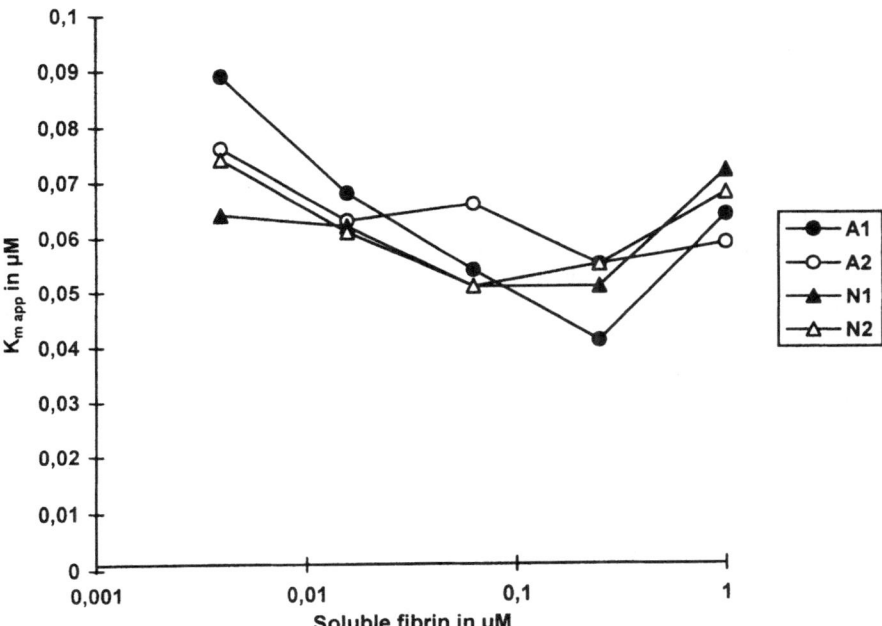

Fig. 1. $K_{m\ app}$ values for t-PA-catalyzed plasminogen activation of various Glu-plasminogen types in the presence of increasing concentrations of SF. *A1*, adult Glu-plasminogen type 1; *A2*, adult Glu-plasminogen type 2; *N1*, fetal Glu-plasminogen type 1; *N2*, fetal Glu-plasminogen type 2

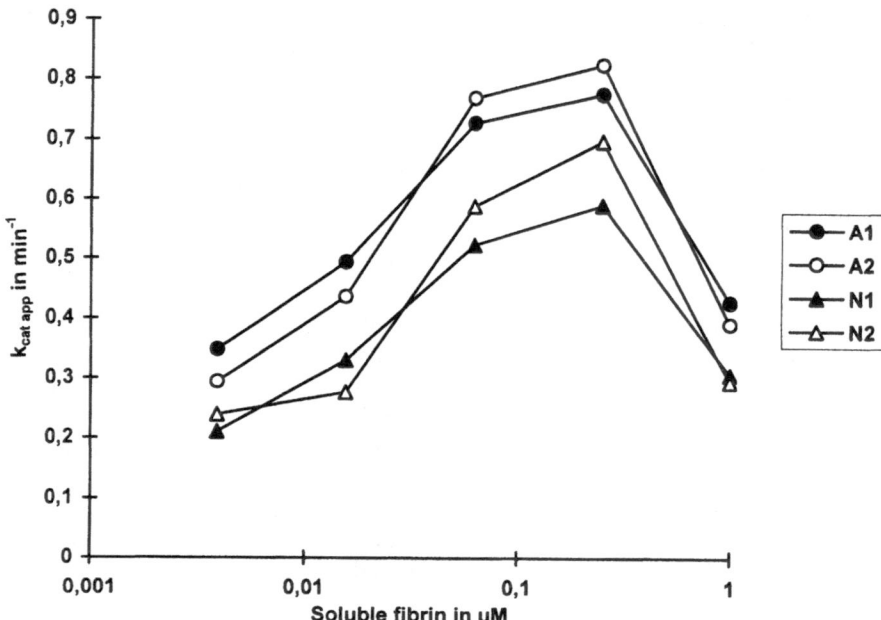

Fig. 2. Values for $k_{\text{cat app}}$ for t-PA-catalyzed plasminogen activation of various Glu-plasminogen types in the presence of increasing concentrations of SF

We compared the influence of fetal and adult fibrin (SF) on plasminogen activation kinetics. No differences were observed when fetal and adult SF were compared for their function as effectors for t-PA-catalyzed plasminogen activation (data not shown).

When plasmin formation is monitored continuously from the beginning of the reaction, maximal effector-mediated increase in plasmin formation is seen only after a lag period [35, 36]. This lag phase is dependent on the initial action of plasmin on fibrin/fibrinogen fragments. This phase was longer in adult and fetal Glu-plasminogen types 1 compared to adult and fetal Glu-plasminogen types 2, and it was prolonged in both fetal plasminogen types compared to the respective adult types (Fig. 5 for CNBr-fibrinogen fragments as an effector). When SF was used as a stimulating protein, this lag phase was much shorter and became evident only at the highest SF concentration used, indicating that most effector sites are already exposed at the earliest phase of the reaction.

Effects of Fetal and Adult Aα-, Bβ-, and γ-Chains on t-PA-Catalyzed Activation of Various Plasminogen Types

Further investigations were undertaken to compare fetal and adult polypeptide chains in stimulating t-PA-catalyzed plasminogen activation. No substantial diffe-

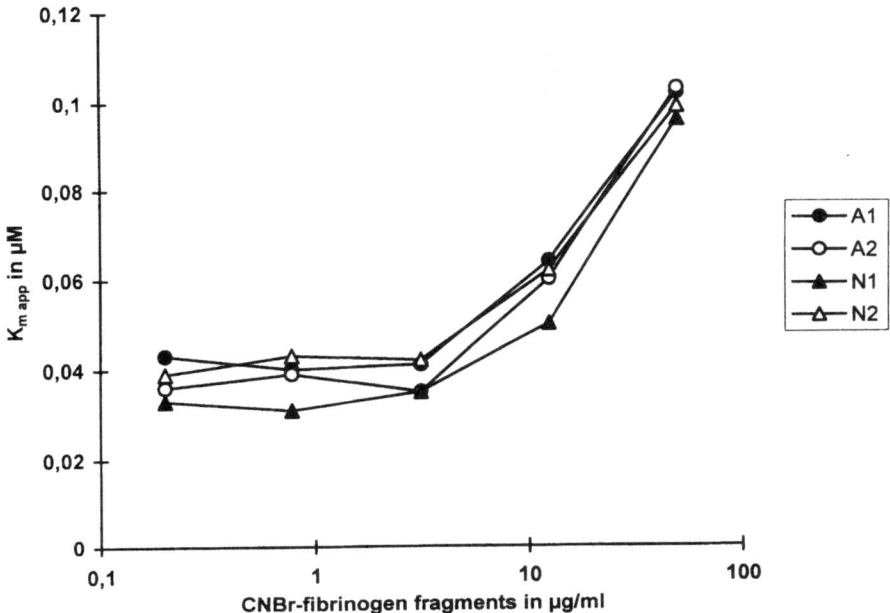

Fig. 3. $K_{m\ app}$ values for t-PA-catalyzed plasminogen activation various all Glu-plasminogen types in the presence of increasing concentrations of CNBr-fibrinogen fragments

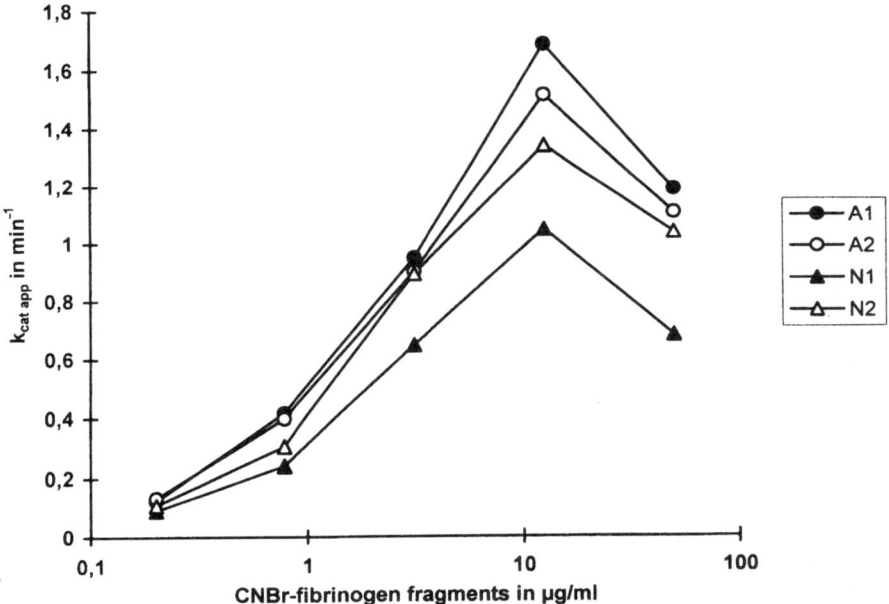

Fig. 4. Values for $k_{cat\ app}$ for t-PA-catalyzed plasminogen activation of various Glu-plasminogen types in the presence of increasing concentrations of CNBr-fibrinogen fragments

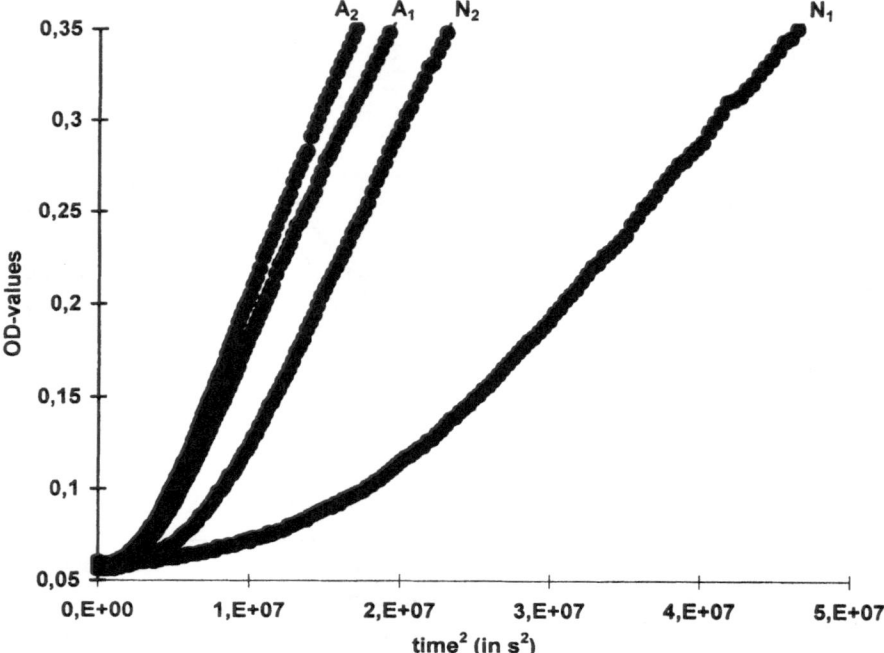

Fig. 5. Plasmin formation by t-PA in the presence of CNBr-fibrinogen fragments. The obtained OD changes are plotted against the incubation time^2. Note the prolonged transition time from the lag phase to the period of maximal and constant plasmin formation in both fetal types compared to the respective adult types

rences could be seen between fetal and adult Aα- and γ-chains as an effector (data not shown). The Bβ-chains had no stimulating effects.

Carbohydrate Data

N-glycosylation has been described to occur only in type 1 plasminogen at Asn[288], whereas both plasminogen types contain the O-glycosylation at Thr[345]. Adult plasminogen type 1 contained a range of complex biantennary structures bearing 0, 1, or 2 sialic acid residues. The major N-glycan present in fetal plasminogen type 1 was a complex disialylated biantennary structure. Fetal plasminogen type 1 revealed a higher level of truncated N-glycans compared to the adult (Fig. 6). The pattern of O-linked carbohydrate was consistent in all fetal and adult plasminogen samples, a single monosialylated trisaccharide being the major component (data not shown). Only minor differences were observed between N-glycans of fetal and adult α_2-antiplasmin, a disialylated biantennary structure being the major component in both the fetal and adult material.

N-glycosylation of fibrinogen has been described to occur in Bβ-chains at Asn[364] and in γ-chains at Asn[52]. In our studies, the major N-glycan present in adult fibrinogen Bβ-chains and γ-chains as well as fetal γ-chains is a monosialylated biantennary structure. In contrast, fetal Bβ-chains contained also a considerable amount of the disialylated form of this biantennary structure (Fig. 7).

Discussion

Throughout childhood, hemostasis is a dynamic, evolving system. Marked differences compared with adults have been reported especially in premature babies and neonates. Most levels of coagulation and fibrinolysis factors are lower than those of the adult [for review see 2]. In normal pregnancy and perinatal period, bleeding and thromboembolic complications are rare events, indicating that coagulation and fibrinolysis are well regulated. Therefore, hemostasis in neonates must be considered physiologically adequate.

In all proteins involved in fibrinolysis and in the coagulation cascade, a number of post-translational modifications occur. These post-translational modifications can affect secretion, binding properties, and plasma half-life and may be important for functional activity of the protein [13, 14].

Although the two major glycoforms of plasminogen have been extensively studied, the mechanism by which glycosylation alters plasminogen structure and function remains unclear. Plasminogen is a multidomainal protein consisting of five kringle regions and a serine proteinase domain. It is a mixture of two major glycoforms. Both contain an O-glycosylation site at Thr[345], while type 1 plasminogen contains an additional N-glycosylation site at Asn[288] [38–40]. Recently, an additional O-glycosylation site has been found at Ser[248] in plasminogen type 2 [41]. Electrophoretic analyses revealed the same molecular weight for fetal and adult plasminogen. In addition, amino-acid composition and partial amino-acid sequencing revealed no differences between the plasminogen forms 1 and 2 of neonates and adults [5, 10]. However, composition analyses of carbohydrate showed marked differences between fetal and adult glycoforms. Fetal plasminogen contained more mannose, N-acetylglucosamine, and sialic acid as well as less galactose than the respective adult glycoforms, while plasminogen activation kinetics with tissue-type plasminogen activator in the presence of CNBr-fibrinogen fragments have been found to be slower for both glycoforms compared to adult plasminogen [5]. In addition, it could be demonstrated [5] that fetal plasminogen does not bind as well to cellular receptors as adult plasminogen.

Our data on N-linked carbohydrate residues in adults are in agreement with the data reported in the literature [38, 39]. Most carbohydrate residues are mono- or disialylated biantennary structures. Mass spectrometric analyses of the glycans present on plasminogen revealed a higher level of truncated N-glycans on the fetal material compared to the adult. Here it has to be mentioned that our data on carbohydrate analysis are not completely in agreement with the compositional analyses of Edelberg et al. [5], who have found much higher amounts of mannose and sialic acid and less galactose per mol of protein than can be predicted from our

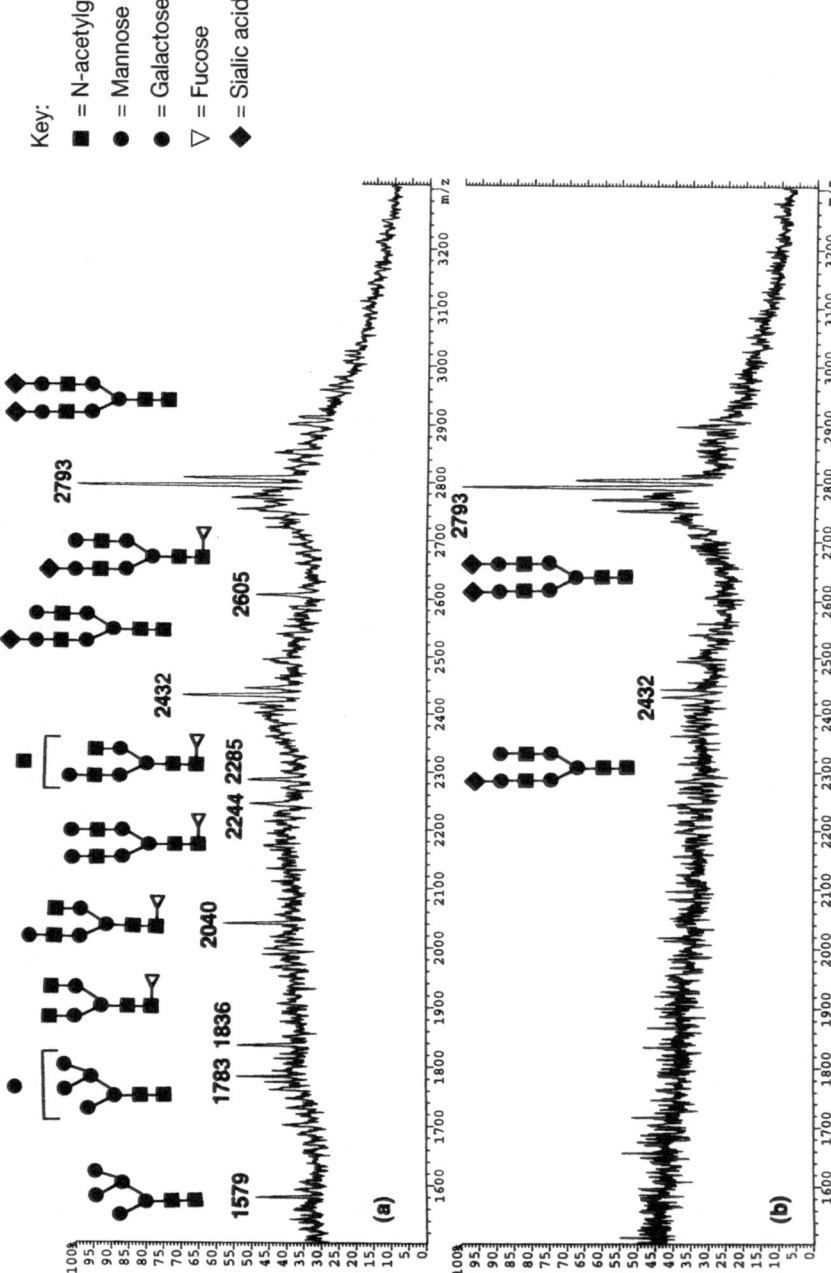

Fig. 6. Comparison of neonatal (a) and adult (b) permethylated N-glycans from plasminogen type 1

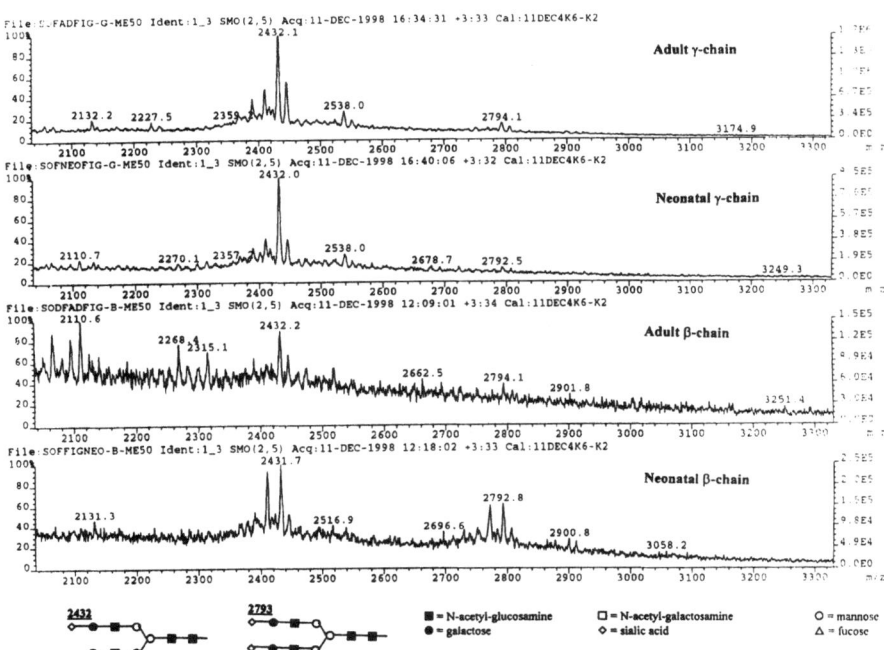

Fig. 7. Carbohydrate structures of both adult and fetal Bβ- and γ-chains. Adult and fetal γ-chains as well as adult Bβ-chains contain almost only the monosialylated biantennary structure (position 2432). Note that fetal Bβ-chain also contains a considerable amount of the disialylated form of this biantennary structure (position 2793)

carbohydrate structures (Fig. 6). O-linked carbohydrate analyses revealed no major differences between all fetal and adult plasmin types. The pattern was consistent in all of the samples, a single monosialylated trisaccharide being the major component. In addition, only minor differences were observed between N-glycans of fetal and adult α_2-antiplasmin, disialylated biantennary structures being the major component in both the fetal and adult material.

Analyses of carbohydrate sequence demonstrated a monosialylated biantennary structure in adult Bβ- and γ-chains as well as in fetal γ-chains. In contrast, fetal Bβ-chains contained also a considerable amount of the disialylated form of this biantennary structure (Fig. 7).

In the absence of SF and CNBr-fibrinogen fragments, no substantial differences in the rate of plasmin formation could be seen between the fetal and adult plasminogen forms. When SF and CNBr-fibrinogen fragments were added, a significant enhancement of the catalytic efficiency could be obtained. In the presence of both effectors, fetal Glu-plasminogen types 1 and 2 revealed lower values for $k_{cat\ app}$ with higher differences between fetal and adult Glu-plasminogen types 1 than between both Glu-plasminogen types 2. No differences could be seen in the values for $K_{m\ app}$. Resulting values for catalytic efficiency $k_{cat\ app}/K_{m\ app}$ revealed, therefore, lower values for all fetal plasminogen types (Figs. 1–4). However, these differences were much smaller than previously reported [5]. In a purified system, maximal enhancement of plasmin formation by SF or CNBr-fibrinogen fragments occurs with a delay after an initial phase of slow plasmin formation (lag phase). When CNBr-fibrinogen fragments were used as an effector, this initial phase was longer in both fetal Glu-plasminogen types compared to their respective adult glycoforms with more abundant differences between both Glu-plasminogen types 1 (Fig. 5). This indicates a slower plasmin-induced modification of CNBr-fibrinogen fragments by both fetal plasmin types. When SF was used as the stimulating protein, this lag phase was much shorter and became evident only at the highest SF concentration used. This suggests that most effector sites have already been exposed during the preparation procedure. No differences could be seen in the function of fetal and adult SF as well as fetal and adult $A\alpha$- and γ-chains as an effector of t-PA-catalyzed plasminogen activation. This indicates that the differences between fetal and adult fibrinogen (phosphorylation and glycosylation) have no influence on the effector region of t-PA-catalyzed plasminogen activation.

Concerning the results of catalytic constants of the various plasmin types with chromogenic substrate S-2251, it is most interesting that fetal plasmin type 1 has a much lower catalytic efficiency (k_{cat}/K_m) than adult plasmin type 1, whereas differences between fetal plasmin type 2 and adult plasmin type 2 were much smaller (Table 1). The differences in catalytic efficiency were mainly due to a lower k_{cat}, while values for K_m were similar in all plasmin types. This is rather unexpected since differences in carbohydrate composition between adult plasmin type 1, type 2, and mini-plasmin and in various recombinant plasminogens have not revealed huge differences in catalytic constants of the plasmin types [42, 43]. However, Edelberg et al. [5] have found an even lower k_{cat} for neonatal plasmin type 1 (only 31% of the k_{cat} of adult plasmin type 1). In addition, fetal plasmin (not separated into the two glycoforms) revealed a much lower hydrolysis of chromogenic substrate S-2251 after activation to plasmin with urokinase [3, 4]. Therefore, the data for catalytic constants of the various plasmin types can be considered in accordance with previous reports.

α_2-Antiplasmin can inhibit various serine proteinases. Because of its high affinity for plasmin, it works in plasma mainly as a plasmin inhibitor. Although there are other plasmin inhibitors like α_2-macroglobulin, α_1-antitrypsin, C_1-esterase inhibitor, and antithrombin III, plasmin is inhibited mainly by α_2-antiplasmin [44]. Thus the plasmin-α_2-antiplasmin reaction can be considered as a key event in regulation of the fibrinolytic system. When α_2-antiplasmin reacts with plasmin, it forms a very stable stoichiometric 1:1 complex with plasmin. The reaction proceeds in two steps. In the first step, α_2-antiplasmin rapidly forms a reversible complex with plasmin, involving both the LBS on plasmin and their complementary sites on α_2-antiplasmin. This step can be competitively inhibited by plasminogen fragments containing LBS or by lysine analogues. It is well to remember that these LBS in plasmin are located in the kringle structure where the only known structural differences exist in the attached carbohydrate moieties. The second step, initially thought to be irreversible, results in a tightly bound complex. However, by use of slow-binding kinetics, this step demonstrates reversibility as well [24]. In our analyses, all curves followed the same pattern, indicating reversible slow-binding inhibition. Therefore, fetal plasmin types 1 and 2 react with α_2-antiplasmin in the same manner to that of adult plasmin types with a first complex formation dependent on LBS interactions followed by a much tighter second complex in a slow reaction step. Detailed kinetic analyses of plasmin-α_2-antiplasmin reaction showed that the differences between fetal and adult plasmin reactions were solely due to the initial loose complex. At 37°C, initial K_i values were 1.5 and 1.6 nM for fetal plasmin types 1 and 2, respectively; compared with 0.3 and 0.7 nM for the corresponding adult types. Our data demonstrate a variation in kinetic behavior between fetal plasmin (type 1 and 2) and α_2-antiplasmin compared to the reaction with adult plasmin types. The knowledge of this difference contributes to further understanding of fibrinolysis in the fetus and neonate. It gives some explanation for the increased overall fibrinolytic activity in fetal plasma measured by gross functional assays such as fibrin plates or plasma clot lysis [15–16] despite relatively low levels and slower activation kinetics of fetal plasminogen, and also for the findings in clot-lysis experiments after adding purified α_2-antiplasmin [45]. We assume that the properties of fetal plasminogen (slower activation kinetics and slower inactivation of fetal plasmin by α_2-antiplasmin) are physiologically relevant and explain an adequate fibrinolytic activity without consumption of large amounts of plasminogen and α_2-antiplasmin, both produced by the fetal liver. The elucidation of the primary carbohydrate structures of fetal plasminogen and fibrinogen provides a rational basis for future investigations of carbohydrate found in different factors of coagulation and fibrinolysis to understand the role of carbohydrate in regulation of hemostasis in the fetus and neonate.

Acknowledgements. This work was supported by a grant from the Deutsche Forschungsgemeinschaft (RI 956/2–1)

References

1. Collen D, Lijnen HR. Basic and clinical aspects of fibrinolysis and thrombolysis. Blood 1991; 78: 3114–3124
2. Andrew M: Developmental hemostasis: relevance to thromboembolic complications in pediatric patients. Thromb Haemost 1995; 74: 415–425
3. Benavent A, Estellés A, Aznar J, Martinez-Sales V, Gilabert J, Fornas E. Dysfunctional plasminogen in full term newborn – Study of active site of plasmin. Thromb Haemost 1984; 51: 67–70
4. Estelles A, Aznar J, Gilabert J, Parrilla JJ. Dysfunctional plasminogen in full-term newborn. Pediatr Res 1980; 14: 1180–1185
5. Edelberg JM, Enghild JJ, Pizzo SV, Gonzalez-Gronow M. Neonatal plasminogen displays altered cell surface binding and activation kinetics. Correlation with increased glycosylation of the protein. J Clin Invest 1990; 86: 107–112
6. Galanakis DK, Mossesson MW. Evaluation of the role of in vivo proteolysis (fibrinogenolysis) in prolonging the thrombin time of human umbilical cord fibrinogen. Blood 1976; 48: 109–118
7. Francis JL, Armstrong DJ. Sialic acid and enzymatic desialation of cord blood fibrinogen. Haemostasis 1982; 11: 223–228
8. Künzer W. Fetales Fibrinogen. Klin Wochenschr 1961; 39: 536–542

9. Ries M. Molecular and functional properties of fetal plasminogen and its possible influence on clot lysis in the neonatal period. Semin Thromb Haemost 1997; 23:247-252
10. Summaria L. Comparison of human normal, full-term, fetal and adult plasminogen by physical and chemical analyses. Haemostasis 1989; 19: 266-273
11. Witt I, Müller H. Phosphorus and hexose content of human foetal fibrinogen. Biochim Biophys Acta 1970; 221: 402-404
12. Witt I, Müller H, Künzer W. Evidence for the existence of foetal fibrinogen. Thromb Diath Hemorrh 1969; 22: 101-109
13. Cumming DA. Physiological relevance of protein glycosylation. Develop Biol Standard 1992; 76: 83-94
14. Kaufman RJ. Post-translational modifications required for coagulation factor secretion and function. Thromb Haemost 1998; 19: 1068-1079
15. Ekelund H, Hedner U, Nilsson IM. Fibrinolysis in newborns. Acta Paediatr Scand 1970; 59: 33-43
16. Phillips LL, Skrodelis V. A comparison of the fibrinolytic enzyme system in maternal and umbilical-cord blood. Pediatrics 1958; 22: 715-726
17. Ries M, Zenker M, Klinge J, Keuper H, Harms D. Age related differences in a clot lysis assay after adding different plasminogen activators in a plasma milieu in vitro. J Pediatr Hematol Oncol 1995; 17: 260-264
18. Ries M, Klinge J, Rauch R, Trusen B, Zenker M, Keuper H, Harms D. In vitro fibrinolysis after adding low doses of plasminogen activators and plasmin generation with and without oxidative inactivation of plasmin inhibitors in newborns and adults. J Pediatr Hematol Oncol 1996; 18: 346-351
19. Robbins KC, Summaria L, Hsieh B, Shah RJ. The peptide chains of human plasmin. Mechanism of activation of human plasminogen to plasmin. J Biol Chem 1967; 242: 2333-2342
20. Christensen U, Clemmensen I. Kinetic properties of the primary inhibitor of plasmin from human plasma. Biochem J 1977; 163: 389-391
21. Christensen U, Clemmensen I. Purification and reaction mechanisms of the primary inhibitor of plasmin from human plasma. Biochem J 1978; 175: 635-641
22. Christensen S, Sottrup-Jensen L, Christensen U. Stopped-flow fluorescence kinetics of bovine α_2-antiplasmin inhibition of bovine midiplasmin. Biochem J 1995; 305: 97-102
23. Wiman B, Collen D. On the kinetics of the reaction between human antiplasmin and plasmin. Eur J Biochem 1978; 84: 573-578
24. Longstaff C, Gaffney PJ. Serpin-serine protease binding kinetics: α_2-antiplasmin as a model inhibitor. Biochemistry 1991; 30: 979-986
25. Christensen U, Bangert K, Thorsen S. Reaction of human α_2-antiplasmin and plasmin. Stopped-flow fluorescence kinetics. FEBS Letters 1996; 387: 58-62
26. Deutsch DG, Mertz ET. Plasminogen: Purification from human plasma by affinity chromatography. Science 1970; 170: 1095-1096
27. Brockway WJ, Castellino FJ. Measurement of the binding of antifibrinolytic amino acids to various plasminogens. Arch Biochem Biophys 1972; 151: 194-199
28. Wallen P, Wiman B. Characterization of human plasminogen. I. On the relationship between different molecular forms of plasminogen demonstrated in plasma and found in purified preparations. Biochim Biophys Acta 1970; 221: 20-30
29. Jameson GW, Roberts DV, Adams RWA, Kyle WSA, Elmore DT. Determination of the operational molarity of solutions of bovine alpha-chymotrypsin, trypsin, thrombin and factor Xa by spectrofluorimetric titration. Biochem J 1973; 131: 107-117
30. Wiman B. Affinity-chromatographic purification of human α_2-antiplasmin. Biochem J 1980; 191: 229-232
31. Jakobsen E, Kierulf P. A modified beta-alanine precipitation procedure to prepare fibrinogen free of antithrombin III and plasminogen. Thromb Res 1973; 3: 145-159
32. Blombäck B, Blombäck M. Purification of human and bovine fibrinogen. Ark Kemi 1956; 10: 415-443

33. Raut S, Corran PH, Gaffney PJ. Ultra-rapid preparation of milligram quantities of the puri-fied polypeptide chains of human fibrinogen. J Chromatogr B Biomed Appl 1994; 660: 390–394
34. Blombäck B, Blombäck M, Henschen A, Hessel B, Iwanaga S, Woods KR. N-terminal disul-phide knot of human fibrinogen. Nature 1968; 218: 130–134
35. Beckmann R, Geiger M, Binder BR. Plasminogen activation by tissue plasminogen activa-tor in the presence of stimulating CNBr fragment FCB-2 of fibrinogen is a two-phase reac-tion. Kinetic analysis of the initial phase of slow plasmin formation. J Biol Chem 1988; 263: 7176–7180
36. Norrman B, Wallen P, Ranby M. Fibrinolysis mediated by tissue plasminogen activator. Disclosure of a kinetic transition. Eur J Biochem 1985; 149: 193–200
37. Dell A, Khoo KH, Panico M, McDowell RA, Etienne AT, Reason AJ, Morris HR. FAB-MS and ES-MS of glycoproteins. In: Glycobiology: A Practical Approach, Eds Fukuda M, Kobata A, 1993, IRL Press, pp. 189–222
38. Hayes ML, Castellino FJ. Carbohydrate of the human plasminogen variants. I. Carbohydrate composition, glycopeptide isolation, and characterization. J Biol Chem 1979; 254: 8768–8771
39. Hayes ML, Castellino FJ. Carbohydrate of the human plasminogen variants. II. Structure of the asparagine-linked oligosaccharide unit. J Biol Chem 1979; 254: 8772–8776
40. Hayes ML, Castellino FJ. Carbohydrate of the human plasminogen variants. III. Structure of the O-glycosidically linked oligosaccharide unit. J Biol Chem 1979; 254: 8777–8780
41. Pirie-Shepherd SR, Stevens RD, Andon NL, Enghild JJ, Pizzo SV. Evidence for a novel O-linked sialylated trisaccharide on Ser-248 of human plasminogen 2. J Biol Chem 1997; 272: 7408–7411
42. Davidson DJ, Castellino FJ. The influence of the nature of the asparagine 289-linked oligo-saccharide on the activation by urokinase and lysine binding properties of natural and recombinant human plasminogens. J Clin Invest 1993; 92: 249–254
43. Morris JP, Blatt S, Powell JR, Strickland DK, Castellino FJ. Role of lysine binding regions in the kinetic properties of human plasmin. Biochemistry 1981; 20: 4811–4816
44. Levi M, Roem D, Kamp AM, de Boer JP, Hack CE, ten Cate JW. Assessment of the relative contribution of different protease inhibitors to the inhibition of plasmin in vivo. Thromb Haemost 1993; 69: 141–146
45. Ries M, Klinge J, Rauch R, Keuper H, Harms D. The role of α_2-antiplasmin in the inhibition of clot lysis in newborns and adults. Biol Neonate 1996; 69: 298–306

Hereditary Thrombophilic Risk Profiles in Children with Spontaneous Venous Thromboembolism

A. Kosch, R. Junker, K. Auberger, R. Schobess, H.-G. Koch, U. Nowak-Göttl

Introduction

Since the recent discovery of activated protein C resistance [6], in the majority of cases due to the factor (FV) G1691A gene mutation [2], evidence has been accumulating that venous thromboembolism is a multigenetic disorder [24]. Besides antithrombin deficiency and deficiencies within the protein C pathway, the 20210A allele within the 3'-untranslated region of the prothrombin (PT) gene is discussed as a common but mild risk factor of venous thrombosis in children and adults [13, 22]. Finally, the C677T mutation in the methylenetetrahydrofolate reductase (MTHFR) gene facilitates the manifestation of hyperhomocysteinemia especially in individuals with low folate intake, and has been discussed to be involved not only in arterial vascular disease but also in venous thromboembolism [11, 23]. The latter is still a matter of controversial discussion [1]. Combinations between the established prothrombotic risk factors mentioned greatly increase the risk of thrombosis in adults [4, 5, 9, 14, 23, 25].

Pediatric venous thromboembolism is being increasingly viewed as a multifactorial disorder as well [8]; however, information on the role of combined hemostatic defects in childhood thrombosis is limited. Very recently we have shown elevated lipoprotein Lp(a), the heterozygous state for the FV G1691A mutation and the prothrombin G20210A mutation, and deficiencies of protein C and antithrombin to be risk factors of childhood thromboembolism [8, 13, 17, 19, 20]. A decreased fibrinolysis due to enhanced levels of the plasminogen activator inhibitor (PAI)-1 concomitant with low activity of tissue-type plasminogen activator has, moreover, been shown in childhood carriers of the FV G1691A gene mutation who suffered a thrombotic event [16]. In addition, evidence is given that elevated PAI-1 levels are associated with the 4G/4G genotype of the recently described deletion/insertion 4G/5G polymorphism in the PAI-1 gene [7, 10, 12].

The present multicenter study has been undertaken to test the hypothesis that genetic prothrombotic risk profiles in children with early onset spontaneous venous thromboembolism (SVT) differ from the carrier status of their first-degree family members, especially if relatively mild thrombophilic polymorphisms not leading to thrombosis in the parents cause a more severe clinical expression when coinherited with an established prothrombotic risk factor. This question does not only raise a scientific issue, but also an ethical one, when considering to what extent a screening of genetic factors is justified in symptomatic patients during childhood and adolescence not associated with a positive family history of a disease, and in particular, if this screening should also be performed in siblings not suffering yet from a symptomatic disease.

I. Scharrer/W. Schramm (Ed.)
30th Hemophilia Symposium Hamburg 1999
© Springer-Verlag Berlin Heidelberg 2001

Patients, Materials, and Methods

Ethics

The present study is part of a prospective multicenter case-control study. It was performed in accordance with the ethical standards laid down in a relevant version of the 1964 Declaration of Helsinki and approved by the medical ethics committee at the Westfälische Wilhelms-University, Münster, Germany.

Patients and First-Degree Family Members

Inclusion criteria: Infants and children (neonate to 18 years old) with first onset SVT confirmed by standard imaging methods (venography, compression sonography, computed tomography, magnetic resonance imaging), whose biological parents were both available for a complete diagnostic work-up including prothrombotic risk factors, were defined as study patients. From September 1995 to September 1999, 48 consecutive Caucasian patients (median age at first thrombotic onset 0.5 years, range neonate to 18 years old, male/female ratio 1:1.1) with clinically and imaging confirmed SVT were recruited from different geographic catchment areas of Germany [13,19]. Exclusion criteria: Childhood patients with potential triggering acquired risk factors, i.e., malignancies, central venous lines, immobilization, surgery, trauma, plaster casts, rheumatic diseases, severe infections, and use of oral contraceptives, were not enrolled in the present study.

At acute onset of SVT, the majority of patients presented with isolated vascular occlusion of the inferior caval vein ($n=9$), combined femoral and iliac vein thrombosis ($n=8$), cerebral vein thrombosis ($n=8$), isolated calf thrombosis ($n=5$), renal venous thrombosis ($n=5$), femoral vein thrombosis concomitant with pulmonary embolism ($n=4$), intracardial thrombus formation ($n=4$), femoral vein thrombosis ($n=3$), and vascular thrombosis of the portal vein ($n=2$).

With their informed consent, 96 biological parents with a median (range) age of 32 years (23–51 years) were investigated. No thromboembolism has occurred so far in 70 of the 72 first-degree family members with at least one prothrombotic gene mutation or thrombophilic polymorphism. However, in a 32-year-old woman with elevated Lp(a) and protein C deficiency, type I first venous thrombosis occurred during pregnancy, and deep venous thrombosis with pulmonary embolism was noted in a 23-year-old male with antithrombin deficiency type I concomitant with immobilization and severe nicotine abuse.

Blood Samples

With informed parental consent, blood samples were collected 6 weeks to 3 months after the acute SVT by peripheral venipuncture into plastic tubes containing 1/10 by volume of 3.8% trisodium citrate or into plastic tubes without additives (Sarstedt, Nümbrecht, Germany). Citrated blood was placed immediately on melting ice. Platelet-poor plasma and serum were prepared by centrifugation at 3000 g for

20 min at 4°C, or at room temperature, aliquoted in polystyrene tubes, stored at
−70°C, and thawed immediately before the assay procedure. For genetic analysis we
obtained venous blood in EDTA-treated sample tubes (Sarstedt, Nümbrecht,
Germany), from which cells were separated by centrifugation at 3000 g for 15 min.
The buffy coat layer was then removed and stored at −70°C pending DNA extraction
by a spin column procedure (Quiagen, Hilden, Germany).

Laboratory Analyses

The MTHFR C677T, FV G1691A, and prothrombin G20210A genotypes were
determined by polymerase chain reaction and analysis of restriction fragments as
previously reported [2, 11, 22]. The PAI-1 4G/5G genotype was detected by allele-
specific polymerase chain reaction [10].

Amidolytic protein C and antithrombin activities were measured on an ACL 300
analyzer (Instrumentation Laboratory, Germany) using chromogenic substrates
(Chromogenix, Sweden). Free protein S antigen, total protein S, and protein C antigen
were measured using commercially available ELISA kits (Stago, France). Partigen
plates (radial immunodiffusion) used to determine antithrombin concentrations
were purchased from Behring Diagnostics, Germany. In addition, crossed immuno-
electrophoresis (Behring Diagnostics, Germany; Dako, Denmark) was performed in
patients with antithrombin deficiency. Lp(a) was determined with the COALIZA
Lp(a) assay kit (Chromogenix, Sweden). The laboratory staff was blind to whether
the blood samples originated from a patient or from a first-degree family member.

A heterozygous type I deficiency state (protein C, antithrombin) was diagnosed
when functional plasma activity and immunological antigen concentration of a protein were 50% below normal of the lower age-related limit [8]. A homozygous state
was defined if activity levels and antigen concentrations were less than 10% of normal. A type II deficiency was diagnosed with repeatedly low functional activity levels
along with normal antigen concentrations. The diagnosis of protein S deficiency was
based on reduced free protein S antigen levels combined with decreased or normal
total protein S antigen concentrations. Criteria for the hereditary nature of a hemostatic defect were its presence in at least one further first- or second-degree family
member and/or the identification of a causative gene mutation [8, 19, 22].

Statistics

Prevalences of prothrombotic risk factors in childhood patients and first-degree
relatives were compared by the chi-square test. The significance level was set at 0.05.
All statistical analyses were performed using the MedCalc software package
(MedCalc, Mariakerke, Belgium).

Results

Of the 48 symptomatic childhood patients, 46 were carriers of prothrombotic risk
factors, whereas no thrombophilia could be detected in 2 of them. In 19 of the 48

patients (39.6%), at least one risk factor was found compared with 55 of the 96 first-degree family members (57.3%). Single prothrombotic risk factors in childhood patients and their first-degree family members are shown in Table 1.

Table 1. Single prothrombotic risk factors in childhood patients and their first-degree family members. In all cases, protein deficiencies were type I

Prothrombotic risk factor	Patients n=48	Father n=48	Mother n=48	Both parents n=96
Factor V G1691A	3 (6.3%)	5 (10.4%)	6 (12.5%)	11 (11.5%)
Prothrombin G20210A	2 (4.2%)	2 (4.2%)	1 (2.1%)	3 (3.1%)
PAI-1 4G/4G	3 (6.3%)	8 (16.7%)	4 (8.3%)	12 (12.5%)
MTHFR T677T	1 (2.1%)	5 (10.4%)	2 (4.2%)	7 (7.3%)
Lipoprotein (a) >30 mg/dl	10 (20.8%)	7 (14.6%)	11 (23%)	18 (18.8%)
Protein C deficiency	–	1 (2.1%)	1 (2.1%)	2 (2.1%)
Protein S deficiency	–	–	–	–
Antithrombin deficiency	–	1 (2.1%)	1 (2.1%)	2 (2.1%)
Total	19 (39.6%)	29 (60.4%)	26 (54.2%)	55 (57.3%)

Table 2. Combined or homozygous prothrombotic risk factors in childhood patients and their first-degree family members. In all cases, protein deficiencies were type I

Prothrombotic risk factors	Patients n=48	Father n=48	Mother n=48	Both parents n=96
Factor V G1691A and:				
Lipoprotein (a) >30 mg/dl	6 (12.5%)	–	2 (4.2%)	2 (2.1%)
PAI-1 4G/4G	3 (6.3%)	4 (8.3%)	2 (4.2%)	6 (6.3%)
MTHFR T677T	2 (4.2%)	–	–	–
Prothrombin G20210A	–	–	1 (2.1%)	1 (1%)
Factor V A1691A (homozygous) and:				
No further risk factor	2 (4.2%)	–	–	–
Prothrombin G20210A	1 (2.1%)	–	–	–
Lipoprotein (a) >30 mg/dl and:				
PAI-1 4G/4G	6 (12.5%)	1 (2.1%)	2 (4.2%)	3 (3.1%)
MTHFR T677T	2 (4.2%)	–	1 (2.1%)	1 (1%)
Antithrombin deficiency	1 (2.1%)	–	–	–
Protein C deficiency	1 (2.1%)	–	–	–
Prothrombin G20210A	–	–	2 (4.2%)	2 (2.1%)
Protein S deficiency	–	1 (2.1%)	–	1 (1%)
Prothrombin G20210A & MTHFR T677T	1 (2.1%)	–	–	–
Prothrombin A20210A & MTHFR T677T & Protein S deficiency	1 (2.1%)	–	–	–
PAI-1 4G/4G and:				
Prothrombin G20210A	–	–	1 (2.1%)	1 (1%)
MTHFR T677T	1 (2.1%)	–	–	–
Total	27 (56.3%)	6 (12.5%)	11 (23.1%)	17 (17.6%)

Of the 48 patients, 27 (56.3%) had two or more genetic risk factors compared with 17 double defects found in the 96 first-degree family members (17.7%). More than two defective alleles, i.e., the homozygous FV A1691A genotype combined with the PT G20210A variant, elevated Lp(a) (>30 mg/dl) along with the PT G20210A variant and the MTHFR T677T genotype, and the homozygous PT A20210A genotype with the MTHFR T677T variant, elevated Lp(a), and protein S type I deficiency were found in 3 further symptomatic subjects. The overall rate of two or more prothrombotic risk factors/polymorphisms (Table 2) was significantly higher in symptomatic childhood patients compared with their parents (P=0.0004).

Discussion

Results of the present family study show that symptomatic children with spontaneous venous thromboembolism have a significantly higher rate of combined genetic prothrombotic risk factors than their first-degree family members. Established prothrombotic risk factors such as the factor V gene G1691A mutation, the prothrombin G20210A variant, deficiency states of protein C, protein S or antithrombin, and increased levels of Lp(a) were found along with further genetic polymorphisms, i.e., the homozygous MTHFR T667T variant and the PAI-1 4G/4G genotype. We wish to point out that 13 of the 27T combined risk profiles (48%) were due to different combinations within established defects of the protein C pathway, the PT gene variant, antithrombin deficiency, or elevated Lp(a), the latter recently shown to be an inherited and independent risk factor of childhood venous thrombosis [3, 19]. In contrast, only 6 out of 17 asymptomatic first-degree family members (35.3%) had a prothrombotic risk profile of two defects within the protein C pathway, the PT gene mutation, and elevated Lp(a), and only twice were similar to the affected children. However, no first-degree family member had more than two combined thrombophilias. A smaller proportion of children with SVT (39.6%) was suffering from only one prothrombotic risk factor. However, no isolated deficiencies of protein C, protein S, or antithrombin were diagnosed in the symptomatic childhood population studied.

Based on various trials, evidence is accumulating that familial thrombophilia, defined as a genetically determined tendency to thrombosis, may be due to a combination of clotting defects [4, 5, 8, 9, 14, 23–25]. In particular, there is evidence that inheritance of FV G1691A combined with deficiencies of protein C [14], S, and antithrombin [4, 25], as well as with the PT G20210A variant [9], the MTHFR T677T genotype in some studies [5, 23], the PAI-1 4G/4G variant [12], or enhanced Lp(a) concentrations [17, 19], further increases the manifestation of early vascular accidents in children and young adults. We suggest from the data presented here that the combination between genetic polymorphisms which are not necessarily independent risk factor for venous thrombosis, such as the MTHFR T677T genotype or the homozygous PAI-1 4G/4G polymorphism, and established prothrombotic risk factors further increases the risk of symptomatic vascular accidents in the subjects affected [12, 23]. This is similar to childhood patients suffering at least one established thrombophilia along with acquired risk factors, i.e., central venous lines or chemotherapy in childhood leukemia [13, 18, 19, 21].

On the one hand, children not only differ from adults anatomically and physiologically, they also differ in the types of diseases from which they suffer and the manifestation of diseases they have in common with adults. Therefore, it is not only a scientific question but also an ethical issue whether a comprehensive screening of genetic factors is justified in symptomatic childhood patients with a negative family history of a disease, and in particular whether this screening is to be also recommended in non-symptomatic siblings. On the other hand, data presented here along with results from recently published controlled studies in childhood thrombophilia give evidence [12, 19, 20] that the risk of a symptomatic thrombotic event during childhood is enhanced in these patients carrying at least one prothrombotic risk factor. Based on the Mendelian theory of inheritance, siblings of a symptomatic childhood patient affected with a combined prothrombotic defect carry, in approximately 50% of cases, a single thrombophilia, and two or more gene mutations or polymorphisms in 25% of cases. Thus, based on the fact that primary anticoagulant prophylaxis is available as a therapeutic option in carriers of prothrombotic risk factors, childhood family members of symptomatic patients will possibly benefit from the screening procedure [15].

Summary

The present study was designed to assess to what extent single and combined clotting abnormalities influence spontaneous thrombophilic onset in pediatric patients and how the children affected differ in their thrombophilic risk profiles from their biological first-degree family members, especially if relatively mild thrombophilic polymorphisms not leading to thrombosis in the parents cause severe clinical expression when coinherited with an established prothrombotic risk factor. Factor V (FV) G1691A mutation, the prothrombin (PT) G20210A variant, the methylenetetrahydrofolate reductase (MTHFR) T677T genotype, the plasminogen activator inhibitor (PAI)-1 promoter polymorphism, lipoprotein Lp(a), antithrombin, protein C, and protein S were investigated in 48 childhood patients, neonate to 18 years old (median 0.5 years), with spontaneous venous thromboembolism (SVT) compared with the carrier status of their first-degree family members. In 19 of the 48 patients (39.6%), one prothrombotic risk factor was diagnosed, and in 27 of the 48 subjects (56.3%) at least two prothrombotic defects/alleles. In the majority of cases with SVT, the FV G1691A mutation was involved either with a second mutated allele ($n=2$) or combined with elevated Lp(a) ($n=6$), the 4G/4G genotype of the PAI-1 promoter polymorphism ($n=3$), and the T677T MTHFR genotype ($n=2$). In addition, the homozygous FV A1691A genotype was combined once with the PT variant. Elevated Lp(a) was combined with the PAI-1 4G/4G genotype ($n=6$), homozygous MTHFR T677T genotype ($n=2$), the PT G20210A mutation and MTHFR T677T variant ($n=1$), protein C ($n=1$), and antithrombin deficiency ($n=1$). Additionally, elevated Lp(a) was combined with the PT A20210A/MTHFR T677T genotypes and protein S deficiency type I ($n=1$). The MTHFR T677T genotype was found in one patient along with the PAI-1 4G/4G genotype. The rate of combined prothrombotic risk factors was significantly higher in childhood patients compared with their parents

(P=0.0004). In conclusion, based on the data presented here, we suggest that early onset SVT in childhood patients is mainly caused by combinations of at least two prothrombotic risk factors. Based on the fact that primary anticoagulant prophylaxis is available, a comprehensive screening for prothrombotic risk factors is not only indicated in childhood patients with SVT but also in their brothers and sisters.

Acknowledgements. The authors thank all technicians from the participating laboratories, in particular Doris Böckelmann, Margit Käse and Anke Reinkemeier, for excellent technical assistance. In addition, they thank Susan Griesbach for help in editing the manuscript.
    *Coinvestigators of the Childhood Thrombophilia Study Group were as follows: U. Göbel, W. Nürnberger (Pediatric Hematology and Oncology, Heinrich-Heine-University Düsseldorf), S. Ehrenforth (Department of Internal Medicine, University Hospital Frankfurt/Main), S. Becker, C. Heller, W. Kreuz (Department of Pediatric Hematology and Oncology, University Hospital Frankfurt/Main), S. Eber (Pediatric Hematology and Oncology, University Hospital Göttingen), N. Münchow (Department of Pediatric Hematology and Oncology, University Hospital Hamburg-Eppendorf), M. Sauer (University Children Hospital Jena), H. Pollmann (Department of Pediatrics, Westphalian Wilhelms-University Münster).

References

1. Alenc-Gelas M, Arnaud E, Nicaud V, Aubry ML, Fiessinger JN, Aiach M, Emmrich J. Venous thromboembolic disease and the prothrombin, methylene tetrahydrofolate reductase and factor V genes. Thromb Haemost 1999; 81: 506–10
2. Bertina RM, Koeleman BPC, Koster T, Rosendaal FR, Dirven RJ, de Ronde H, van der Velde PA, Reitsma PH. Mutation in blood coagulation factor V associated with resistance to activated protein C. Nature 1994; 369: 64–7
3. Boerwinkle E, Leffert CC, Lin J, Lackner C, Chiesa G, Hobbs HH. Apolipoprotein (a) gene accounts for greater than 90% of the variation in plasma lipoprotein (a) concentrations. J Clin Invest 1992: 90, 52–60
4. Boven van HA, Reitsma PH, Rosendaal FR, Baiston TA, Chowdhury V, Bauer KA, Scharrer I, Conard J, Lane DA. Factor V Leiden (FVR506Q) in families with inherited antithrombin deficiency. Thromb Haemost 1996; 75: 417–21
5. Cattaneo M, Tsai MY, Bucciarelli P, Taioli E, Zighetti ML, Bignell M, Mannucci PM. A common mutation in the methylenetetrahydrofolate reductase gene (C677 T) increases the risk for deep-vein thrombosis in patients with mutant factor V (Factor V:Q506). Arterioscler Thromb Vasc Biol 1997; 17: 1662–6
6. Dahlbäck B, Carlsson M, Svensson PJ. Familial thrombophilia due to a previously unrecognized mechanism characterized by poor anticoagulant response to activated protein C: prediction of a cofactor to activated protein C. Proc Natl Acad Sci USA 1993; 90: 1004–8
7. Dawson SJ, Wiman B, Hamsten A, Green F, Humphries S, Henney AM. The two allele sequences of a common polymorphism in the promoter of the plasminogen activator inhibitor (PAI-1) gene respond differently to interleukin-1 in HepG2 cells. J Chem Biol 1993; 268: 10739–45
8. Ehrenforth S, Junker R, Koch HG, Kreuz W, Münchow N, Scharrer I, Nowak-Göttl U. Multicenter evaluation of combined prothrombotic defects associated with thrombophilia in childhood. Eur J Pediatr 1999; 158: 97–104

9. Ehrenforth S, von Depka Prondsinski M, Aygören-Pürsün E, Nowak-Göttl U, Scharrer I, Ganser A. Study of the prothrombin gene 20210 GA variant in FV:Q506 carriers in relationship to the presence or absence of juvenile venous thromboembolism. Arterioscler Thromb Vasc Biol 1999; 19: 276–80

10. Falk G, Almquist A, Nordenhem A, Svensson H, Wiman B. Allele specific PCR for detection of a sequence polymorphism in the promoter region of the plasminogen activator inhibitor-1 (PAI-1) gene. Fibrinolysis 1995; 9: 170–4

11. Frosst P, Blom HJ, Milos R, Goyette P, Sheppard CA, Matthews RG, Boers GJH, den Heijer M, Kluitmans LAJ, van den Heuvel LP, Rozen R. A candidate genetic risk factor for vascular disease: a common mutation in methylenetetrahydrofolate reductase. Nature Genetics 1995; 10: 111–3

12. Junker R, Bäumer R, Koch HG, Schettler C, Weber D, Nowak-Göttl U. Heterozygous FV R506Q mutation in childhood thrombosis: A possible link to the plasminogen activator inhibitor-1 (PAI-1) 4G/4G genotype and elevated lipoprotein (a) – preliminary results of a single center pilot study. Fibrinolysis & Proteolysis 1999; 13: 26–9

13. Junker R, Koch HG, Auberger K, Münchow N, Ehrenforth S, Nowak-Göttl U. Prothrombin G20210 A gene mutation and further prothrombotic risk factors in childhood thrombophilia. Arterioscler Thromb Vasc Biol 1999; 19: 2568–72

14. Koelemann BPC, Reitsma PH, Allaart CF, Bertina RM. Activated protein C resistance as an additional risk factor for thrombosis in protein C-deficient families. Blood 1994; 84: 1031–5

15. Lane DA, Mannucci PM, Bertina RM, Bochkov NP, Bouljenkov V, Chandy M, Dahlbäck B, Ginter EK, Miletich JP, Rosendaal FR, Seligsohn U. Inherited thrombophilia: Part 2. Thromb Haemost 1996; 76: 824–34

16. Nowak-Göttl U, Binder M, Dübbers A, Kehrel B, Koch HG, Veltmann H, Vielhaber H. Arg to Gln mutation in the factor V gene causes poor fibrinolytic response in children after venous occlusion. Thromb Haemost 1997; 78: 1115–18

17. Nowak-Göttl U, Debus O, Findeisen M, Kassenböhmer R, Koch HG, Pollmann H, Postler C, Weber P, Vielhaber H. Lipoprotein (a): Its role in childhood thromboembolism. Pediatrics 1997; 99(6). URL: http://www.pediatrics.org/cgi/content/full/99/6/e11

18. Nowak-Göttl U, Dübbers A, Kececioglu D, Koch HG, Kotthoff S, Runde J, Vielhaber H. Factor V Leiden, protein C, and lipoprotein (a) in catheter-related thrombosis in childhood: a prospective study. J Pediatr 1997: 131, 608–12

19. Nowak-Göttl U, Junker R, Hartmeier M, Koch HG, Münchow N, Assmann G, von Eckardstein A. Increased lipoprotein (a) is an important risk factor for venous thrombosis in childhood. Circulation 1999; 100: 743–8

20. Nowak-Göttl U, Sträter R, Heinecke A, Junker R, Koch HG, Schuierer G, von Eckardstein A. Lipoprotein (a) and genetic polymorphisms of clotting factor V, prothrombin, and methylenetetrahydrofolate reductase are risk factors of spontaneous ischemic stroke in childhood. Blood 1999; 94: 3678–82

21. Nowak-Göttl U, Wermes C, Junker R, Koch HG, Schobess R, Fleischhack G, Schwabe D, Ehrenforth S. Prospective evaluation of the thrombotic risk in children with acute lymphoblastic leukemia carrying the MTHFR TT677 genotype, the prothrombin G20210 A variant, and further prothrombotic risk factors. Blood 1999; 93: 1595–99

22. Poort SR, Rosendaal FR, Reitsma PH, Bertina RM. A common genetic variation in the 3'-untranslated region of the prothrombin gene is associated with elevated plasma prothrombin levels and an increase in venous thrombosis. Blood 1996; 88: 3698–03

23. Salomon O, Steinberg DM, Zivelin A, Gitel S, Dardik R, Rosenberg N, Berliner S, Inbal A, Many A, Lubetsky A, Varon D, Martinowitz U, Seligsohn U. Single and combined prothrombotic factors in patients with idiopathic venous thromboembolism – Prevalence and risk assessment. Arteriol Thromb Vasc Biol 1999; 19: 511–8

24. Seligsohn U, Zivelin A: Thrombophilia as a multigenic disorder. Thromb Haemost 1997; 78: 297–1

25. Zöller B, Berntsdotter A, Frutos de PG, Dahlbäck B: Resistance to activated protein C as an additional genetic risk factor in hereditary deficiency of protein S. Blood 1995; 85: 3518–23

Inhibitor Development in Previously Untreated Patients with Hemophilia A and B: A Prospective 23-Year Follow-Up

C. Escuriola Ettingshausen, A. Zyschka, J. Oldenburg,
I. Martinez Saguer, S. Ehrenforth, W. Kreuz

Introduction

Progress in biotechnical methods of purification and virus inactivation as well as the introduction of recombinant FVIII and IX concentrates have improved dramatically the treatment of hemophiliacs. However, the development of neutralizing antibodies against FVIII or IX remains one of the most serious complication of repeated FVIII or IX replacement therapy, occurring in 22–52% of patients with severe hemophilia A and to a lesser extent (5.3–12.5%) in those with moderate hemophilia [1, 2, 4]. These conflicting data indicate that the reported frequency of inhibitor development is influenced by a number of variables caused by different study designs and study duration. One critical factor which may contribute to the wide-ranging data in many prospective studies on previously untreated patients (PUPs) may be an insufficient observation period and a low exposure status to FVIII or IX concentrates in a considerable number of patients. We, therefore, conducted a prospective long-term study, started in 1976, on inhibitor development in PUPs with hemophilia A or B treated with a single plasma-derived or recombinant FVIII or IX concentrate.

Patients and Methods

Since January 1976, a total of 92 PUPs with severe (<1%) and moderate (1–5%) hemophilia A and B have been enrolled in this prospective study (Table 1). All patients were at least once exposed to factor concentrate. Of the 92 patients, 91 were Caucasian and 1 was from African descent. All patients were managed at the outpatient clinic of the University Hospital Frankfurt/Main, Department of Pediatrics.

Table 1. Patients' demographics – type and severity of hemophilia (update January/1999)

	Hemophilia A	Hemophilia B
Residual activity <1%	48	8
Residual activity 1–5%	24	12
Total	72	20

I. Scharrer/W. Schramm (Ed.)
30th Hemophilia Symposium Hamburg 1999
© Springer-Verlag Berlin Heidelberg 2001

From 1976 to 1992, inhibitor assays were performed before the first exposure to clotting factor concentrate, thereafter every 20th exposure day (ED) and additionally in any case of suspicion of inhibitor formation.

Since 1993, the frequency of inhibitor testing (modified Bethesda method) has been intensified during the initial phase of replacement therapy: prior to the first ED, during the first 20 EDs every 3rd to 5th ED, and until the 200th ED every 10th ED, thereafter every 3 months. Additional testing should be performed in any case of suspicion of inhibitor development.

Results

During a 23-year study (update January 1999), a total number of 92 patients were enrolled (Table 1) and exposed at least once to a single plasma-derived (hemophilia A n=51, hemophilia B n=20) or recombinant (hemophilia A n=21, hemophilia B n=0) factor concentrate in order to cover bleedings and surgical procedures or for routine prophylaxis. To date, all patients have had 270 EDs (median, range 1–3051). Median age at first exposure was 1 year (range 0.1–9.8 years).

Inhibitor Development in Hemophilia A

Out of 72 hemophilia A patients with severe and moderate disease, 23 (32%) developed an inhibitor after 15 EDs (median, range 4–195). Five patients (22%) were low responders [>0.6–5 Bethesda units (BU)] and 18 patients (78%) were high responders (>5 BU). Among the severely affected hemophilia A patients, inhibitor formation occurred in 44% (21/48 patients), whereas only 8.35% patients with moderate hemophilia A developed an inhibitor. In the plasma-derived treated patients, inhibitors were detected in 37%. The exposure status in the non-inhibitor patients of this group, reflecting the further risk of inhibitor development, is rather high (median 290 EDs). So the risk for further inhibitor formation in this patient group can be considered as extremely low. In the recombinant treatment group, inhibitors have occurred in 19% of patients to date. However, the median ED in the non-inhibitor patients of this group was only 49, therefore presenting still a high risk to develop inhibitors in the future.

The mutation type profile revealed intron 22 inversion (55%), stop mutation (5%), missense mutation (10%), and small deletions (9%). Until now, no large deletion has been found in our hemophilia A patient cohort. The mutation type was not detectable in 8%, while 13% of the samples are still undergoing analysis.

Inhibitor Development in Hemophilia B

None of the 20 severely and moderately affected hemophilia B patients developed an inhibitor.

Discussion

The actual update (January 1999) gained from the 23-year follow-up revealed an inhibitor development in 32% of the previously untreated hemophilia A patients, with FVIII residual activity less than 5% after exposure to clotting factor concentrate, thereby confirming our results reported in 1992 [3]. In addition, the remarkably higher risk for inhibitor formation in severely affected hemophilia A patients (52% in 1992 and 44% in 1999) in comparison to the moderate ones is obvious. The mutation type profile of our hemophilia A patient group is comparable to that reported in other severely and moderately affected hemophilia A cohorts, concluding that there is primarily no higher risk for inhibitor development in our cohort.

The outweighing part of the inhibitor patients were high responders (78%), emphasizing once more the seriousness of this complication during treatment with factor concentrates, particularly in severe hemophilia A. The actual data are based on a frequently exposed PUP patient cohort (median 270 EDs) and should, therefore, be an approach to estimate the true risk of inhibitor development in treated hemophiliacs, since we know that the risk to develop inhibitors after the 200th ED is rather low. However, the patient cohort is too small to make statistically reliable statements. In particular, when the group was subdivided for further evaluations, such as comparison of concentrate types, the following was found: inhibitor formation was detected in 37% of hemophilia A patients (FVIII <5%) who were exclusively treated with plasma-derived concentrates, whereas only 19% of the recombinant group developed an inhibitor. However, there is a remarkable difference regarding the exposure status of both groups (median 290 EDs in plasma-derived treated patients vs median 49 EDs in the recombinant treated patients), which must surely contribute to the widely ranging preliminary results.

Comparison to data of recent retrospective as well as prospective plasma-derived and recombinant studies implies that there are slight, but not substantial, differences regarding frequency of inhibitor formation and distribution between high and low responders [1, 4, 5, 6, 7]. This may be caused by several variables of the study design. In particular, the patient cohort (PUPs, severity of hemophilia) and the study duration or better exposure status of each non-inhibitor patient plays an important role [1].

Therefore, standardized protocols considering the long-term observation of present cohorts seem to be imperative in order to assess the true risk of inhibitor formation.

No inhibitor formation was observed in hemophilia B patients, thereby confirming the low risk for this complication.

Summary

In order to assess inhibitor development in previously untreated patients (PUPs) with severe and moderate hemophilia A and B, a prospective study was initiated in 1976. During a 23-year study period, 92 severely (<1%) and moderately (1–5%)

affected hemophilia A and B patients were frequently exposed to FVIII or IX concentrates (median 270 EDs) and tested for inhibitor formation at regular intervals. In 72 hemophilia A patients (FVIII<5%), inhibitor development occurred in 32%. Most patients were high responders (>5 Bethesda Units, 78%). The severely affected patients showed a significantly higher frequency of inhibitor formation (44%) than the moderately affected ones (8.35%).

To date, none of 20 hemophilia B patients has developed an inhibitor.

References

1. Kreuz W, Escuriola Ettingshausen C, Martinez Saguer I, Güngör T, Kornhuber B: Epidemiology of inhibitors in haemophilia A. Vox Sang 1996; 70 (Suppl 1): 2–8
2. Brettler DB: Inhibitors in congenital haemophilia. Ball Clin Haematol 1996; 9(2): 319–29
3. Ehrenforth S, Kreuz W, Scharrer I, Linde R, Funk M, Güngör T, Krackhardt B, Kornhuber B: Incidence of development of factor VIII and IX inhibitors in haemophiliacs. Lancet 1992; 339: 594–98
4. Pasi KJ: Previously untreated patients and recombinant factor VIII concentrate studies. Blood Coag & Fibrinolysis: 1997; 8 (Suppl 1): 29–32
5. Lusher J, Arkin S, Hurst D et al.: Recombinant FVIII (Kogenate™) treatment in previously untreated patients (PUPs) with haemophilia A: Update of safety, efficacy and inhibitor development after seven study years. Thromb Haemost 1997; ISTH Florence Abstract 663
6. Gruppo R, Bray GL, Schroth P, Perry M, Gomperts ED: Safety and immunogenicity of recombinant factor VIII (Recombinate™) in previously untreated patients (PUPs): a 6.5 year update. Thromb Haemost, ISTH Florence Abstract 664
7. Addiego J, Kasper C, Abildgaard C, Hilgartner M, Lusher J, Glader B, Aledort L: Frequency of inhibitor development in haemophiliacs treated with low purity factor VIII. Lancet 1993; 342: 462–64

HIT Type II without Thrombocytopenia in a 15-Year-Old Boy with Protein S Deficiency and Recurrent Deep Vein Thrombosis

T. Severin, R. Ensenauer, A. Wiedensohler, K.-G. Fischer, B. Zieger, A. Greinacher, M. Brandis, A.H. Sutor

Background

Patients receiving heparin therapy can develop heparin-induced thrombocytopenia (HIT). In HIT type I, a nonimmunological interaction of heparin and thrombocytes causes a reduction in platelet count with minor clinical implication. HIT type II, however, is considered to be a serious complication of heparin therapy. Antibodies against complexes of heparin and platelet factor 4 (PF-4) lead to an activation of thrombocytes and endothelial cells and an increase in thrombin production resulting in thrombocytopenia. In severe cases, life-threatening thromboembolic complications occur (review in [1]).

In pediatric patients, HIT type II was described both in newborns [2] and in case reports regarding children and juveniles [3–10]. After diagnosis of HIT type II, heparin treatment has to be stopped; further anticoagulation, however, is necessary. In pediatric patients danaparoid-sodium was used as alternative anti-coagulant [3, 6, 7, 8, 10]. In one case published, a boy was treated with hirudin [9]. We report on a 15-year-old boy with an unusual form of HIT type II, since thrombocytopenia was absent, and clinical improvement occurred after lysis and hirudin treatment.

Case Report

History

A 15-year-old boy developed pain and a swelling of the right leg on the second day after appendectomy. Deep vein thrombosis was suspected.

Diagnostics

Duplex sonography revealed thrombosis of the deep pelvic and femoral veins on the right side. In the patient's family, protein S deficiency was diagnosed (patient, mother, one of two twin sisters). An uncle had developed a deep vein thrombosis at the age of 19 years. The patient further carried a heterozygous MTHFR mutation.

I. Scharrer/W. Schramm (Ed.)
30th Hemophilia Symposium Hamburg 1999
© Springer-Verlag Berlin Heidelberg 2001

Clinical Course

The patient was treated with unfractionated heparin (UFH). A high heparin dosage up to 38 IU/kg per hour was necessary to reach a sufficient increase of aPTT. Thrombocytes were within the normal range (minimum 228,000/µl).

After 1 week of anticoagulation with UFH, the patient developed pain and an increase in circumference of the opposite left leg. Duplex sonography showed a thrombus in the inferior caval vein, and thromboses in the external iliac vein and femoral veins on both sides. Although the platelet count was normal, the following factors were suggestive of HIT type II: new thromboses under full-dose heparin-anticoagulation, high heparin doses necessary to reach the target aPTT, and lack of clinical improvement despite lysis with urokinase and rt-PA. Diagnosis was confirmed by detection of antibodies against heparin/PF-4 complexes (ELISA).

Heparin was replaced by recombinant hirudin (lepirudin, Refludan, Aventis Pharma, Frankfurt, Germany) and overlapping phenprocoumon therapy was started. Although clinical symptoms improved, sonography constantly showed thrombosis in the pelvic veins with collateral vessels. The patient was almost free of symptoms 6 months after the first thrombotic event.

Discussion

In pediatric patients, heparin is used for prophylaxis and therapy of thrombosis, in neonatology and intensive care units up to several weeks. As in adults, in pediatric patients, HIT type II represents a potentially dangerous complication of heparin therapy.

In case of a decrease in platelet count, or continuation or occurrence of a new thrombosis under heparin therapy, HIT should be included in differential diagnosis. An increase in the heparin dose to reach the desired aPTT can also lead towards the diagnosis. Lack of thrombocytopenia may delay the diagnosis of HIT type II, but was described in adults [11, 12] and in a juvenile [3].

Only a few reports published address HIT type II in pediatric patients. In a study on 34 newborns with clinical assumption of HIT type II, antibodies against heparin/PF-4-complexes were detected in 14 patients. In this group of newborns, 11 patients developed thrombosis in the aorta. In older children and adolescents, thrombosis and embolism are also described as complications of HIT type II during heparin therapy [3–10]. In the majority of these reports, treatment was continued with danaparoid-sodium (Orgaran) as an alternative to heparin [3, 6–8, 10].

Prospective multicenter studies, addressing the thrombin inhibitor hirudin in adults with HIT type II, revealed an effective anticoagulation and a reduced incidence of HIT-related complications [13, 14]. So far, hirudin therapy in pediatric patients with HIT type II has been described in one other case of a patient with deep vein thrombosis and embolism of the left femoral artery [9].

Further experience in pediatric patients will reveal whether hirudin proves to be a therapeutic option in pediatric HIT patients.

Summary

The case of a 15-year-old boy with recurrent thrombosis under heparin therapy is presented. Although platelet count was normal, an increasing need of heparin to reach the desired aPTT led to the assumption of HIT type II. After antibody detection against heparin/PF-4 complexes, diagnosis of HIT type II without thrombocytopenia was confirmed. In addition, an underlying familial protein S deficiency and a heterozygous MTHFR mutation were found. After lysis and treatment with recombinant hirudin and phenprocoumon, the patient's condition improved. Six months after initial diagnosis of thrombosis he is almost free of symptoms.

References

1. Greinacher A (1999) Heparin-induzierte Thrombozytopenie – Pathogenese und Behandlung. Hämostaseologie 19:1–12.
2. Spadone D, Clark F, James E, Laster J, Hoch J, Silver D (1992) Heparin-induced thrombocytopenia in the newborn. J Vasc Surg 15:306–312.
3. Klement D, Rammos S, v. Kries R, Kirschke W, Kniemeyer H-W, Greinacher A (1996) Heparin as a cause of thrombus progression. Eur J Ped 155:11–14.
4. Potter C, Gill JC, Scott JP, McFarland JG (1992) Heparin-induced thrombocytopenia in a child. J Pediatr. 121:135–138.
5. Murdoch IA, Beattie RM, Silver DM (1993) Heparin-induced thrombocytopenia in children. Acta Paediatr 82:495–497.
6. Saxon BR, Black MD, Edgell D, Noel D, Leaker MT (1999) Pediatric heparin-induced thrombocytopenia: management with danaparoid (Orgaran). Ann Thorac Surg. 68: 1076–1078.
7. Sauer M, Gruhn B, Fuchs D, Altermann W, Zintl F (1998) Heparin-induzierte Thrombozytopenie Typ II im Rahmen einer Hochdosis-Chemotherapie mit anschließender Stammzellrescue. Klin. Pädiatr. 210:102–103.
8. Ranze O, Ranze P, Magnani HN, Greinacher A (1999) Heparin-induced thrombocytopenia in paediatric patients – a review of the literature and a new case treated with danaparoid sodium. Eur J Pediatr 158 [Suppl 3]:S130–S133.
9. Schiffmann H, Unterhalt M, Harms K, Figulla HR, Völpel H, Greinacher A (1997) Erfolgreiche Behandlung einer Heparin-induzierten Thrombozytopenie Typ II im Kindesalter mit rekombinantem Hirudin. Monatsschr Kinderheilkd 145:606–612.
10. Wilhelm MJ, Schmid C, Kececioglu D, Möllhoff T, Ostermann H, Scheld H (1996) Cardiopulmonary bypass in patients with heparin-induced thrombocytopenia using Org 10172. Ann Thorac Surg 61:920–924.
11. Phelan BK (1983) Heparin-associated thrombosis without thrombocytopenia. Ann Intern Med 99:637–638.
12. Hach-Wunderle V, Kainer K, Krug B, Müller-Berghaus G, Pötzsch B (1994) Heparin-associated thrombosis despite normal platelet counts. Lancet 344:469–470.
13. Greinacher A (1999) Rekombinantes Hirudin zur weiteren Antikoagulation bei Heparin-induzierter Thrombozytopenie. Hämostaseologie 19:19–29.
14. Greinacher A, Völpel H, Janssens U, Hach-Wunderle V, Kemkes-Matthes B, Eichler P, Mueller-Velten HG, Pötzsch B (1999) Recombinant hirudin (Lepirudin) provides safe and effective anticoagulation in patients with heparin-induced thrombocytopenia. Circulation 99:73–80.

VII. Free Lectures

Chairmen:

H. LENK (Leipzig)
E. O. MEILI (Zurich)

Modified Bonn-Malmö Protocol

L. Hess, H. Zeitler, C. Unkrig, W. Nettekoven, W. Effenberger,
P. Hanfland, H. Vetter, H.-H. Brackmann

Patients with an acquired inhibitor – usually directed against factor VIII – generally represent a medical emergency by the time the inhibitor is diagnosed. Emergency treatment or long-term management of such patients is one of the most cost-intensive therapies in medicine [2, 4, 5, 6, 8, 9].

In the following paper, we present an update of our experience with the modified Bonn-Malmö protocol (MBM protocol) in the treatment of acquired factor VIII (or V) inhibitors on the basis of a more extensive patient population.

The MBM protocol combines the experience gained with the Malmö and Bonn protocols [1, 3, 11, 12, 13]. The primary indication for use of the Bonn-Malmö protocol is in patients with acquired inhibitors who display life-threatening decompensation of the coagulation system. The treatment protocol is also suitable for use in patients with acquired chronic inhibitor disease and acute decompensation of coagulation.

Method

The 7-day treatment cycle is repeated a number of times depending on the clinical situation and coagulation response:
1. Long-term immunoadsorption from day 1–5 (adsorption of 2.5 times the plasma volume per day).
2. Stimulation of immune response by administration of factor VIII every 6 h (100–200 U/kg body weight, depending on the clinical response). Optimal dose reduction is done in consideration of the achieved factor VIII recovery values of 50–80% and on the basis of clinical signs throughout the therapy cycle.
3. Immunoglobulin substitution on treatment days 5 and 6 (IgG 0.3 g/kg body weight per day i.v.).
4. Administration of cyclophosphamide (2 mg/kg body weight per day) in combination with prednisolone (1 mg/kg body weight per day).

Initial therapy with recombinant factor VIIa or Feiba may be necessary while the patient is being transported or while an apheresis facility is being prepared.

Immunoadsorption was done using a Baxter Ig Therasorb column, which features Sepharose-bound polyclonal sheep antibodies with an IgG binding capacity of 4 g.

I. Scharrer/W. Schramm (Ed.)
30th Hemophilia Symposium Hamburg 1999
© Springer-Verlag Berlin Heidelberg 2001

Patients

We initiated treatment according to the MBM protocol in 18 patients (9 women, 9 men), all of whom displayed high-titer inhibitors, in most cases anti-factor VIII. One patient had high-titer factor V inhibitors. The mean age was 65.4 years (median 69, maximum 89, minimum 30). The mean inhibitor titer level was 585 Bethesda units (maximum 8400, median 63, minimum 16). All patients presented with Hb-relevant life-threatening bleeding.

Clinically, there were Hb-relevant hemorrhages alongside extensive hematomas frequently resulting in compartment syndromes or respiratory tract displacement, depending on the localization. Retroperitoneal and urogenital bleeding was also seen. Typically, hemarthrosis was seen in only two patients (see Table 1).

Diagnosis was confirmed on the basis of individual factor analysis, specifically by measuring factor VIII in at least two measuring systems: by a chromogenic measuring technique (supplied by Baxter) and using a one-stage clotting test with naturally deficient plasma (supplied by Immuno). The factor VIII inhibitor was assayed using the Bethesda and Nijmegen technique. To rule out lupus inhibitors, we performed a plasma dilution test, lupus aPTT, DRVVT (Diluted Russel Viper Venom Test), and additionally determined kaolin clotting time.

We diagnosed three postpartum processes, two cases of neoplastic disease (carcinoma of the prostate and lung), and two cases of collagen disease as the inhibitor-associated disease (see Table 1).

Results

Treatment according to the MBM protocol was initiated in January 1996. We treated 18 patients from then until November 1999. All 18 patients responded well to the MBM protocol, and were out of danger after 1 or 2 days of apheresis treatment.

Four patients were unable to complete the treatment protocol because of secondary disease. Severe cardiopulmonary, vascular, and neoplastic underlying diseases were the main factors. Fourteen patients were treated consequently according to the complete MBM-Protocol. Patients showed negative inhibitor test after a mean of 5.6 day of apheresis. Clotting factor products were no longer required after only 15.4 days of apheresis treatment. Six patients required a mean of 2 additional days of apheresis (maximum 5, median 2, minimum 0) after discontinuation of exogenous clotting factors. Based on 14 patients, the total duration of treatment was 17.4 apheresis treatment days until permanent inhibitor elimination (see Fig. 1).

A sample case is that of a 31-year-old female patient who developed a postpartum anti-factor VIII inhibitor. Her inhibitor titer measured 16 Bethesda units. The patient had to undergo emergency hysterectomy at another hospital because of a rapidly decompensating coagulation situation. Upon transfer, the patient's situation was still critical. In Fig. 2, the bars show her declining inhibitor titers and the line displays her factor VIII values on the MBM protocol. She tested inhibitor-negative after only 5 days of apheresis. Exogenous factor VIII units were no longer necessary

Table 1. Patients treated according to the modified Bonn-Malmö Protocol

Number	Patients' initials	Age	Sex	Maximum inhibitor titer	Indication for MBM protocol	Therapy completed?
1	RA	62	M	33	Bleeding from knee joint, hematuria, bleeding from soft tissues and extremities	Yes
2	HW	34	F	298	Postpartum bleeding from extremities, operative hematoma evacuation	Yes
3	MU	87	F	8400	Operative pleurodesis in presence of recurrent malignant pleural effusion	No
4	PK	79	F	67	Retroperitoneal bleeding, compartment syndrome, intra-abdominal bleeding after hematoma aspiration	Yes
5	HG	35	F	70	Postpartum retroperitoneal bleeding	Yes
6	MG	76	M	33	Intrathoracic bleeding after jugular vein centesis	Yes
7	SH	59	M	665	Retroperitoneal bleeding and bleeding from the extremities	Yes
8	WS	89	M	49	Multiple bleeding sites, extremities	No
9	KF	60	F	32	Bleeding from extremities and trunk, peritoneal bleeding	Yes
10	GF	74	F	22	Bleeding from knee joint and extremities	Yes
11	HH	81	F	15	Bleeding from extremities and trunk	No
12	HE	76	M	135	Urogenital bleeding, intrathoracic bleeding after jugular vein centesis	No
13	WH	68	M	59	Bleeding from extremities and trunk, iliopsoas muscle bleeding and leg paralysis	Yes
14	SE	68	M	327	Multiple bleeding sites, upper and lower extremities	Yes
15	MG	70	F	128	Multiple bleeding sites, upper and lower extremities	Yes
16	TS	30	F	16	Postpartum uterine bleeding mandating emergency hysterectomy	Yes
17	ME	53	M	110	Head and lower leg hematoma, fasciotomy in presence of compartment syndrome, lower leg	Yes
18	HW	66	M	76 (Factor V)	Retroperitoneal bleeding, hematuria	Yes

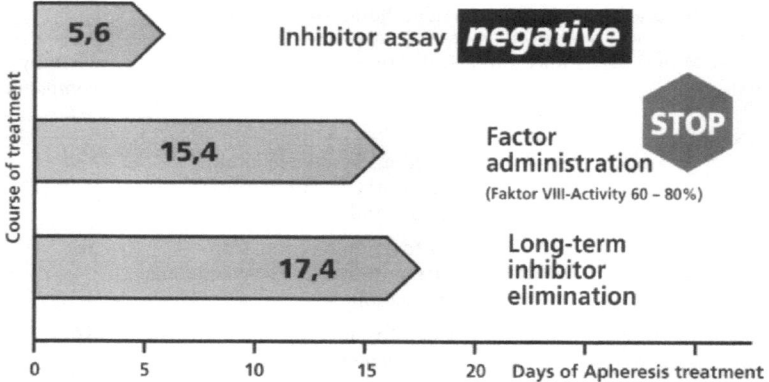

Fig. 1. Treatment response in the MBM protocol (average number of apheresis treatment days in 14 patients)

after 10 days of apheresis treatment. We required 365,000 factor VIII units for the treatment cycle presented.

Another exemplary treatment course is shown in Fig. 3. This 68-year-old male patient developed a factor VIII inhibitor at a titer of 327 Bethesda units, resulting in multiple soft-tissue bleeding sites in the upper and lower extremities. The bar elements in Fig. 3 represent the factor VIII units administered. Exogenous factor VIII was discontinued completely as early as day 13 of apheresis treatment. The

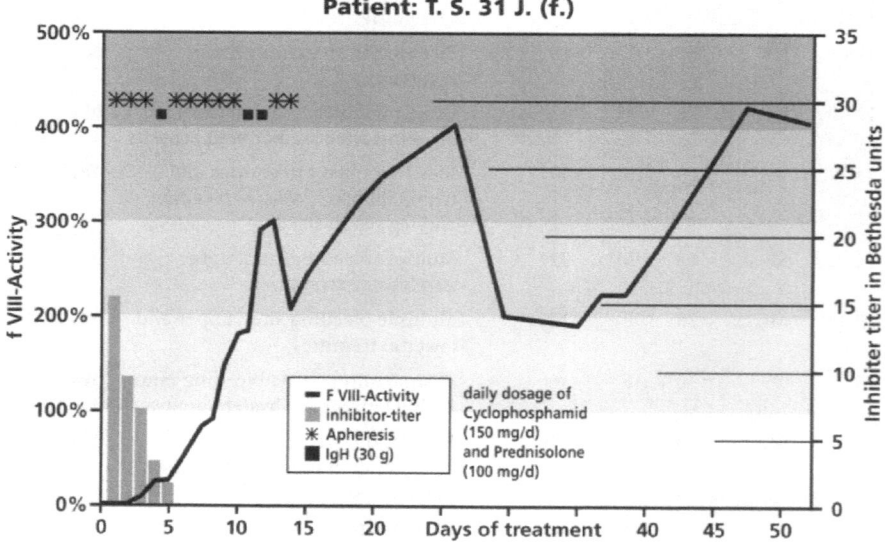

Fig. 2. Course of treatment in a 31-year-old female patient (for details see text)

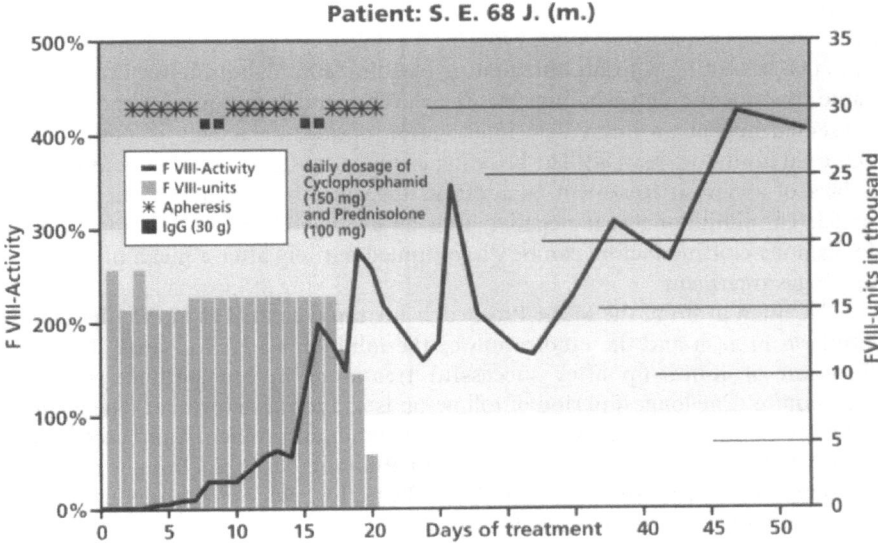

Fig. 3. Course of treatment in a 68-year-old male patient (for details see text)

patient required 340,000 units of factor VIII in total. No additional factor VIIa or FEIBA was necessary in the treatment courses presented here.

Our patients (n=14) have now been followed up for a mean of 20.6 months after completion of treatment by the MBM protocol. To date, one (male) patient's coagulation system has been stable without supportive therapy for 42 months (the median is 19.5 months, the shortest period of follow-up in November 1999 was 0.5 months).

Only one patient demonstrated declining factor VIII levels during follow-up. He required repeat apheresis treatment for an average of 6 days on two occasions. As the patient had residual factor VIII activities of 10% and 50%, we were able to do without exogenous clotting factors. This patient has now been stable at follow-up for the past 2 years.

Supportive treatment with Novo Seven or FEIBA was indicated in only six patients. The supportive treatment was not required after the fifth day of apheresis treatment. The mean was 3.3 days (median 3, minimum 0).

We administered 29,000 KIU of recombinant FVIIa (Novo Seven) solely for hemostasis in the treatment of the high-titer factor V inhibitor already referred to. It was clear that the administration of FVIII in this case was not appropriate.

The cost of treatment is largely attributable to the use of clotting factors, of which 1/2 million units were used on average to date (median 384,000, maximum 2 million, minimum 181,000 units). The maximum of 2 million units featured here is definitely an isolated case.

Discussion

Patients presenting with life-threatening bleeding and high inhibitor titers require rapid therapeutic intervention [8, 9, 10]. The updated Bonn-Malmö protocol presented here is an immediate intervention option for acutely ill patients with acquired inhibitors [6, 7, 15]. The bleeding is under control after 1 day, or at the most 2 days, of apheresis treatment. In addition, the causative inhibitor disease is eliminated. The inhibitor test is negative after an average of only 5 days of apheresis. Exogenous clotting factors can be discontinued entirely after a mean of 17 days of apheresis treatment.

The main profit of the MBM-Protocol is the rapid control of the life threatening situation in 24 h and the eradication of the inhibitor so far for years. The mean duration of follow-up after successful treatment in our patients ($n=14$) is 19.5 months. The longest period of follow-up is 42 months at present. The evidence suggests that we have a lifelong solution to the inhibitor problem. Undoubtedly, continued follow-up and a larger patient population are desirable. In view of the low incidence of inhibitor disease (1:1 million), the performance of a randomized trial is hardly possible at this time [4, 9, 10].

We believe a rapid allocation procedure could reduce the treatment costs, which are largely due to the use of clotting factors (mean 0.5 million units).

The median factor VIII consumption is 384,000 units, reflecting the trend toward reduced factor consumption in patients on the MBM Protocol.

We consider immunostimulation by presentation of antigen factor VIII to be an indispensable part of treatment [6, 7]. An insuffcient FVIII dosis entail a prolongation of the overall treatment protocol.

References

1. Brackmann HH (1984) Induced immunotolerance in factor VIII inhibitor patients. Prog Clin Biol 150: 181–185
2. Brackmann HH, Formsen J (1977) Massive factor VIII infusion in hemophilic patients with factor VIII inhibitor. Lancet II 933
3. Brackmann HH, Oldenburg J, Schwaab R (1996) Immune tolerance for the treatment of factor VIII inhibitors – Twenty years' 'Bonn Protocol'. Vox Sang 70: 30–35
4. Green D, Lechner K (1981) A survey of 215 non-hemophilic patients with inhibitors to factor VIII. Thromb Haemost 45: 200–203
5. Kessler, CM (1991) Acquired factor VIII inhibitors in the nonhemophiliac: Historical perspectives, current therapies, and future approaches. Am J Med 91 (5A): 1S-48S
6. Hess L, Unkrig C, Zeitler H, Effenberger W, Nettekoven W, Stier S, Hanfland P, Vetter H, Brackmann HH (1998) Modifiziertes Bonn- und Malmö-Protokoll: Behandlung erworbener Hemmkörper bei Nichthämophilen. 29. Hämophilie-Symposium Hamburg (1998), 44–49
7. Huth-Kühne A, Zimmermann R (1999) New Therapeutic Options In Acquired Hemophilia. Abstract, Vortrag 43, Jahrestagung GTH Mannheim
8. Lottenberg R, Kentro TB, Kitchins CS (1987) Acquired Haemophilia: A natural history study of 16 patients with factor VIII inhibitor receiving little or no therapy. Arch Intern Med 147: 1077–1081
9. Ludlam CA, Morrison AE, Kessler C (1994) Treatment of acquired hemophilia. Semin Hematol 31 2(4): 16–19

10. Morrison AE (1995) Acquired haemophilia and its management. British Journal of Haematology 89: 231–236
11. Nilsson IM, Berntorp E, Zettervall O (1988) Induction of immune tolerance in patients with hemophilia and antibodies to factor VIII by combined treatment with intravenous IgG, Cyclophosphamide, and Factor VIII. N Engl J Med 318: 947–50
12. Nilsson IM, Freiburghaus C (1993) Treatment of patients with factor VII and IX inhibitors. Thromb Haemost 79: 56–9
13. Nilsson IM, Freiburghaus C (1995) Apheresis Inhibitors to Coagulation Factors. Plenum Press, New York
14. Zeitler H, Unkrig C, Brackmann HH, Effenberger W, Hanfland P, Ko Y, Vetter H (1997) An immunomodulatory treatment of acquired hemophilia A with long-term IgG immunoadsorption, immunosuppression, and antigen substitution – A modified Bonn-protocol inducing immunotolerance. 39th ASH Meeting (Abstract)

A Novel Type of Mutation at the Propeptide Cleavage Site (Ala+1Thr) Causing Symptomatic Protein C Type II Deficiency

R. Dodojacek, G. Höfler, B. Leschnik, W. Muntean

Protein C is a precursor of a vitamin K-dependent serine protease that plays an important role in the regulation of blood coagulation [1]. The nucleotide sequence of the protein C gene is composed of nine exons that span over 11.2 kb. The nucleotides in this manuscript are numbered according to Foster et. al. [2,3]. Protein C is synthesized by hepatocytes as a polypeptide of 462 amino acids and undergoes several posttranslational modifications prior to secretion. The family of vitamin K-dependent coagulation proteins have two domains with marked sequence homology, the propeptide and the Gla domain. Glutamic acids in the Gla domain are converted during posttranslational processing to gamma-carboxyglutamic acid in a reaction that requires vitamin K as a cofactor [4,5]. After completion of gamma-carboxylation, the propeptides are cleaved off [6]. The two-chain mature protein is formed by removal of an internal dipeptide Lys156-Arg157 and consists of a light chain (155 amino acids) and a heavy chain (262 amino acids), held together by a disulfide bond [7]. Vitamin K-dependent proteins undergo a conformational transition upon metal ion binding, but only calcium ion mediates the binding of the Gla residues to phospholipid membranes, where the proteins exert their biological functions. Protein C is activated by thrombin in the presence of an endothelial cofactor, thrombomodulin, through the proteolytic removal of a dodecapeptide (the activation peptide) from the heavy chain [8]. The resulting activated protein C (APC) degrades the procoagulant cofactors Va and VIIIa in the presence of protein S, Ca^{2+} and phospholipids [9]. Individuals with hereditary protein C deficiency tend to have an increased risk of thromboembolism [10].

Hereditary protein C deficiency has been classified into two types. In type I both the level of activity and antigen of protein C are decreased, while in type II the level of anticoagulant activity is decreased although the protein C antigen level remains normal.

In this study we aimed to characterize the gene defect of a family with type II protein C deficiency. Several different mutations leading to protein C deficiency, in the majority point mutations, have been published in a database [11]. Almost all of the mutations associated with type II protein C deficiency described in this database are located either in exon III in the Gla domain or around the propeptide cleavage site or in exon IX clustered around the active site, the thrombomodulin binding or the substrate binding site. For this reason we investigated exon III and IX of the protein C gene and found a novel point mutation (G1390 A) at the propeptide cleavage site.

I. Scharrer/W. Schramm (Ed.)
30th Hemophilia Symposium Hamburg 1999
© Springer-Verlag Berlin Heidelberg 2001

Materials and Methods

Molecular Biology Methods

Genomic DNA was extracted from peripheral blood leukocytes of family members according to standard protocols.

PCR

The 5' end of exon III of the protein C gene was amplified by PCR, using oligonucleotide primers PRC 3 A, GC-PRC 3 as described [12]. Purification of primers containing a GC-clamp suitable for DGGE was performed using OPC columns (Applied Biosystem, Foster City, USA). For sequence analysis of exon III PCR was repeated using primer PRC-3, identical in sequence to GC PRC-3 except for the GC-clamp. PCR amplification of the 5' end of exon III was carried as described by Saiki et al. [13] out on a Hybaid Omnigene Thermalcycler (Teddington, UK) under the following conditions: 0.5 µg of genomic DNA was amplified in 100 µl of a solution containing 100 pmol/l of each primer, 0,2 mmol/l of each dNTP (Phamacia, Uppsala, Sweden), 10 mmol/l Tris-HCl pH 8.3, 50 mmol/l KCL, 1.15 mmol/l $MgCl_2$. After an initial denaturation step of 5 min at 94°C, 5 U of Ampli Taq DNA Polymerase (Perkin Elmer Cetus, Norwalk, Conn., USA) were added to each tube and 35 PCR cycles were performed with denaturation for 1 min at 94°C, annealing for 1 min at 58°C, and extension for 2 min at 72°C. A final extension step of 10 min at 72°C was followed by 10 min. denaturation at 94°C and 30 min annealing at 55°C to allow heteroduplex formation. PCR products were checked by electrophoresis on a 3% agarose gel.

Amplification of the 5' end of exon IX was done using described primers PRC 9A1 and GC-PRC 9A2 under the same conditions, except that the annealing temperature was 63°C.

DGGE

DGGE was performed essentially as described by Attree et al. [14]. Briefly 15 µl of PCR product were loaded on a 6.5% acrylamide gel containing a 30–80% denaturing gradient [100% denaturant =7 mol/l urea and 40% formamide in TAE buffer (40 mmol/l Tris, 20 mmol/l Na-acetate, 1 mmol/l EDTA, pH 7.4)] and run for 7 h at 160 V in a DGGE System 2000 (C.B.S Scientific, Del Mar, USA).

Cloning and plasmid preparation: PCR products of exon III without GC-clamp were amplified with primers PRC 3 and PRC 3 A and cloned into vector PCR II using TA Cloning Kit (Invitrogen, Groningen, The Netherlands). Preparation of the vector from bacterial culture was performed with Plasmid Maxi Kit (Quiagen, Valencia, USA).

Sequencing

Sequence analysis was performed using an ALF Automated DNA Sequencer (Pharmacia) and the Auto Cycle Sequencing Kit (Pharmacia). All commercial kits were applied in accordance with the manufacturers protocols.

RFLP

PCR products of Exon III without a GC-clamp were digested by the restriction endonuclease Rsa I under the following conditions: 14 µl PCR product and 10 Units of Rsa I (Boehringer Mannheim, Germany, Vienna, Austria) were incubated at 37°C overnight and electrophoresed on a 3% agarose gel. As the activity of Rsa I in the PCR mixture was high enough to digest the DNA complete, purification of the PCR products and use of the buffer recommended by the manufacturer was not necessary.

Blood Coagulation

Protein C antigen, amidolytic and anticoagulant activity were determined according to standard methods (Elisa, Boehringer Mannheim; and Asserachrom Protein C, Stago) [15].

Immunoblot Analysis

Protein C from normal plasma or from patients was purified by means of immmunoadsorption using a goat anti human protein C antibody attached to protein A sepharose CL-4B (Pharmacia). The material retained was electrophoresed on 4–20% gradient SDS-polyacrylamide gels, transferred to 0.2 µm nitrocellulose sheets (Bio Rad, Vienna, Austria) and incubated with blotto. Protein C bands were visualized using rabbit immunoglobulins against human protein C (Enzyme Research Labs, South Bend, Ind., USA) diluted 1:1000 and alkaline phosphatase-conjugated goat anti-rabbit antibody (Bio Rad) in a dilution of 1:300.

Results

Clinical and Blood Coagulation Investigations

The mother had experienced her first thrombosis, a deep venous thrombosis of the leg, at the age of 20 years, after minor trauma to the leg. Recurrences without obvious triggering causes occurred at the age of 43 years and 45 years, respectively. Her two sons, now 16 years and 19 years old, so far had not experienced thromboembolic events, as has her husband.

Protein C antigen in the mother was 90%, protein C amidolytic activity 66%, anticoagulant activity 50%. In her sons antigen was 86% and 88%, respectively; amidolytic activity was 65% and 63%, and anticoagulant activity was 46% in both. Values in mother and sons are compatible with the diagnosis of protein C deficiency, type II. In the father, all protein C values were within the normal range.

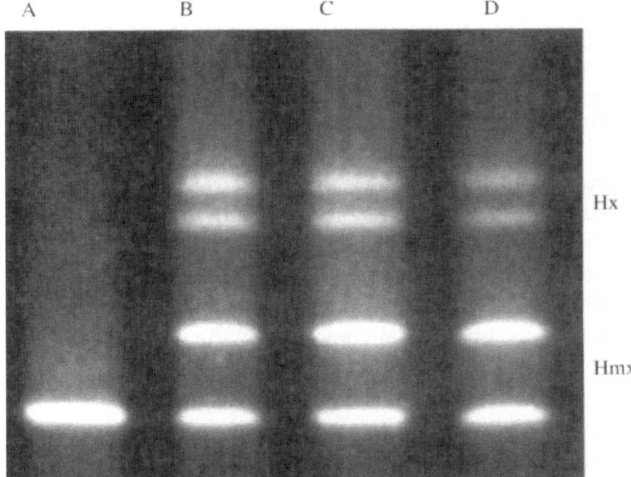

Fig. 1. DGGE patterns obtained with the amplified 5' end of exon III. *Lane A*: father, *Lane B*: mother, *Lanes C,D*: sons

Identification of Protein C Mutations

Exon III and IX of protein C, where most previously described mutations leading to type II Protein-C deficiency are located, were amplified and submitted to DGGE analysis. Fragments corresponding to the 5' end of exon III from the mother and her two sons showed abnormal migration, typical for heterozygous subjects. The father was found to be homozygous for the wild type (Fig. 1). PCR products without a GC-clamp were sequenced after subcloning, and a change of G to A at nucleotide number 1390 was detected by all family members showing abnormal patterns in the DGGE. This mutation was confirmed by digestion with Rsa I restriction endonuclease, as the mutation creates a new recognition site (GTAC) for this enzyme. To rule out a neutral

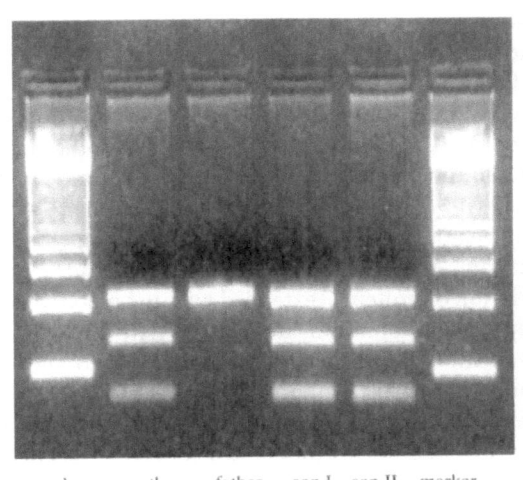

Fig. 2. PCR product of the 5' end of exon III digested with the endonuclease Rsa I: Rsa I did not cleave the PCR product of the normal allele, but cleaved that of the mutant allele into fragments of 135 and 76 pb

polymorphism we also investigated 70 healthy individuals for the presence of this restriction site. None of them exhibited a pattern indicative for this mutation (Fig. 2).

SDS-PAGE and Western Blotting

Immunoblotting of material analyzed by SDS-Page showed normal migration of the mutant and the wild type protein C antigen both under reducing and nonreducing electrophoresis conditions (Fig. 3). Furthermore, the proportions of the three components α, β and γ were apparently identical in control and patient plasmas [16]. Therefore the mutation Ala +1 to Thr of the protein C gene does not lead to secretion of a protein C form elongated by the propeptide.

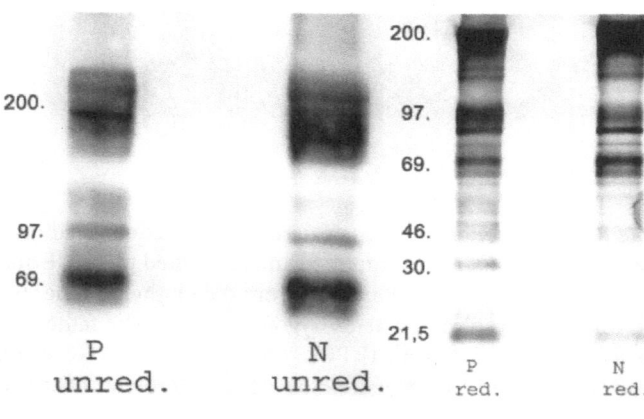

Fig. 3. Western blot of normal (*N*) and patient (*P*) protein C under nonreducing (*left two panels*) and reducing (*right two panels*) conditions

Discussion

We characterized the genetic defect in a patient with hereditary protein C type II deficiency and thromboembolic complications. The mutation detected is located in exon III of the protein C gene at the propeptide cleavage site. The G to A change at nucleotide number 1390 results in the substitution of Thr for Ala at amino acid position +1. A possible impairment of the processing of protein C by the mutation leading to the secretion of protein C circulating with the propeptide was excluded by Western blotting. This finding is compatible to results of earlier studies investigating the influence of mutations at amino acid position −1 (Arg to Ser [17], Arg to His [18] and Arg to Cys [12, 19]) on the propeptide cleavage. All these mutations lead to secretion of protein C extended with the mutated amino acid, due to a shift of the propeptidase recognition site Arg^{-5}-Ile-Arg-Lys-Arg^{-1} to Arg^{-5}-Ile-Arg-Lys^{-2} resulting in a shift of the propeptidase cleavage site to a new position, between amino acid position −2 and −1. As the mutation described here seems not to affect the propeptidase recognition site and the defective protein C is not secreted with the whole propeptide, the substitution of Thr for Ala +1 might lead to the secretion of a dysfunctional protein C without an influence on the processing of the propeptide.

References

1. Esmon CT. Protein-C: Biochemistry, physiology, and clinical implications. Blood 1983; 62: 1155-8.
2. Foster DC, Yoshitake S, Davie EW. The nucleotide sequence of the gene for human protein C. Proc Natl Acad Sci USA 1985; 82: 4673-7.
3. Plutzky J, Hoskins JH, Long GL, Crabtree GR. Evolution and organization of the human protein C gene. Proc Natl Acad Sci USA 1986; 83: 546-50.
4. Furie B, Furie BC: Molecular basis of vitamin K-dependent γ-carboxylation. Blood 1990; 75: 1753.
5. Foster DC, Rudinski MS, Schach BC, Berkner KL, Kumar AA, Hagen FS, Sprecher CA, Insley MY, Davie EW. Propeptide of human protein C is necessary for γ-carboxylation. Biochemistry 1987; 26: 7003-11.
6. Davie EW, Kawabata S: A microsomal endopeptidase from liver with substrate specificity for processing proproteins such as the vitamin K-dependent proteins in plasma. J Biol Chem 1992; 267: 10331.
7. Beckmann RJ, Schmidt RJ, Santerre RF, Plutzky J, Crabtree GR, Long GL. The structure and evolution of a 461 amino acid human protein C precursor and its messenger RNA, based upon the DNA sequence of cloned human liver cDNAs. Nucleic Acids Res 1985; 13: 5233-47.
8. Esmon CT. The regulation of natural anticoagulant pathways. Science 1987; 235: 1348-52.
9. Kisiel W, Canfield WM, Ericsson LH, Davie EW. Anticoagulant properties of bovine plasma protein C following activation by thrombin. Biochemistry 1977; 16: 5824-31.
10. Griffin JH, Evatt B, Zimmermann TS, Kleiss AJ, Wideman C. Deficiency of protein C in congenital thrombotic disease. J Clin Invest 1981; 68: 1370-3.
11. Reitsma PH, Poort SR, Bernardi F, Gandrille S, Long G, Sala N, Cooper DN. Protein C deficiency: a database of mutations, 1995 update. Thromb Haemost 1995; 73: 876-89.
12. Gandrille S, Alhenc-Gelas M, Gaussern P, Aillaud MF, Dupuy E, Aiach M. Five novel mutations located in exon III and IX of the protein C gene in patients presenting with defective protein C anticoagulant activity. Blood 1993; 82: 159-68.
13. Saiki RK, Gelfand DH, Stoffel S, Scharf SJ, Higuchi R, Horn GT, Mullis KB, Herlich HA. Primer-direct amplification of DNA with a thermostable DNA polymerase. Science 1988; 239: 489-91.
14. Attree O, Vidaud D, Vidaud M, Amselm S, Lavergne JM, Goossens M. Mutations in the catalytic domain of human coagulation factor IX: Rapid characterization by direct genomic sequencing of DNA fragments displaying an altered melting behaviour. Genomics 1989; 4: 266-72.
15. Sturk A, Morrien-Salomons WM, Huisman MV, Borm JJ, Buller HR, ten Cate JW. Analytical and clinical evaluation of commercial protein C assays. Clin Chim Acta 1987; 165: 263-70.
16. Greffe BS, Manco-Johnson MJ, Marlar RA. Molecular forms of human protein C: Comparison and distribution in human adult plasma. Thromb Haemost 1989; 62: 902.
17. Miyata T, Zheng YZ, Sakata T, Kato H. Protein C Osaka 10 with aberrant propeptide processing: loss of anticoagulant activity due to amino acid substitution in the protein C precursor. Thromb Haemost 1995; 74: 1003-8.
18. Lind B, Johnson AH, Thorsen S. Naturally occurring Arg-1 to His mutation in protein C leads to aberrant propeptide processing and secretion of dysfunctional protein C. Blood 1997; 89: 2807-16.
19. Girolami A, Simioni P, Girolami B, Marchiori A, Millar DS, Bignell P, Kakkar VV, Cooper DN. A novel dysfunctional protein C (Protein C Padua 2) associated with a thrombotic tendency: Substitution of Cys for Arg-1 results in a strongly reduced affinity for binding of Ca^{++}. Br J Haematol 1993; 85: 521

Lithuanian Hemophilia A and B Register Comprising Phenotypic and Genotypic Data

V. Ivaskevicius, R. Jurgutis, S. Rost, A. Müller, C. Schmitt, K. Wulff, F.H. Herrmann, C.R. Müller, R. Schwaab, J. Oldenburg

Introduction

Hemophilia A (HA) and B (HB) are two X-linked recessive bleeding disorders caused by deficiencies of the corresponding coagulation factors VIII (FVIII) and IX (FIX). Affected individuals develop a variable degree of hemorrhaging, predominantly in joints and muscles. The severity of bleeding symptoms relates to the residual activity of clotting factors. Thus, patients with severe disease (FVIII:C/FIX:C<0.01 IU/dl) usually experience recurrent spontaneous bleeding episodes while mildly affected patients (FVIII:C/FIX:C >0.05 IU/dl) only bleed upon provocation.

HA and HB are caused by heterogeneous mutations in the FVIII and FIX genes, respectively. In severe HA the most prevalent mutation is the intron 22 inversion that accounts for about 35–50% of the mutations (Lakich et al. 1993; Naylor et al. 1993; Becker et al. 1996), while in non-severe HA almost all gene defects are missense mutations (Schwaab et al. 1995). The large size of the FVIII gene (186 kb, 26 exons and 9 kb mRNA) has complicated molecular diagnostics of HA for years. Nowadays, screening methods, such as Single-Strand Conformation Polymorphism (SSCP), Denaturing Gradient Gel Electrophoresis (DGGE), Chemical Mismatch Cleavage (CMC) and Temperature Modulated Heteroduplex Chromatography (TMHC) provide efficient tools for the analysis of large genes like FVIII. The smaller FIX gene spans 34 kb of DNA and consists of eight exons. FIX mRNA is 2.8 kb of which 1.4 kb code for the FIX protein. Mutations in the FIX gene are mainly detected by direct sequencing. As reported by Giannelli et al. (1998) the most prevalent gene defects in HB are missense mutations (68%), followed by nonsense mutations (14%) and splice site mutations (6%).

Lithuania is one of the Baltic states and has a population of 3.7 million people. Until 1990, when Lithuania restored its independence, very little attention was given to congenital coagulation disorders. From 1990, Lithuanian hematologists started improving diagnostic and treatment facilities for those patients. In April 1994, the Lithuanian Hemophilia Association (LHA) entered the World Federation of Hemophilia. A hemophilia center was established in Klaipeda and further specialized units for hemophilia care became available in the hematological departments of the Vilnius and Kaunas university clinics.

In the present study, we compiled phenotypic and genotypic data from 71 unrelated HA and HB families that comprise about 80% of the Lithuanian patients. This data will be instrumental for a National Hemophilia Register that will considerably improve the medical care of hemophilia families in Lithuania with respect to treatment and genetic counseling.

I. Scharrer/W. Schramm (Ed.)
30th Hemophilia Symposium Hamburg 1999
© Springer-Verlag Berlin Heidelberg 2001

Patients, Materials and Methods

Patients and Relatives

From March 1998 to October 1998 data and blood samples of the Lithuanian hemophilia patients and their relatives were collected. Some of these data were already obtained by the hemophilia center in Klaipeda. From the hemophilic index patients information on name, date of birth, type of hemophilia, degree of severity, level of FVIII/FIX activity and inhibitor status were registered. From the relatives name, date of birth, relationship to index patient (sister, brother, mother, etc.) and pedigree information comprising three generations were taken. Blood samples consisted of 10 ml EDTA blood for genetic analysis and 5 ml citrate blood for coagulation assays. EDTA blood was stored frozen at –20°C. Citrate blood was centrifuged, aliquoted in 2–3 portions of about 1 ml in plastic tubes and stored frozen at –40°C. In November 1998 stored plasma and EDTA blood samples were sent on dry ice to Wuerzburg/ Germany for further analysis.

Coagulation Assays

Coagulation assays were performed at the Hemophilia Center Bonn. FVIII:C was measured by a chromogenic assay (Baxter Diagnostic, Deerfield, USA) and a one-stage assay based on natural FVIII-deficient plasma purchased from Baxter Immuno (Vienna, Austria). FVIII:Ag determination was carried out using a highly sensitive FVIII-ELISA (Schmitt et al. 1997). FVIII inhibitors were determined according to the Bethesda method with the Nijmegen modification (Verbruggen et al. 1995). FIX:C was measured using a one-stage assay applied by DADE Diagnostic, USA. Von Willebrand factor (vWF:RiCoF) was analyzed according to Macfarlane et al. (1975) and von Willebrand factor antigen (vWF:Ag) according to Cejka (1982).

Southern Blot Analysis for the Detection of Intron 22 Inversions

Genomic DNA was prepared from frozen EDTA blood leukocytes by standard procedure (Miller et al 1988). All HA patients were screened by Southern Blot for the presence of an intron 22 inversion. An intron 22-specific hybridization probe was generated as described by Becker et al. (1996), labeled with 32P and hybridized to a Southern blot of BclI – digested DNA using standard conditions (Lakich et al. 1993).

FVIII Gene Mutation Screening

The FVIII gene of patients that were negative for intron 22 inversion were screened for mutations in a subsequent procedure by DGGE, CMC and TMHC. For DGGE analysis of the FVIII gene, exons 1–13 and exons 15–26 were amplified individually by PCR according to Schwaab et al. (1995). Three small regions of exon 14 that code for the thrombin cleavage sites (nt2116 to nt2324 and nt4893 to nt5219) and a mutation hotspot encompassing an adenin run (nt3543 to nt3691) were amplified by PCR with the following primer pairs Intron13F(GC-clamp)-GTAACCAGAGTCT TATTCTT and nt2346R-TTCTGGAATTGTGGTGGCATTA, nt3523F (GC-clamp)-GA ATTTACAAAGGACGTAGG and nt3710R-GTCACTGTATGTATCTGAGG, nt4983F (GC-clamp)-CTTGAAACGCCATCAACGGG A and Intron14R-AGCAGAGCAAAG GAATAACCA. DGGE conditions were chosen according to Oldenburg et al. (2000, submitted) to allow for a high throughput mutation analysis. For PCR an uniform annealing temperature of 55°C could be applied to all exons except exons 20 and 21 (T_a=50°C) and exon 26 (T_a=60°C). Conditions for polyacrylamide gel electrophoresis were standardized for all fragments (formamide gradient 0–80%, T=60°C, U=150 V, t=3.5 h).

In patients that showed no mutation by DGGE analysis, the whole exon 14 (nt2116–5220) was amplified in two overlapping fragments (nt2116–3769 and nt3513–5220) and subjected to CMC according to Schwaab et al. (1995).

In nine patients in whom no mutations could be found by DGGE and CMC, the whole coding regions of the FVIII gene were additionally screened by a highly sensitive Temperature Modulated Heteroduplex Chromatography using the WAVE System (Transgenomics) according to Oldenburg et al. (2000, submitted). By this technique heteroduplex DNA strands are separated from homoduplexes by ion-pair reverse-phase liquid chromatography according to their difference in melting behavior. The different retention times on the DNA[Sep] column allow for a highly sensitive detection of changes in the DNA sequence (Kunkel et al. 1997).

All aberrant DNA fragments detected by the various screening techniques were sequenced by the dideoxynucleotide chain termination method and the sequenase version 2.0 DNA sequencing kit (US Biochemical).

FIX Gene Mutation Screening

All exons of the FIX gene were individually amplified by PCR and directly sequenced according to Wulff et al. (1995).

Haplotype Analysis

Haplotype-analysis of HA families was carried out by PCR-based polymorphisms of two intragenic VNTRs in intron 13 and intron 22, respectively (Lalloz et al. 1994) and one extragenic VNTR DXS52, (Richards et al. 1991).

Results

Hemophilia A Phenotype

In 63 unrelated HA families 50 (79.4%) patients had severe disease, 8 (12.7%) had moderate and 5 (7.9%) had mild disease. Five (7.9%) of 63 patients were Cross

Reacting Material Positive (CRM+), indicating that FVIII:C is at least 30% lower than the corresponding FVIII:Ag. Three (6%) of 50 patients with severe HA had developed inhibitors ranging from 20 to 64 Bethesda units (BU). No significant vWF:RiCoF and vWF:Ag decrease could be found in anyone of the patients.

Genotypes of Hemophilia A Patients

The prevalent intron 22 inversion was investigated by Southern Blot. Point mutations, splice site mutations and small deletions or insertions of the FVIII gene were detected by a step-wise strategy starting with DGGE, followed by CMC of exon 14 and TMHC (Wave System). Large deletions were identified indirectly by failure of PCR amplification of the lost exons and in two patients directly by Southern Blot (loss of the intragenic FVIII signal).

In severe HA, 24 (48%) of 50 patients had an intron 22 inversion. Twenty of these patients (83.4%) showed the distal and 4 patients (16.6%) the proximal type. Application of the screening methods revealed a mutation in 25 of the remaining 26 patients. The mutations identified comprised 6 (12%) nonsense mutations, 6 (12%) missense mutations, 5 (10%) small deletions, 3 (6%) small insertions, 4 (8%) large deletions and 1 (2%) splice site mutation (see Table 1). Overall in 49 (98%) of 50 patients with severe HA the molecular defect in the FVIII gene could be detected by our screening strategy.

In non-severe HA we found 11 (84.6%) missense mutations and 1 (7.7%) small deletion. One (7.7%) mutation remained undetected (see Table 1). Altogether, in only 2 of all HA patients no mutation could be identified.

A detailed description of the mutations and the corresponding phenotypes is given in Table 2. Seven (29.2%) of the 24 identified point mutations occurred at

Table 1. Mutation profiles of severe HA and non-severe HA

Mutation Type	Mutation Frequency
Severe hemophilia A (n=50)	
Intron 22 inversion	24 (48.0%)
Distal	20 (83.4%)
Proximal	4 (16.6%)
Nonsense	6 (12.0%)
Missense	6 (12.0%)
Small deletion	5 (10.0%)
Small insertion	3 (6.0%)
Large deletion	4 (8.0%)
Splice site	1 (2.0%)
Mutation unknown	1 (2.0%)
Non-severe hemophilia A (n=13)	
Missense	11 (84.6%)
Small deletion	1 (7.7%)
Mutation unknown	1 (7.7%)

Table 2. Detailed list of mutations and phenotypes in Lithuanian HA patients

ID	Mutation	Amino acid change	CpG	Domain	FVIII:C (IU/dl)	FVIII:Ag (IU/dl)
A. Large Del						
LT1	Exon 1	Large del	–	A1	<0.01	<0.003
LT2	Exon 15–22	Large del	–	A3–C1	<0.01	<0.003
LT3	Exon 15–22	Large del	–	A3–C1	<0.01	n.d.
LT4	Exon 19–21	Large del	–	A3–C1	<0.01	<0.003
B. Small Del						
LT5	202-207del[a]	T49-50del	–	A1	<0.01	<0.003
LT6	1579-1601del[a]	I(Ile)508-15del	–	A2	<0.01	<0.003
LT7	3637delA	E1191-94del	–	B	<0.01–<0.01	0.005–0.007
LT8	3701-3704del[a]	I(Ile)1214-16del	–	B	<0.01	0.006
LT9	4379delA	K1439-41del	–	B	<0.01–<0.02	0.004
LT10	6595delA[a]	G2179-80del	–	C2	<0.01–<0.01	<0.003
C. Small Ins						
LT11	2373insG[a]	F773ins	–	B	<0.01	<0.003
LT12	4379insA	N1439-41ins	–	B	<0.01–0.01	<0.003
LT13	4379insA	N1439-41ins	–	B	<0.01–0.01	<0.003
D. Nonsense						
LT14	871G>T[a]	E272X	–	A1	<0.01	n.d.
LT15	1357G>T[a]	E434X	–	A2	<0.01	<0.003
LT16	2246T>A[a]	L730X	–	A2	<0.01	<0.003
LT17	2440C>T	R795X	CpG	B	<0.01	<0.003
LT18	2443C>T[a]	Q796X	–	B	<0.01	<0.003
LT19	3392C>T[a]	Q1079X	–	B	<0.01	n.d.
E. Missense						
LT20	764G>A[a]	G236D	–	A1	<0.01	<0.003
LT21	968G>A[a]	G304E	–	A1	<0.01	<0.003
LT22	1171C>T	R372C	CpG	A2	0.01–0.02	0.14–0.16
LT23	1648C>T	R531C	CpG	A2	0.07	0.19
LT24	1756A>G[a]	M567V	–	A2	0.11–0.22	1.04
LT25	5122C>T	R1689C	CpG	B	0.01–0.02	0.16–0.24
LT26	5398C>T	R1781C	CpG	A3	0.02–0.03	0.024
LT27	5825G>C[a]	G1923A	–	A3	0.01–0.02	0.02–0.03
LT28	5888T>C[a]	L1944P	–	A3	<0.01	0.01
LT29	6107A>G[a]	Y2017C	–	A3	0.02–0.04	0.047
LT30	6371A>G	Y2105C	–	C1	0.05–0.08	0.09
LT31	6515C>G[a]	P2153R	–	C1	<0.01	<0.003
LT32	6544C>T	R2163C	CpG	C1	<0.01–0.01	0.09
LT33	6683G>A	R2209Q	CpG	C2	<0.01	0.01
LT34	6920A>C[a]	D2288A	–	C2	0.05–0.09	0.07–0.12
LT35	6920A>C[a]	D2288A	–	C2	0.01–0.02	0.09
LT36	6920A>C[a]	D2288A	–	C2	0.09	0.14
F. Splice site						
LT37	IVS19+1G>A[a]	–	–	A3	<0.01	0.003

[a]Mutations not reported previously

CpG-sites known as mutation hotspots. Eleven mutations, predominantly nonsense mutations, small deletions and insertions, were recognized in exon 14 that codes for the FVIII-B domain. Beside the intron 22 inversion only very few mutations were found in more than one family. Two of the 3 insertions were located at codons 1439–41, within a series of eight adenine nucleotides. In two unrelated families (LT2 and LT3) a large deletion spanning exons 15–22 could be detected (all of them have developed inhibitors) and in three apparently unrelated families the same missense mutation D2288A could be found.

Five missense mutations were CRM+. Two of them (R372C and R1689C) affected the thrombin cleavage sites, another two mutations (R531C and M567V) were situated in the A2 domain and one mutation (R2163C) was found in the C1 domain.

Overall, 19 mutations (8 missense mutations, 5 nonsense mutations, 1 splice site mutation, 4 small deletions and 1 insertion) have not been reported in the International Hemophilia A Mutation Database (HAMSTeRS).

Carrier Diagnosis and Mutation Origin in HA

In 36 (57.1%) families only one hemophiliac was known (isolated HA) while 27 (42.9%) families had a history of the disease (familial HA).

Direct mutation analysis in 55 females from families with isolated HA identified 33 carriers and 22 non-carriers. In familial HA, 8 of 17 females were found to be carriers and 9 non-carriers. Prenatal diagnosis has been performed on chorion biopsies in 2 families (LT3 and LT63) revealing two healthy girls.

In 11 families with isolated HA, we were able to determine the origin of the mutation. Two mutations originated in the mother of the hemophiliac. Interestingly, the P2153R missense mutation turned out to be a mosaic, indicating the emergence of the mutation in early embryogenesis.

Five mutations originated in male germ cells of the healthy maternal grandfather or great-grandfather, respectively. In four families the mutations have occurred in earlier generations not available for analysis (Table 3).

Table 3. Mutation origin in families with isolated HA

No.	ID	Mutation Type	Mutation Origin
1	LT40	Inversion	MGGF
2	LT41	Inversion	MGF
3	LT42	Inversion	MGF
4	LT20	Missense	MGF
5	LT28	Missense	MGF
6	LT43	Inversion	EGT MGM
7	LT44	Inversion	EGT MGM
8	LT45	Inversion	EGT MGM
9	LT13	Insertion	EGT MGM
10	LT31	Missense	M (Mosaicism)
11	LT5	Small deletion	M

M, mother; MGF, maternal grandfather; MGM, maternal grandmother; MGGF, maternal great-grandfather; EGT, earlier generation than.

Hemophilia B Phenotype and Genotype

In HB, all patients had a severe form of the disease. For genetic analysis of the FIX gene all exons were amplified by PCR and directly sequenced. In eight (100%) of eight families the mutations could be found including five missense mutations, one nonsense mutation, and two small (1 bp) deletions (LT64, LT71). The latter two mutations have not been described before (Table 4). Patient LT69 exhibited also a polymorphism within the activation peptide (20422G>A). In two unrelated families (LT65, LT66) the same missense mutation (6364C>T) at a CpG site was detected. Overall four of eight identified mutations occurred at CpG-sites.

Table 4. Detailed list of mutations and phenotypes in Lithuanian HB patients

ID	Base change	Amino Acid Change	CpG	Domain	FIX:C (IU/dl)
LT64	84delC[a]	L(-28)del	–	Signal peptide	<0.01
LT65	6364 C>T	R(-4)W	CpG	Propeptide	<0.01
LT66	6364 C>T	R(-4)W	CpG	Propeptide	<0.01
LT67	6451 G>C	E26Q	–	GLA	<0.01
LT68	6460 C>T	R29X	CpG	GLA	<0.01
LT69	20519 G>A	R180Q	CpG	Activation peptide	<0.01
LT70	31092 A>C	E324P	–	Catalytic	<0.01
LT71	31325delT[a]	S402del	–	Catalytic	<0.01

[a]Mutation not reported previously.

Carrier Diagnosis in HB and Mutation Origin

Carrier diagnosis was done in ten women showing four carriers and six non-carriers of the disease. In four families, only isolated cases of HB were known. In two of these families (LT64 and LT71) a de novo mutation could be found.

Discussion

Phenotype of HA and HB

In order to set up a Lithuanian hemophilia register phenotypic and genotypic data were assessed from 63 unrelated families with HA and 8 families with HB, respectively.

The majority of patients known to have hemophilia in Lithuania are severely affected. In our study, 50 (79.4%) of 63 in HA and 8 (100%) of 8 in HB had a severe form of the disease. Other studies have observed higher proportions of non-severe hemophiliacs. Antonarakis et al. (1995) described the proportion of HA cases that are severe, moderate and mild as 50%, 10%, and 40%, respectively. Soucie et al. (1998) studied the frequency of HA and HB in six US states and found that 43% of HA patients had severe, 26% moderate and 31% mild disease. It may be speculated that the lower proportion of non-severe hemophiliacs in Lithuania is due to lack of diagnosis. In Lithuania the first diagnosis is mainly based on activated partial thromboplastin time (aPTT) that may fail to detect milder FVIII and FIX deficiencies. Single factor measurement in cases of mildly increased aPTT is carried out rarely. Jennings et al. (1998) reported that a higher proportion of hemophilia centers in developing countries failed to identify milder deficiencies of the intrinsic system by aPTT. It may also be speculated that patients in developing countries are taking less care of minor health problems.

Mutation Analysis in HA

Efficacy of Mutation Screening Methods

The availability of PCR based screening methods and the knowledge of the intron 22-inversion mutation (Lakich et al. 1993; Naylor et al. 1993) enabled us to identify the FVIII gene mutations in 61 (96.8%) of 63 families. In most studies reported so far, the FVIII gene mutations could not be identified in 10–15%, independent of whether the patient cohorts contained mildly, moderately or severely affected patients and also independent from the mutation screening method used (Higuchi et al. 1991a; Lin et al. 1993; Pieneman et al. 1995; Schwaab et al. 1995; Becker et al. 1996). Using DGGE and CMC (for exon 14) we identified 85.7% of mutations, i.e., the same efficacy as other studies. The additional application of TMHC in our study increased the detection rate to 96.8%, indicating that the detection of mutations by DGGE is limited by complex melting profiles of some exons (e.g., the exons 7, 12 and 26). Only two studies reported a higher efficacy of mutation screening methods. Waseem et al. (1999) detected 141 of 141 mutations by applying Solid Phase Fluorescent CMC to patients' RNA. However they failed to examine 80 patients because of poor quality of RNA preparation. Using a similar CMC approach Freson et al. (1998) detected a mutation in all of 20 patients. However it is still unknown whether the preselection of analyzing RNA may influence the detection rate of mutations.

Mutation Type Profile in HA

In our study 48% severely affected HA patients exhibited an intron 22 inversion. A similar proportion of inversions in severe HA is reported by several other studies (Collins et al 1994; Goodeve et al 1994; Ljung and Sjörin 1995; Antonarakis et al. 1995). The proportions for distal (83.4%) and proximal (16.6%) inversions observed in our study corresponded well to those of 84.1% and 15.9% described by Antonarakis et al. (1995).

In our study, we detected 24% point mutations (half missense and half nonsense), 16% small deletions/insertions and 8% large deletions. These data also correspond well to those reported from other studies (Higuchi et al. 1991; Lin et al. 1993; Becker et al. 1996) where the proportions of point mutations vary from 20.8% to 32%, small deletions/insertions from 10.9% to 20.8% and large deletions from 3.9% to 7%, respectively.

Mutation Hotspots

In the present study, four mutations could be detected within 2 series of adenines in exon 14 previously described as mutation hotspots (Becker et al. 1996). Three of them (one A-deletion and two A-insertions) are located in codon 1439–1441 (eight adenines) and one A-deletion in codon 1191–1194 (nine adenines). All of these patients had severe HA (FVIII:C<0.01 IU/dl). These small deletions/insertions within in a series of adenines probably are caused by polymerase errors during RNA transcription/DNA replication. Interestingly, the same mechanism causing the mutation also leads to the phenomenon of an unexpected mitigation of the hemophilia phenotype in some patients (Young et al. 1997; Oldenburg et al. 1998).

CpG sites are known to represent another very important mutation hotspot and accounted for 29.2% of point mutations in our study. Cooper et al. (1988) and Pattinson et al. (1990) found that up to 40% of point mutations were localized at CpG sites.

Mutations Within the FVIII-B Domain

The proportion of mutations in exon 14 is of special interest, because exon 14 codes for the B domain that is not essential for coagulation activity of the mature FVIII protein (Pittman et al. 1993). In our study, 6 (66.6%) of 9 small deletions/insertions, 3 of 6 nonsense mutations, and 1 (5.9%) of 17 missense mutations were located in the B domain. Since the B domain accounts for 40% of the FVIII:C DNA the high proportion of small deletions may be due to the hotspot character of the two series of adenine nucleotides at codons 1191–1194 and 1439–1441, respectively. However, missense mutations were significantly underrepresented, likely due to the low functional importance of this region. Our results are mirrored by the HAMSTeRS database in which 48.0% of small deletions/insertions (39.6% of them in one of the two adenine stretches) and 8.6% of missense mutations (72% of them in amino acids 1689 and 1680) were located within the exon 14 (B domain) .

Spectrum of Mutations in CRM+ Positive Hemophilia A

Higher FVIII:Ag values compared to FVIII:C were found in 5 (7.9%) of 63 patients. Four of these mutations (R372C, R531C, R1689C, R2163C) have been reported earlier (Higuchi et al 1991a; Gitschier et al. 1988; Arai et al. 1990; Shima et al 1989; Reiner et al. 1992). We identified a novel CRM+ mutation M567V that was associated with a FVIII:C of 0.11–0.22 IU/dl and a FVIII:Ag of 1.041 IU/dl. Amino acid M567 is located very close to a factor IXa interactive site (residues 558–565). Fay et al. (1994) found that chemically synthesized peptides including FVIII residues 556–564 and 561–569 were inhibitory to FXa generation and thus confirmed their importance for a functional factor X as enzyme complex. The proportion of CRM+ patients found in our study corresponds well to the of 5% that were reported earlier (Lazarchick et al. 1978).

Three of five detected CRM+ mutations were located within the A2 domain. McGinniss et al. (1993) suggested that the A2 domain is critical for the function of FVIII and therefore exhibits a higher number of CRM+ mutations.

Novel Mutations

A total of 19 mutations comprising point mutations, small deletions and insertions have been reported for the first time in our study (Table 2). In three families (LT34, LT35, LT36) with mild to moderate phenotype we identified the same missense mutation in exon 26 (N2288A). Haplotype analysis showed evidence for a founder mutation (data not shown).

Seventy-seven different small deletions were reported so far in HAMSTeRs. Most of these produce frameshifts and consequently abolition of FVIII expression. Almost all of them are associated with a severe form of hemophilia. Interestingly, we detected a 4 bp deletion (3701–3704delATAC) in a 61-years-old patient (LT8) that was associated with a moderate phenotype (residual FVIII:C<0.01 IU/dl). Bleeding from the nose and bruising were main symptoms of the disease in the patient's childhood and adolescence. HA diagnosis was suspected at the age of 32 after several episodes of hematuria. The patient has received only few FVIII substitutions during life and joint function is still quite normal.

Another patient of interest is the oldest Lithuanian hemophiliac, born in 1919. He also has a small deletion (6595delA). Unexpectedly, in spite of a severe form of the disease and limited treatment in the early years of this century he is still alive up to a ripe old age. FVIII gene analysis on the RNA level may help to find an explanation for this unexpected clinical courses of the disease.

Factor IX Gene Analysis

Direct sequencing of the complete FIX gene identified the causative mutation in all of the HB patients. The majority of patients (five of eight) exhibited missense mutations that are known to represent the predominant mutation type in HB. All mutations, except the two small deletions (84delC, 31325delT), have been described before.

Lithuanian Hemophilia Register

The availability of PCR-based screening methods enabled us to identify the causative mutations in 61 of 63 (96.8%) unrelated hemophilia A patients and in 8 of 8 (100%) hemophilia B patients. Together with the detailed phenotype data obtained from almost all of the patients a hemophilia register could be set up in Lithuania.

Such a register is of essential importance for developing countries like Lithuania. Once the mutation in a family has been identified a very safe and fast carrier and prenatal diagnosis can be offered to the affected families. This aspect is of special importance since the supply of clotting factor concentrates in Lithuania is limited and does not allow for a general prophylactic treatment. For the health care system, such a register provides an important tool for the prediction of health costs caused by hemophiliacs. For the physicians, the register allows for a prediction of the clinical course of a patient with respect to concentrate consumption and risk of inhibitor development. We expect this register to grow continuously in the future.

References

Antonarakis SE, Rossiter JP, Young M, Horst J, de Moerloose P, Sommer SS, Ketterling RP, Kazazian HH Jr, Negrier C, Vinciguerra C, et al. (1995) Factor VIII gene inversions in severe hemophilia A: results of an international consortium study. Blood 86, 2206-2012.

Arai M, Higuchi M, Antonarakis SE, Kazazian HH Jr, Philips JA III, Janco RL, Hoyer LW (1990) Characterization of a thrombin cleavage site mutation (Arg1689 to Cys) in the factor VIII gene of two unrelated patients with cross-reacting material-positive hemophilia A. Blood 75, 384

Becker J, Schwaab R, Möller-Taube, Schwaab U, Schmidt W, Brackmann H-H, Grimm T, Olek K, Oldenburg J (1996) Characterization of the Factor VIII Defect in 147 Patients with Sporadic Hemophilia A: Family Studies Indicate a Mutation Type-Dependent Sex Ratio of Mutation Frequencies Am. J. Hum. Genet. 58, 657-670

Cejka J (1982) Enzyme immunoassay for factor VIII-related antigen. Clin Chem 28, 1356

Collins PW, Jenkins PV, Goldman E, Lee CA, Pasi KJ (1994) Inversions in hemophilia A. Lancet 343, 791

Cooper DN, Youssouffian H (1988) The CpG dinucleotide and human genetic disease. Hum. Gen 78, 151-155

Fay PJ, Beattie T, Huggins CF, Regan LM (1994) Factor VIIIa A2 subunit residues 558-565 represent a factor IXa interactive site. J Biol Chem 12, 269:20522-7

Freson K, Peerlink K, Aguirre T, Arnout J, Vermylen J, Cassiman JJ, Matthijs G (1998) Fluorescent chemical cleavage of mismatches for efficient screening of the factor VIII gene. Hum Mut 11, 470-9

Gitschier J, Kogan S, Levinson B, Tuddenham EG (1988) Mutations of factor VIII cleavage sites in hemophilia A. Blood 72, 1022-8

Goodeve AC, Preston FE, Peake IR (1994) Factor VIII gene rearrangements in patients with severe hemophilia A. Lancet 343, 329-30

Higuchi M, Antonarakis SE, Kasch L, Oldenburg J, Economou-Peterson E, Olek K, Inaba H (1991a) Molecular characterization of mild-to-moderate hemophilia A: detection of mutation in 25 of 29 patients by denaturing gradient gel electrophoresis. Proc Natl Acad Sci USA 88, 8307-8311

Higuchi M, Kazazian HH Jr, Kasch L, Warren TC, McGinniss MJ, Phillips JA, Kasper C, Janco R, Antonarakis SE (1991b) Molecular characterization of severe hemophilia A suggests that about half the mutations are not within the coding regions and splice junctions of the factor VIII gene. Proc Natl Acad Sci U S A 88, 7405-9

Jennings I, Kitchen S, Woods TA, Preston FE (1998) Laboratory performance of hemophilia centres in developing countries: 3 years´ experience of the World federation of Hemophilia External Quality Assessment Scheme. Hemophilia 4, 739-46

Kuklin A, Munson K, Gjerde D, Haefele R, Taylor P (1997/98) Detection of Single-Nucleotide Polymorphisms with the WAVE™ DNA Fragment Analysis System. Genetic Testing 1, 201-206

Lakich D, Kazazian HH Jr, Antonarakis SE, Gitschier J Inversions disrupting the factor VIII gene are a common cause of severe hemophilia A. Nat Genet 1993 5, 236-41

Lalloz MRA, Schwaab R, McVey JH, Michaelidis K, Tuddenham EG (1994) Hemophilia A diagnosis by simultaneous analysis of two variable dinucleotide tandem repeats within the factor VIII gene. Br J Haematol 86, 804-809

Lazarchick J, Hoyer LW (1978) Immunoradiometric measurement of the factor VIII procoagulant antigen. J Clin Invest 62, 1048

Lillicrap D (1998) The molecular basis of hemophilia B. Haemophilia 4: 350-357

Lin SW, Lin SR, Shen MC (1993) Characterization of genetic defects of hemophilia A in patients of Chinese origin. Genomics 18, 496-504

Ljung R, Sjörin E (1995) Inversions of the factor VIII gene in Swedish patients with severe hemophilia A. Eur J Haematol 54, 310-313

Macfarlane DE, Stibbe J, Kirby EP, Zucker MB, Grant RA, McPherson J (1975) A method for assaying von Willebrand factor (ristocetin cofactor). Thromb Diath Haemorrh 34, 306–8

McGinniss MJ, Kazazian HH Jr, Hoyer LW, Bi L, Inaba H, Antonarakis SE (1993) Spectrum of Mutations in CRM-Positive and CRM-Reduced Hemophilia A Genomics 15, 392–398

Miller SA, Dykes DD, Polesky HF (1988) A simple salting out procedure for extracting DNA from human nucleated cells. Nucleic Acids Res 16, 1215

Naylor JA, Green PM, Rizza CR, Gianelli F (1993) Analysis of factor VIII mRNA defects in everyone of 28 hemophilia A patients. Hum Mol Genet 2, 11–17

Oldenburg J, Schröder J, Schmitt C, Brackmann H-H, Schwaab R (1998) Small deletion/insertion mutations within poly-A runs of the factor VIII gene mitigate the severe hemophilia A phenotype. Thromb Haemost 79, 452–3

Pattinson JK, McVey JH, Boon M, Ajani A, Tuddenham EG (1990) CRM+ hemophilia A due to a missense mutation (372Cys) at the internal heavy chain thrombin cleavage site. Br J Haematol 75, 73–7

Peake I (1998) The molecular basis of hemophilia A. Haemophilia 4, 346–349

Pieneman WC, Deutz-Terlouw PP, Reitsma PH, Briet E (1995) Screening for mutations in hemophilia A patients by multiplex PCR-SSCP, Southern blotting and RNA analysis: the detection of a genetic abnormality in the factor VIII gene in 30 out of 35 patients. Br J Haematol 90, 442–9

Pittman DD, Alderman EM, Tomkinson KN, Wang JH, Giles AR, Kaufman RJ (1993) Biochemical, immunological, and in vivo functional characterization of B-domain-deleted factor VIII. Blood 81, 2925–35

Reiner AP, Stray SM, Thompson AR (1992) Three missense mutations in Arg codons of the factor VIII genes of mild to moderately severe hemophilia A patients. Thromb Res 66, 93–9

Richards B, Heilig R, Oberle I, Storjohann L, Horn GT (1991) Rapid PCR analysis of the St 14 (DXS52) VNTR. Nucleic Acids Res 19, 1944

Schmitt C, Oldenburg J, Haack A, Poller W, Brackmann H-H, Schwaab R (1997) Investigation of factor VIII-antigen levels of patients with hemophilia A by a new highly sensitive enzyme linked immunosorbent assay (ELISA). Thromb Haemost [Suppl]: PS 120

Schwaab R, Oldenburg J, Schwaab U, Johnson DJD, Schmidt W, Olek K, Brackmann H-H, et al. (1995) Characterization of mutations within the factor VIII Gene of 73 unrelated mild and moderate hemophiliacs. Br J Haematol 91, 458–464

Shima M, Ware J, Yoshioka A, Fukui H, Fulcher CA (1989) An arginine to cysteine amino acid substitution at a critical thrombin cleavage site in a dysfunctional factor VIII molecule. Blood 74, 1612–7

Verbruggen B, Novakova I, Wessels H, Boezeman J, van den Berg M, Mauser-Bunschoten E (1995) The Nyjmegen modification of the Bethesda assay for factor VIII:C inhibitors: improved specificity and reliability. Thromb Haemost 73, 247–251

Waseem NH, Bagnall R, Green PM, Gianelli F (1999) Start of UK confidential hemophilia A database: analysis of 142 patients by solid phase fluorescent chemical cleavage of mismatch. Thromb Haemost 81, 900–5

Wulff K, Stirred W, Wehnert M, Herrmann FH´(1995) Twenty-five novel mutations of the factor IX gene in hemophilia B. Hum Mutat 6, 346–348

Young M, Inaba H, Hoyer LW, Higuchi M, Kazazian HH Jr, Antonarakis SE (1997) Partial correction of a severe molecular defect in hemophilia A, because of errors during expression of the factor VIII gene. Am J Hum Genet 60, 565–73

Greifswald Hemophilia B Study

K. Wulff, W. Schröder, F.H. Herrmann

Hemophilia B is a recessive X-linked bleeding disorder caused by a deficiency of the clotting factor IX (FIX). The FIX gene is located on the long arm of X chromosome at Xq 27 and the genomic sequence was analyzed by Yoshitake et al. (1985).

The product of the FIX gene is a polypeptide of 415 amino acids (aa) preceded by a pre-pro signal peptide. The circulating FIX consists of a gla domain and two epidermal growth factor-like (EGF) domains separated from the serine protease domain by an activation region (Yoshitake et al. 1985).

Hemophilia B is due to multiple defects in the FIX gene. More than 90% of mutants are single substitutions, small additions or small deletions (<30 bp).

The available data (Green et al./Hemophilia B database 2000) clearly indicate that hemophilia B is highly heterozygous at the molecular level. The spectrum of mutations causing hemophilia B is different in the population. Repeated observations in apparently unrelated individuals generally occur at either CpG dinucleotides or by founder effects (Peake 1995; Tuddenham at al. 1994).

In the »Greifswald hemophilia B study« the molecular basis of FIX deficiency was analyzed. In a period of more than 10 years, FIX gene mutations were analyzed in 203 unrelated hemophilia B patients from different clinical centers as a part of an approach to provide an efficient hemophilia B genetic counseling service. The results of the mutation study are summarized here.

Material and Methods

Patients

In the Greifswald hemophilia B study we have investigated more than 220 unrelated patients from different clinical centers in Germany and in Argentina, the Czech Republic, Cuba, Estonia, Hungary, Indian, Lithuania, Poland, Romania, Singapore, and Switzerland (Table 1) with severe, moderate, or mild hemophilia B.

DNA Studies

DNA was isolated from 10 ml EDTA blood, from white blood cells by standard methods (Miller et al. 1988). PCR primer pairs for the FIX gene, derived from the FIX sequence (Yoshitake et al. 1985) and PCR conditions were described previously (Wulff et al. 1995, 1999).

I. Scharrer/W. Schramm (Ed.)
30th Hemophilia Symposium Hamburg 1999
© Springer-Verlag Berlin Heidelberg 2001

Table 1. Greifswald hemophilia B study: origin of the hemophilia B patients

Countries (symbols)	Number of unrelated patients
Germany (G)	109
Poland (P)	63
Argentina (A)	10
Hungary (H)	5
Lithuania (Li)	4
Switzerland (S)	2
India (I)	2
Czech Republic (C)	2
Romania (R)	2
Cuba (Cu)	2
Estonia (E)	1
Singapore (Si)	1

Sequencing

The double-stranded PCR products were purified and concentrated in Microcon 100 concentrators (Amicon). The sequence analysis was performed as a cycle sequencing procedure using the Taq Dye Deoxy-terminator FS sequencing kit PE/Applied Biosystems and the automatic sequencer type 373 A from PE/Applied Biosystems (Wulff et al. 1995).

Results and Discussion

203 unrelated FIX gene mutations were analyzed the »Greifswald hemophilia B study« in a period of more than 10 years. The hemophilia B patients are from different countries (Table 1). Most patients/families were diagnosed as outpatients at German clinics. FIX gene mutations were identified by different techniques, such as amplification and direct sequencing of the FIX gene (Wulff et al. 1995, Wulff et al. 1999) or by Southern analysis (Schröder et al. 1998, 1998a, Wulff et al. 1997, 2000) in cases with large FIX gene abnormalities.

Eight (4%) patients had gross gene lesions (>30 bp) in the FIX gene (Table 2). Six large deletions were identified: three complete FIX gene deletions and three partial deletions encompassed the exons a–e, exons d–h or exons f–h. Three (50%) of the hemophilia B patients with a deletion have developed FIX antibodies (an inhibitor) after replacement therapy.

A large gene insertion, an addition of an Alu repeated element in exon e (Wulff et al. 2000), was analyzed in one patient. In a Polish hemophilia B patient a chromosomal rearrangement was detected (Schröder et al. 1998).

Small FIX gene lesions were detected in 195 (96%) of all hemophiliacs (Bendex et al. 1998; Herrmann et al. 1993, 1996, 1996a, 1997, 1997b, 1998, 1998a, 1999; Schröder et al. 1998; Wulff et al. 1994, 1994a, 1995, 1997, 1997a, 1999).

In the promoter region 5 (3%) mutations were found, in exon regions 179 cases (88%) and in exon splice sites of factor IX gene 10 cases (5%) (Table 3).

Table 2. Greifswald hemophilia B study: mutation analysis in 203 hemophilia B patients

Type of mutations	Number of mutants (%)	Repeated molecular events	Unique molecular events
Missense mutations	136 (67)	29	58
Nonsense mutations	32 (16)	7	8
Promoter mutations	5 (3)	–	5
Splice site mutations	10 (5)	–	10
Deletions (<30 bp)	11 (5)	1	7
Inframe	6	1	2
Outframe	5	–	5
Additions (<30 bp)	–	–	–
Subtotal	195 (96)	37	88
Deletions (>30 bp)	5 (3)	1	3
Complete deletion	3	1	–
Partial deletion	3	–	3
Insertion >30 bp	1 (0.5)	–	1
Gene rearrangements	1 (0.5)	–	1
Total	203 (100)	38	93

Single base caused a stop codon (nonsense mutation) in 32 patients, in 10 cases a splice site variation, in 5 cases a promoter mutation, and in 136 patients an amino acid substitution (missense mutation).

Small deletions of 1, 2, 3, or 6 base pairs were identified in 11 patients.

The 184 single-base substitutions analyzed represent 117 different point mutations. Eighty-one of these mutants were unique molecular events. Thirty-six point mutations were analyzed in more than one hemophilia B family/unrelated patients. In the most patients with identical FIX lesions we could analyze an identical haplotype of the FIX gene (Wulff et al. 1995, 1999). The origin of the mutation is likely to be the same in these patients.

The mutations could influence the FIX function in different ways. The promoter mutation could influence transcription of the factor IX. The position (–26) in the

Table 3. Point mutations and small deletions (<30nt) in the factor IX (FIX) gene analyzed in hemophilia B patients: results of the Greifswald Hemophilia B Study

Patient ID		Clinical severity	Amino acid substitution	Nucleotide substitution	Codon no.	Exon no.
52	(P)	Severe	Promoter	–26GA	–	–
3792	(G)	Moderate	Promoter	–20T→A	–	–
9845	(G)		Promoter	7T→C	–	–
9069	(I)		Promoter	9C→G	–	–
3587	(G)		Promoter	13A→C	–	–
9189	(G)		Ile→Phe	48A→T	–40	–
9169	(G)		Frameshift stop at –27	84 C del	–28	–
43	(P)	Moderate	Cys→Arg	111T→C	–19	a

Table 3. (Continued)

Patient	ID	Clinical severity	Amino acid substitution	Nucleotide substitution	Codon no.	Exon no.
9280	(G)		Val→Ile	117G→A	−17	a
55	(P)	Severe	Donor splice	122G→A	−	−
37	(Si)		Donor splice	121–124 delGTTT	−	−
8205	(R)		Arg→Trp	6364C→T	−4	b
1989	(G)		Arg→Trp	6364C→T	−4	b
9232	(G)		Arg→Trp	6364C→T	−4	b
1784	(P)	Severe	Arg→Gln	6365G→A	−4	b
31	(P)	Severe	Arg→Gln	6365G→A	−4	b
3571	(P)	Severe	Arg→Gln	6365G→A	−4	b
2252	(G)	Severe	Arg→Leu	6365G→T	−4	b
2270	(G)	Severe	Arg→Leu	6365G→T	−4	b
2271	(G)		Arg→Leu	6365G→T	−4	b
8783	(G)		Arg→Leu	6365G→T	−4	b
2269	(G)	Severe	Frameshift	6370–71 delAA	−2	b
14	(P)	Moderate	Arg→Ser	6375G→T	−1	b
3	(P)	Severe	Glu→Val	6395A→T	7	b
44	(P)	Severe	Glu→Asp	6399G→C	7	b
8	(P)	Severe	Glu→Asp	6399G→C	8	b
2705	(G)	Severe	∆Arg, ∆Glu	6420–25 delGAGAGA	16,17	b
3282	(G)	Moderate	Cys→Arg	6427T→C	18	b
2232	(A)	Moderate	Glu→Val	6434A→T	20	b
3408	(G)	Severe	Cys→Arg	6442T→C	23	b
3149	(A)	Severe	Phe→Ser	6449T→C	25	b
9172	(Li)		Glu→Gln	6451G→C	26	b
2133	(H)		Arg→stop	6460C→T	29	b
2225	(A)	Severe	Arg→stop	6460C→T	29	b
2230	(A)	Severe	Arg→stop	6460C→T	29	b
2237	(A)	Moderate	Arg→stop	6460C→T	29	b
3168	(G)	Severe	Arg→stop Inhibitor	6460C→T	29	b
9048	(G)		Arg→stop	6460C→T	29	b
2254	(G)	Severe	Glu→stop	6463G→T	30	c
2309	(Cu)		Acceptor splice	6677G→C	−	−
2249	(G)	Moderate	Tyr→Cys	6697A→G	45	c
1	(P)	Severe	Asp→Asn Donor splice	6702G→A	47	d
1759	(P)	Severe	Donor splice	6706A→G	−	−
53	(P)	Moderate	Donor splice	6707G→A	−	−
2257	(G)	Severe	Tyr→Cys	10458A→G	69	d
2332	(S)	Severe	Cys →Phe	10470G→T	73	d
8135	(G)	Moderate	Cys→Tyr	10497G→A	82	d
2489	(G)	Severe	Acceptor splice	17665T→C	−	−
6	(P)	Severe	Cys→Arg	17677T→C	88	d
2265	(G)	Mild	Ile→Thr	17684T→C	90	e
9182	(Li)		Asn→Asp	17689A→G	92	e
2067	(G)	Severe	Gly→Asp	17693G→A	93	e
8705	(G)		Gly→Asp	17693G→A	93	e
33	(P)	Severe	Cys→Phe	17741G→T	109	e
1760	(P)	Severe	Ser→Pro	17743T→C	110	e
10567	(G)		Ser→Pro	17743T→C	110	e

Table 3. (Continued)

Patient	ID	Clinical severity	Amino acid substitution	Nucleotide substitution	Codon no.	Exon no.
62	(P)	Severe	Ser→Pro	17743T→C	110	e
3551	(G)	Severe	Cys→Arg	17746T→C	111	e
2243	(G)	Mild	Gly→Glu	17756G→A	114	e
2268	(G)	Mild	Gly→Glu	17756G→A	114	e
2059	(G)		Gly→Glu	17756G→A	114	e
9222	(G)		Gly→Arg	17775G→A	114	e
9274	(G)		Arg→Arg	17761C→A	116	e
2228	(A)	Mild	Gln→His	17778G→T	121	e
2235	(A)	Mild	Gln→His	17778G→T	121	e
2367	(A)		Gln→His	17778G→T	121	e
8070	(G)	Severe	Ser→Ser.	17784C→T	123	e
			Cys→Phe.	17786G→T	124	e
			Double mutation			
8744	(G)		Ala→Ala	17796A→G	127	e
3647	(I)		Donor splice	17798G→A	–	–
2276	(G)	Severe	Cys→Trp	20376T→G	132	f
856	(G)	Moderate	Arg→Cys	20413C→T	145	f
8260	(G)		Arg→Cys	20413C→T	145	f
8923	(G)		Arg→Cys	20413C→T	145	f
8720	(G)		Arg→Cys	20413C→T	145	f
2253	(G)		Arg→His	20414G→A	145	f
3997	(G)	Severe	Arg→His	20414G→A	145	f
8987	(G)		Arg→His	20414G→A	145	f
10569	(G)		Arg→His	20414G→A	145	f
64	(P)	Mild	Arg→His	20414G→A	145	f
1763	(P)	Severe	Arg→Trp	20518C→T	180	f
34	(P)	Severe	Arg→Trp	20518C→T	180	f
2130	(H)		Arg→Gln	20519G→A	180	f
2132	(H)		Arg→Gln	20519G→A	180	f
1764	(P)	Severe	Arg→Gln	20519G→A	180	f
8469	(G)		Arg→Gln	20519G→A	180	f
9170	(Li)		Arg→Gln	20519G→A	180	f
10566	(G)		Arg→Pro	20519G→C	180	f
47	(P)	Severe	Val→Phe	20521G→T	181	h
2280	(S)		Val→Asp	20522T→A	181	f
49	(P)	Moderate	Pro→Ser	20557C→T	193	f
2352	(G)	Severe	Gln→Gln	20565G→A	195	f
			Donor splice			
58	(P)	Severe	Gly→Glu	30073G→A	206	g
2308	(Cu)		Gly→Glu	30073G→A	207	g
2274	(G)	Mild	Ala→Thr	30107G→A	219	g
9227	(G)		Ala→Thr	30107G→A	219	g
8711	(G)		Ala→Thr	30150G→A	233	g
2128	(C)		Asn→Asp	30830G→A	237	h
2244	(G)	Severe	ΔGlu	30839–41 delGAG	240	h
2259	(G)	Severe	ΔGlu	30839–41 delGAG	240	h
2260	(G)	Severe	ΔGlu	30839–41 delGAG	240	h
2267	(G)	Severe	ΔGlu	30839–41 delGAG	240	h
3814	(G)		Glu→Lys	30854G→A	245	h

Table 3. (Continued)

Patient ID		Clinical severity	Amino acid substitution	Nucleotide substitution	Codon no.	Exon no.
17	(P)	Severe	Arg→Stop	30863C→T	248	h
952	(G)	Severe	Arg→Gly	30863C→G	248	h
9141	(G)		Arg→stop	30863C→T	248	h
2273	(G)	Moderate	Arg→Gln	30864G→A	248	h
3328	(G)	Mild	Arg→Gln	30864G→A	248	h
19	(P)	Severe	Arg→Leu	30864G→T	248	h
3146	(G)	Severe	Arg→stop	30875C→T	252	h
8459	(G)		Arg→stop	30875C→T	252	h
3867	(E)	Moderate	Arg→stop	30875C→T	252	h
9056	(G)		Arg→stop	30875C→T	252	h
8948	(G)		Arg→stop	30875C→T	252	h
54	(P)	Severe	Arg→stop	30875C→T	252	h
8426	(G)		His→Tyr	30890C→T	257	h
2131	(H)		Frameshift stop codon 279	del 30892 C	257	h
1986	(P)	Severe	Tyr→stop	30919C→A	266	h
51	(P)	Severe	Tyr→stop	30919C→A	266	h
10	(P)	Severe	Asp→Val	30927A→T	269	h
3969	(G)	Severe	Ala→Asp	30933C→A	271	h
3147	(G)	Severe	Leu→Gln	30945T→A	275	h
2266	(G)	Severe	Frameshift stop codon 308	del 30968 A	283	h
8839	(G)	Severe	Frameshift stop codon 308	del 30968 A	283	h
2234	(A)	Mild	Pro→His	30981C→A	287	h
8832	(G)		Cys→Arg	30986C→T	289	h
1757	(P)	Severe	Tyr→stop	31006C→G	295	h
40	(P)	Severe	Tyr→stop	31006C→G	295	h
2121	(C)	Moderate	Frameshift stop codon 308	del 31007 A	296	h
1758	(P)	Severe	Thr→Met	31008C→T	296	h
2256	(G)	Moderate	Thr→Met	31008C→T	296	h
27	(P)	Mild	Thr→Met	31008C→T	296	h
2722	(G)	Mild	Thr→Lys	31008C→A	296	h
8711	(G)		Thr→Met	31008C→T	296	
8954	(G)		Thr→Met	31008C→T	296	h
9113	(G)		Thr→Met	31008C→T	296	h
1765	(P)	Severe	Trp→Arg	31049T→A	310	h
61	(P)	Severe	Trp→Arg	31049T→A	310	h
10568	(G)		Trp→Arg	31049T→A	310	h
3913	(G)	Mild	Trp→Leu	31050G→T	310	h
9195	(G)		Trp→Leu	31050G→T	310	h
2223	(A)	Severe	Trp→Cys	31051G→T	310	h
41	(P)	Severe	Gly→Arg	31052G→A	311	h
3371	(G)	Severe	Gly→Arg	31052G→A	311	h
50	(P)	Severe	Gly→stop	31052G→T	311	h
830	(G)	Moderate	Lys→Glu	31067A→G	316	h
1761	(G)	Severe	Frameshift stop codon 321	del 31069 A	317	h

Table 3. (Continued)

Patient ID		Clinical severity	Amino acid substitution	Nucleotide substitution	Codon no.	Exon no.
4	(P)	Severe	Gln→Pro	31092A→C	324	h
9168	(Li)		Gln→Pro	31092A→C	324	h
26	(P)	Severe	Tyr→stop	31096C→A	325	h
8095	(G)		Val→Phe	31103G→T	328	h
1984	(P)	Severe	ΔLeu	31113–15 delTTG	331	h
1766	(P)	Severe	Arg→stop	31118C→T	333	h
41	(P)	Severe	Arg→stop	31118C→T	333	h
3549	(P)	Severe	Arg→stop	31118C→T	333	h
3294	(G)	Moderate	Arg→Gln	31119G→A	333	h
1756	(P)	Severe	Arg→Gln	31119G→A	333	h
25	(P)	Severe	Cys→Arg	31127T→C	336	h
1990	(P)	Severe	Arg→stop	31133C→T	338	h
29	(P)	Severe	Arg→stop	31133C→T	338	h
16	(P)	Severe	Arg→stop	31133C→T	338	h
37	(P)	Mild	Ser→Pro	31136C→T	339	h
2245	(G)	Moderate	lle→Phe	31151A→T	344	h
2261	(G)	Severe	lle→Phe	31151A→T	344	h
2120	(G)		Tyr→stop	31156T→A	345	h
8433	(G)		Phe→Tyr	31167T→A	349	h
45	(P)	Severe	Cys→Arg	31169T→C	350	h
965	(G)	Severe	Cys→Ser	31170G→C	350	h
42	(P)	Severe	Gly→Asp	31176G→A	352	h
2248	(G)	Severe	Cys→Ser	31202T→A	361	h
9	(P)	Severe	Cys→Gly	31202T→G	361	h
1780	(P)	Severe	Ser→Asn	31215G→A	365	h
35	(P)	Severe	Pro→His	31224C→A	368	h
1762	(P)	Severe	Pro→His	31224C→A	368	h
3299	(G)	Severe	Glu→stop	31241G→T	374	h
8712	(G)		Leu→stop	31257T→G	379	h
59	(P)	Mild	Ser→Cys	31271A→T	384	h
3591	(H)		Ser→Arg	31273C→G	384	h
2227	(A)	Moderate	Trp→Arg	31202T→A	385	h
2251	(G)	Severe	Gly→Ser	31277G→A	386	h
3633	(G)		Gly→Ala	31278G→C	386	h
8787	(G)		Gly→Ala	31278G→C	386	h
36	(P)	Moderate	Glu→Lys	31280G→A	387	h
10565	(G)		Glu→Lys	31280G→A	387	h
63	(P)	Severe	Glu→Lys	31280G→A	387	h
3625	(G)		Glu→Ala	31281A→C	387	h
8200	(R)	Moderate	Glu→Ala	31281A→C	387	h
39	(P)	Severe	Cys→Tyr	31287G→A	389	h
1987	(P)	Severe	Cys→Tyr	31287G→A	389	h
8878	(G)		Gly→Val	31308G→T	396	h
2229	(G)	Mild	Arg→Trp	31328C→T	403	h
22	(P)	Severe	Trp→stop	31342G→A	407	h
28	(P)	Severe	Trp→stop	31342G→A	407	h
8027	(G)	Mild	Trp→Cys	31342G→C	407	h

Origin of patients: A, Argentina; C, Czech Republic; Cu, Cuba; E, Estonia; G, Germany; H, Hungary; I, India; Li, Lithuania; P, Poland; R, Romania; Si, Singapore; S, Switzerland

promoter is located in the liver-enriched transcription factor HNF4 and caused severe hemophilia B (Peak 1995; Green et al./Hemophilia B database 2000).

Point mutations in position −23 to 13 in the promoter could lead to the hemophilia B type Leiden. This factor IX variant is characterized by severe childhood hemophilia which is ameliorated at puberty. In the »Greifswald hemophilia B study« a point mutation in the promoter region was identified in four patients in positions −20, 7, 9, and 13.

Splice-site mutations were analyzed in ten unrelated patients. In a study of Polish hemophilia B patients we could show that in all cases the splice mutation led to severe disease with phenotype CMR⁻ (Triplett et al. 1985) − a reduction of FIX activity (FIX: C) with similarly reduced antigen level (FIX:Ag), and the absence of dysfunctional FIX molecules in the plasma (Wulff et al. 1999).

Nonsense mutations (point mutations which caused the substitution of an amino acid codon by a stop codon) were detected in 32 unrelated patients in 15 different codons. In one of these patients an inhibitor was analyzed (Table 3).

Most of the lesions in the FIX gene − 136 (67%) of all 203 mutants − are missense mutations, the substitution of one amino acid by another. Missense mutations cause hemophilia B, varying from severe to mild phenotype (Table 3). In one patient a two-point mutation was detected (double mutation) in exon e of the FIX allele, the silent mutation Ser123 Ser and the missense mutation Cys124 Phe (Table 3).

Hemophilia B is caused by a large number of different mutations in the region of the FIX gene. Hemophilia B is mostly due to small changes in the FIX gene affecting either the transcription, the mRNA maturation, the mRNA translation or the fine structure of the FIX. To date, over 689 unique molecular mutations have been analyzed from 1918 unrelated patients (Green et al./Hemophilia B database 2000). Only 2–3% of the patients showed gross deletions (>30 bp) or rearrangements. Repeat observations in apparently unrelated individuals generally applied at either CpG dinucleotides or founder effects (Peak 1995).

Direct sequencing of individually PCR-amplified FIX exon sequences has emerged as a relatively rapid and accurate method of diagnostic analysis in hemophilia B families (Herrmann et al. 1990, 1993, 1994, 1995, 1996, 1997, 1997a, 1998). The practical application to genetic analysis of the FIX genes are accurate carrier detection and prenatal diagnosis. Counseling of potential carriers and their relatives is an extremely important part of the procedure.

References

Bendix M, Schröder W, Wulff K, Aumann V, Barthels M, Bratanoff B, Bergmann F, Eberl W, Haubold E, Hempelmann L, Kirsten K, Kreuz W, Lenk H, Niekrenz C, Pollmann H, Prager S, Scheel H, Schmeltzer B, Wendisch J, Wenzel E, Wollina K, Zeitler P, Herrmann FH (1998) Genomische Diagnostik in deutschen Familien mit Hämophilie B. Von der RFLP-Analyse zum Mutationsnachweis. In: I. Scharrer, W. Schramm (ed.) 27. Hämophilie-Symposion Hamburg 1996. Springer, Berlin Heidelberg New York, pp 340–343

Green PM, Giannelli F, Sommer S, Poon M-C, Ludwig M, Schwaab R, Reitsma PH, Goossens M, Yoshioka A, Figueiredo MS, Brownlee GG (2000) Hemophilia B: Database of point mutations and short additions and deletions. 9th Edn. http://www.uwcm.ac.uk/molgen/haem Bdatabase.htm

Herrman FH, Wulff K, Wehnert M (1990) Results and experiences of the genomic diagnosis in classic phenylketonuria, Duchenne muscular dystrophy and hemophilia A and B. In: Henke J, Kömpf J, Drisel AJ (Eds) Advances in molecular genetics. DNA polymorphism in forensic medicine. Hüthig Buch Verlag, Heidelberg pp 17–31

Herrmann FH, Wulff K, Schröder W, Machill G, Wehnert M (1993) Molecular genetics and genomic diagnosis of X-linked disorders in the man. Genet Live Sci Adv. 12: 43–53

Herrmann FH, Schröder W, Wehnert M, Wulff K (1994) Zur genomischen Diagnostik von Hämophilie A und B in den fünf neuen Bundesländern. In: A. Kurme, Klose HJ, Beer H-J (Eds) Psychosoziale Aspekte bei Hämophilie und HIV. Georg Thieme Verlag, Stuttgart New York pp 222–231.

Herrmann FH, Scharrer I (1995) Humangenetische Beratung bei Hämophilie A und B. In: Deutsche Hämophiliegesellschaft, Hamburg (Ed) Mitteilungen der Deutschen Hämophiliegesellschaft zur Bekämpfung von Blutungskrankheiten e.V. Hamburg 3–30 (Sonderdruck 2/95)

Herrmann FH, Wulff K, Schröder W, Wehnert M, Machill G, Ebener U (1995a) Molekulargenetik und genomische Diagnostik bei Hämophilie A und B. Med. Genetik 7: 376–381

Herrmann FH, Schröder W, Wulff K, Wehnert M (1996) Neue Ergebnisse zur Mutationscharakterisierung bei Hämophilie A und B In: I. Scharrer, W. Schramm (Eds) 25. Hämophilie-Symposion. Springer, Berlin Heidelberg New York, pp 235–246

Herrmann FH (1996a) Genomische Diagnostik bei Hämophilie B (1). mta 11; 12: 958–963

Herrmann FH, Schröder W, Wulff K, Bendix M, Wehnert M, Anders O, Aumann V, Bratanoff E, Ebener U, Franke D, Güldenring A, Heinrichs Ch, Lenk H, Mitulla B, Pindur G, Seyfert UT, Thiele G, Vogel G, Weippert M, Wendisch J, Wenzel E (1997) Genomische Diagnostik bei Hämophilie A und B – Ergebnisse einer multizentrischen zehnjährigen Zusammenarbeit. In: I. Scharrer, W. Schramm (Eds) 26. Hämophilie-Symposion. Springer, Berlin Heidelberg New York, pp 261–267

Herrmann FH (1997a) Genomische Diagnostik bei Hämophilie B (2). mta 12; 1: 15–18

Herrmann FH (1997b) Genomische (DNA) Diagnostik bei Hämophilie A und B – DNA-Analyse zur Konduktorinnendiagnostik. Hautnah Pädiatrie 9, 479–487

Herrmann FH, Vogel G (1998) Molekulargenetik hereditärer Hämostasedefekte In: Ganten D, Ruckpaul K.: Handbuch der molekularen Medizin, Band 3. Herz Kreislauf-Erkrankungen. Springer, Berlin Heidelberg New York, pp 223–287

Herrmann FH, Wulff K (1998a) Molekulare Genanalyse und Gendiagnostik bei Hämophilie B und Faktor VII Mangel. Hämostaseologie. 3, 129–139.

Herrmann FH, Scharrer I (1999) Humangenetische Beratung bei Hämophilie A und B In: Deutsche Hämophiliegesellschaft, Hamburg (Ed) Mitteilungen der Deutschen Hämophiliegesellschaft zur Bekämpfung von Blutungskrankheiten e.V.: Hamburg 3–33 (Sonderdruck 1/99), 2nd edn

Miller M, Dykes DD, Polesky HF (1988) A simple salting out procedure for extracting DNA from human nucleated cells. Nucleic Acids Res 16, 121

Peake I (1995) Molecular genetics and counseling in hemophilia. Thromb Haemostasis 74, 40–44

Schröder W, Wulff K, Wollina K, Herrmann FH (1997) Hemophilia B in female twins caused by a point mutation in one Factor IX gene and nonrandom inactivation patterns of the X-chromosomes Thromb Haemost 78: 1347–51

Schröder W, Wollina K, Wulff K, Herrmann FH (1998) Unbalancierte X-Chromosomen-Inaktivierung in weiblichen Zwillingen mit Hämophilie B In: I. Scharrer, W. Schramm (Eds) 27. Hämophilie-Symposion, Hamburg 1996. Springer, Berlin Heidelberg New York, pp 306–313

Schröder W, Poetsch M, Gazda H, Werner W, Reichelt T, Knoll W, Robicka-Milewska R, Zieleniewka B (1998a) A de novo translocation 46,X(X15) causing haemophilia B in a girl: a case report. Br J Haemotol 100: 750–757

Triplett DA, Brandt JT, McGann, Batard MA, Schaeffer Dixon JL, Fair DS (1985) Hereditary factor VII deficiency: Heterogeneity defined by combined functional and immunochemical analysis. Blood 66, 1284–1287.

Tuddenham EGD, Cooper DN (1994) The molecular genetics of hemostasis and its inherited disorders. pp 78–110, Oxford University Press, New York Tokyo

Wulff K, Schröder W, Blanco A, Wehnert M, Herrmann FH (1994) Factor IX structural gene mutations in haemophilia B patients from Argentina. Rev Iberoamer Thromb Hemostasia 7: 256–258

Wulff K, Wehnert M, Schröder W, Herrmann FH (1994a) Mutationen im Strukturgen des Faktor IX In: I. Scharrer, W. Schramm (eds.) 24. Hämophilie-Symposion Springer, Berlin Heidelberg New York, pp 130–134

Wulff K, Schröder W, Wehnert M, Herrmann FH (1995) Twenty-five novel mutations of the factor IX gene in haemophilia B. Hum Mutat. 6, 346 –348.

Wulff K, Gazda H, Schröder W, Robicka-Milewska R, Herrmann FH (1997) Mutationsanalyse bei 27 Hämophilie B-Patienten aus Polen In: Scharrer I, Schramm W. 28. Hämophilie-Symposion Hamburg 1997. Springer, Berlin Heidelberg New York, pp 157–162

Wulff K, Schröder W, Herrmann FH (1997a) Molekulare Defekte bei 116 Hämophilie B (Faktor IX Mangel) Patienten und bei Patienten mit Faktor VII Mangel In: Herrmann F.H. (ed) Molekulargenetik hereditärer Hämostasedefekte pp 157–162, Pabst-Verlag

Wulff K, Bykowska K, Lopaciuk S, Herrmann FH (1999) Molecular analysis of hemophilia B in Poland: 12 novel mutations of the factor IX gene. Acta Biochimica Polonica 721–726

Wulff K, Gazda H, Schröder W, Robicka-Milewska R, Herrmann FH (2000) Identification of a novel F9 gene mutation – an insertion of an Alu repeated element in exon e of the factor IX gene. Hum Mutat 15, Report 99 (1999) Online

Yoshitake S, Schach BG, Foster DC, Davie EW, Kurachi K (1985) Nucleotide sequence of the gene of human factor IX (hemophilia factor B). Biochemistry 24, 3736–3750.

Successful Treatment of Patients with von Willebrand Disease Using a High-Purity Double Virus Inactivated FVIII/vWF Concentrate (IMMUNATE)

G. Auerswald, B. Eberspächer, W. Kreuz, A. Nimtz, G. Pindur, H. Scheel, H.-H. Wolf

A multicenter trial was started in Germany in September 1998 using a high-purity FVIII/vWF concentrate (IMMUNATE, Baxter Deutschland) for the treatment of patients with von Willebrand Disease (vWD).

In a prospective, phase III, open-label, single-armed study the clinical efficacy of IMMUNATE in the management of acute bleeding episodes and in surgical prophylaxis in vWD patients is documented. In addition, the product's safety with respect to adverse experiences is monitored and data on its pharmacokinetics in vWD patients are collected.

Material and Methods

IMMUNATE is a high-purity double virus inactivated FVIII/vWF concentrate manufactured from human plasma. All plasma units are obtained exclusively from licensed plasmapheresis centers in Europe and the USA. Only plasma units that have alanine transaminase (ALT) levels not exceeding twice the upper limit of normal and that are found non-reactive for hepatitis B surface antigen (HBsAg) and antibodies against HCV, HIV-1 and HIV-2 are used. All donors and individual plasma units are screened for viral markers. Each plasma pool is PCR tested for the absence of selected genomic sequences of HIV, HBV and HCV. Viruses are partitioned during manufacture and inactivated by initial treatment with polysorbate 80 followed by vapor heating for 10 h.

Inclusion Criteria

Patients, 6 years or older, with all types of inherited vWD who have acute hemorrhages of mucous membranes, gums, muscles and soft tissue, central nervous system (CNS), or joints or are facing elective surgery, who have received vaccination against hepatitis B and provide written informed consent are included.

Exclusion Criteria

Patients who received coagulation factor concentrates, the vasopressin analogue DDAVP or acetylsalicylic acid preparations within 15 days prior to study entry, in

I. Scharrer/W. Schramm (Ed.)
30th Hemophilia Symposium Hamburg 1999
© Springer-Verlag Berlin Heidelberg 2001

whom treatment with DDAVP is considered sufficient, who have a FVIII inhibitor, suffer from AIDS or the AIDS-related complex (ARC), or who are participating in another clinical study are not eligible for study participation. Pregnancy also is an exclusion criterion.

Administration of Concentrate

Patients treated for acute bleeding receive IMMUNATE by intravenous (i.v.) injection at a dose of 80–100 IU FVIII per kg body weight at intervals of 12 h. For surgical prophylaxis patients receive the concentrate either by i.v. injection at the same dose beginning 1 h prior to surgical intervention or by continuous i.v. infusion (CI). In the latter case a bolus of 80 IU FVIII/kg b.w. is given 1 h prior to surgery followed by perioperative administration of 4–8 IU FVIII/kg per hour. Patients receive treatment for one period of acute bleeding or perioperative prophylaxis only.

Patient Monitoring

In patients with acute hemorrhages, bleeding is evaluated at baseline and every 3 h until cessation of bleeding; rebleeding is noted. In patients receiving prophylaxis for elective surgery, the extent of intra- and postoperative bleeding is assessed and patients are monitored for bleeding complications and for the occurrence of adverse experiences.

Laboratory Assessments

Samples for central testing of hemostasis parameters (FVIII:C, vWF:Ag, vWF:RCo, CBA, aPTT, and vW-multimers) are drawn at baseline and at several intervals until 48 h after the first injection or initiation of continuous infusion. Sampling is discontinued upon administration of a second injection. The test results are used for pharmacokinetic analyses.

Tests for hematological parameters (blood group, platelets, WBC, RBC, hemoglobin, hematocrit) are performed locally on samples drawn at baseline and at predetermined intervals after the first injection or initiation of continuous infusion.

Results

Six patients with von Willebrand Disease from five treatment centers have been treated so far (Table 1). One patient (patient 02/0001) with hypermenorrhea received one single bolus to reduce bleeding. The other patients were substituted perioperatively for surgical prophylaxis (bolus+CI).

Figures 1–6 show the behavior of hemostasis parameters in different patients with vWD.

Table 1. Patients with vWD treated with IMMUNATE

Patient	Sex	vW-Type	Indication	Bolus (IU/kg b.w.)	Cont. Infusion Initial dose (IU/kg b.w./h)
02/0001	F	2	Hypermenorrhea	78.4	–
03/0001	F	3	Knee replacement	86.5	9.6
04/0001	F	2	Tooth extraction (4x), Frenotomy	75.8	3.8
06/0001	M	1	Tympanoplasty	88.2	4.9
06/0002	F	2	Tooth extraction	71.4	9.4
12/0001	F	3	Conization	83.3	8.3

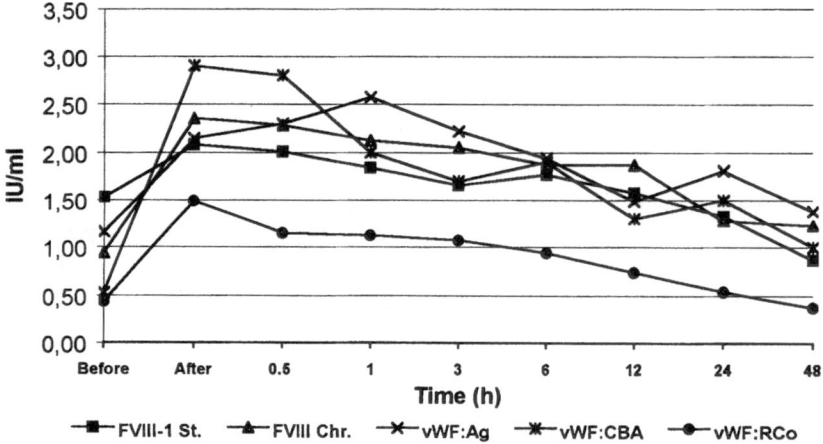

Fig. 1. Patient 02/0001, vWD Type 2, Hypermenorrhea, Bolus (1x)

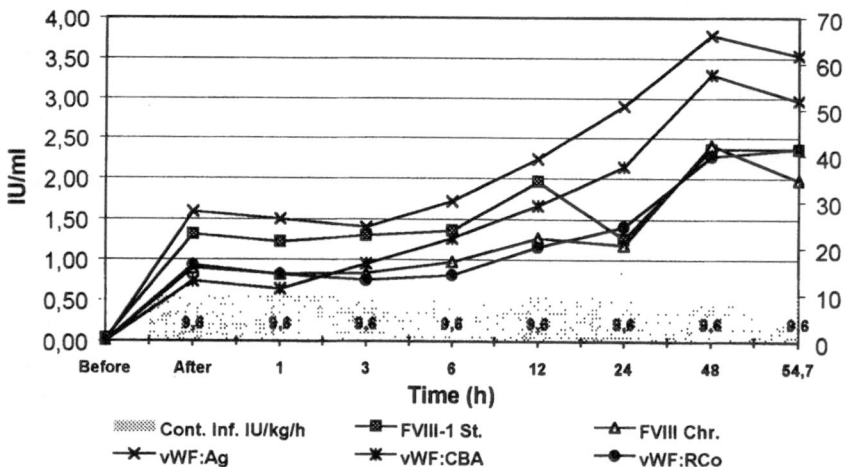

Fig. 2. Patient 03/0001, vWD Type 3, Knee Replacement, Cont. Inf

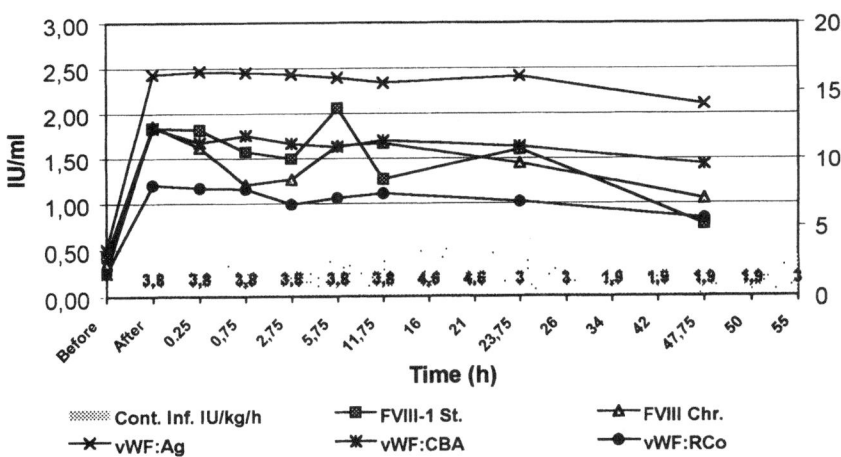

Fig. 3. Patient 04/0001, vWD Type 2, Tooth Extraction (4x), Frenotomy, Cont. Inf

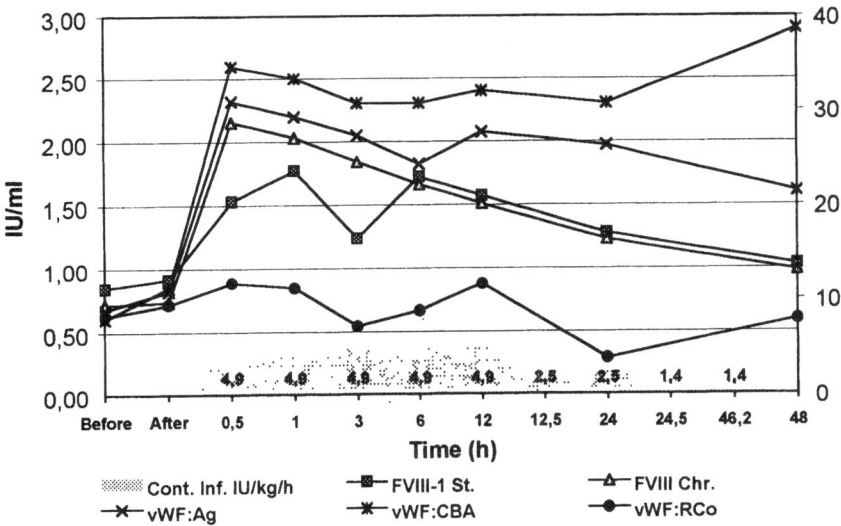

Fig. 4. Patient 06/0001, vWD Type 1, Tympanoplasty, Cont. Inf

Table 2. IMMUNATE pharmacokinetics in patients with vWD

Parameter	Incremental Recovery (IU/dl/IU/kg)	In vivo Recovery (%)	Half-Life (h) Patient 02/0001
FVIII:C 1-Stage	1.69 (0.78–2.08)	84.1 (45.6–110.6)	6.5
FVIII:C Chromogenic	1.57 (1.08–2.09)	82.7 (54.5–109.4)	23.2
vWF:Ag	1.54 (1.39–2.17)	78.8 (68.9–103.9)	19.8
vWF:RCo	1.57 (0.43–1.81)	77.0 (19.8–105.1)	7.5
vWF:CBA	2.58 (1.12–5.17)	125.2 (56.9–252.3)	34.2

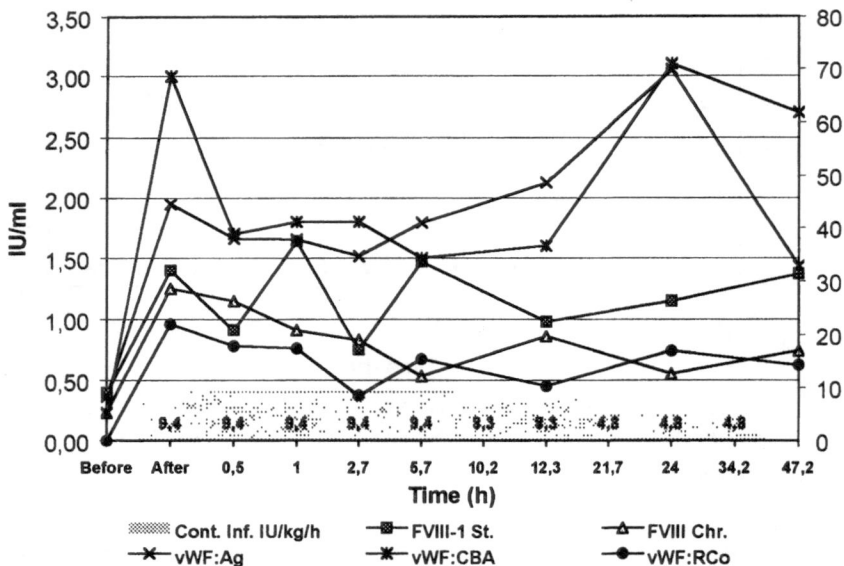

Fig. 5. Patient 06/0002, vWD Type 2, Tooth Extraction, Cont. Inf

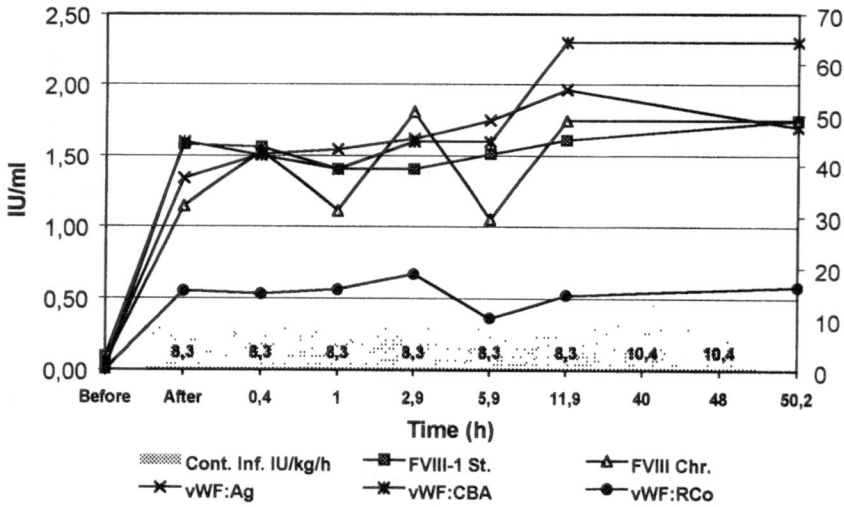

Fig. 6. Patient 12/0001, vWD Type 3, Conization, Cont. Inf

Pharmacokinetic results obtained with IMMUNATE in patients with vWD so far are given in Table 2. Values listed refer to median and range.

Clinical efficacy of IMMUNATE was rated excellent or good in all cases. The multimere pattern was normalized in both type 3 patients (Figures 7, 8).

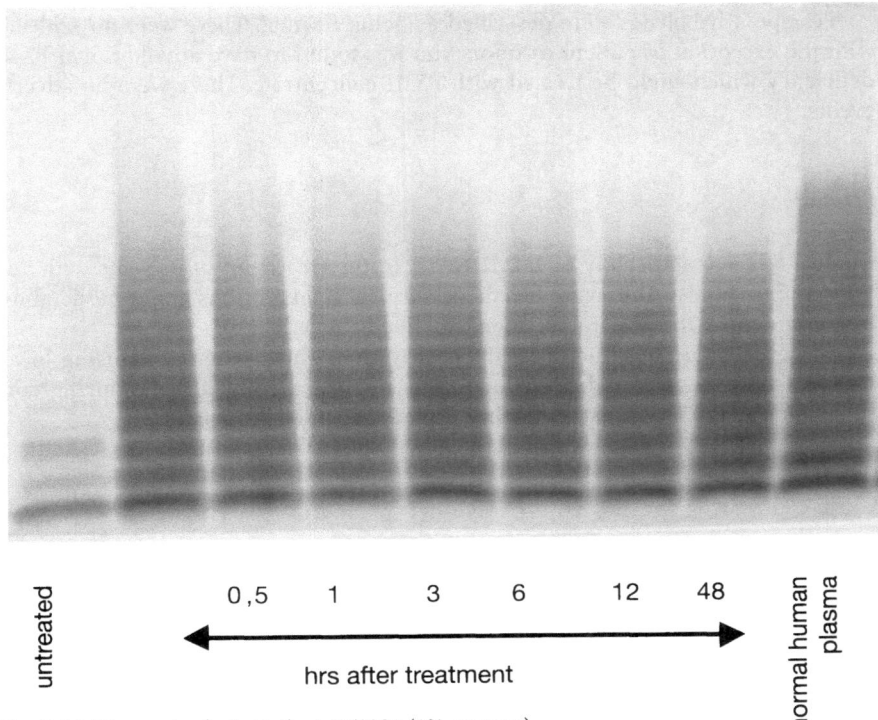

untreated

0,5   1   3   6   12   48

hrs after treatment

normal human plasma

Fig. 7. Multimere Analysis, Patient 12/0001 (1% agarose)

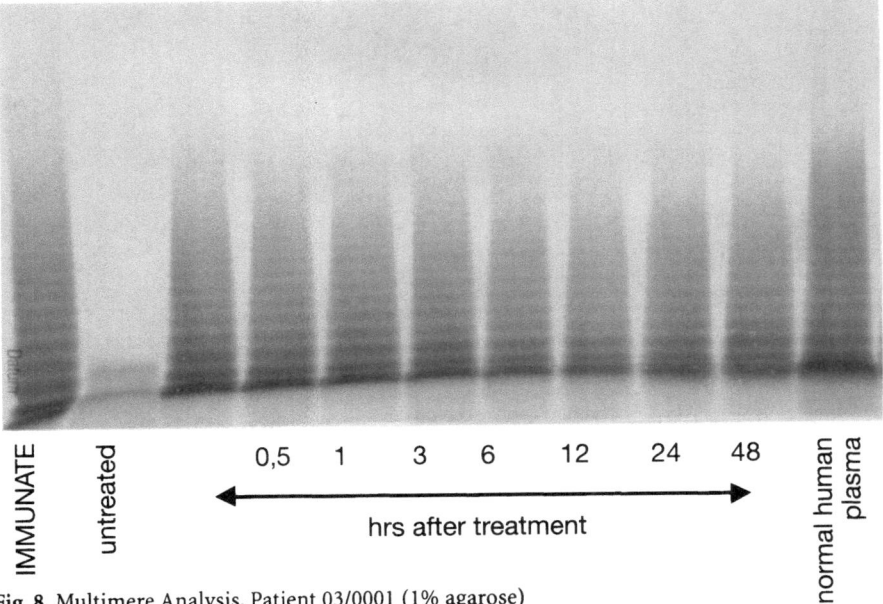

IMMUNATE

untreated

0,5   1   3   6   12   24   48

hrs after treatment

normal human plasma

Fig. 8. Multimere Analysis, Patient 03/0001 (1% agarose)

Perioperative bleeds were described as being normal. There were no rebleeds with the exception of patient 03/0001, who was found to have an additional FXIII deficiency which could be treated with FXIII concentrate. There were no adverse events.

Conclusion

Clinical efficacy and safety of IMMUNATE in the treatment of patients with von Willebrand Disease and acute bleeds or surgical interventions could be demonstrated under the therapeutic regimen described above.

However, pharmacokinetic results clearly show the possibility of using lower doses of boluses and/or dose reduction at an earlier point of time during continuous infusion. This must be further explored in upcoming patients.

VIII. Research Cooperation

Chairmen:

I. SCHARRER (Frankfurt/Main)
W. SCHRAMM (Munich)

Industry Sponsoring and Acceptance of Benefit by Hospital Officials: Opportunities and Limits of Third-Party Funding

K. Ulsenheimer

I.

Industry sponsoring and acceptance of benefit by hospital officials caught the public imagination in May 1994 following the publication of a report entitled »Heart Valve Scandal« in the weekly news magazine »Spiegel« alleging that deliberate overcharging was standard practice in the sale of artificial heart valves. The article sparked off widespread discussion centering on the untapped rationalization potentials in the healthcare system, and brought to light the many forms that »industry sponsoring« can assume. The whistleblower, a former employee of a US-based company that sold artificial heart valves and pacemakers in Germany, claimed that prices of these products were being artificially maintained at a high level and that the financial resources thus generated were mainly used as kickbacks to persuade decision-makers to buy the product. We are talking about the »greatest bribery scandal in the German healthcare system«, »fixed commissions« per heart valve for senior physicians and heads of administration, generous gifts of holidays and cars, payments to foreign bank accounts, »millions of marks'-worth of corruption«, fraud and embezzlement, damages amounting to millions of marks, and more than 1800 court cases – after some 900 cases were thrown out for »lack of relevance in criminal law«.

The mood engendered by the media has affected state prosecutors and the courts and made bribery offenses a very dangerous area for anyone to get involved in. To incur *suspicion* is enough. Suspicion alone is grounds enough for a preliminary investigation and gives probable cause for a police raid, search and confiscation at the hospital and/or home of the suspicious party, although section 152, subsection 2 of the German Code of Criminal Procedure (StPO) states that there must be evidence to back up a suspicion.

It is little comfort to know that some authors in criminal law journals have urged legislators to keep a sense of proportion in tightening up anti-bribery legislation and have stressed the importance of medical *research*, which needs *clinical trials* of new medical devices and medicinal products and relies on collaboration with the industry. It is also of little help when authors point – quite rightly – to forces and politicians that are blatantly encouraging hospital managers and physicians to »collect« money for scientific research and hospitals from the industry and even intend to pass laws to make allocation of public funds dependent upon hospital »self financing« by means of third-party funding. Those concerned

I. Scharrer/W. Schramm (Ed.)
30th Hemophilia Symposium Hamburg 1999
© Springer-Verlag Berlin Heidelberg 2001

are also not helped by the knowledge that medical equipment, other medical devices and drugs must be tested by law in clinical trials – in return for suitable compensation – and that such activities therefore cannot be rendered punishable in criminal law. It is a fact that many activities hitherto undertaken in full innocence may, objectively speaking, qualify as the granting of an undue advantage and as such provide grounds for preliminary intervention by the state prosecutor, with all the unpleasantness, distress, annoyance and possible hostility that this would involve.

1. To shed some light on the problems that can arise in association with sponsoring activities such as:
– Study contracts (postmarketing)
– Consulting contracts
– Gratuitous hire contracts
– Transfer of equipment possession contracts
– Transfer of possession of equipment for clinical trials
– Test contracts
– Invitations to conferences
– Research contracts
– Detailer fees
– Payment of travel expenses and attendance fees
in the course of collaboration between the industry and hospitals, I intend to explore what constitutes the offense that is called the »acceptance of benefit by public officials« (the other side of the coin, from the industry's point of view, is the offense called the »granting of undue advantage«) and describe its characteristic features. »Acceptance of benefit by public officials« assumes that a »public official solicits, accepts a promise of, or accepts a benefit for himself or a third party for the discharge of a duty«. In accordance with section 331, subsection 3 of the Penal Code (StGB), acceptance of benefit by public officials is *not* liable to prosecution »if the competent authorities, acting on the powers vested in them, approved the *acceptance* of an – unsolicited – benefit by the recipient *beforehand* or did so upon *prompt notification* by the recipient«. In contrast, the offenses of corruptibility and bribery (sections 332, 334 StGB) are primarily characterized by the acceptance of benefit by a public official *in violation of duty*, and therefore by definition cannot have been approved beforehand.

It is important, however, to note the following: Chiefs of staff and attending physicians often have a large say in the selection and proliferation of orders for drugs. The law therefore looks upon them as »officials entitled to decide at their own discretion«. A public official of this category is guilty of corruptibility pursuant to section 332 subsection 3 no. 2 StGB if he »shows himself willing« to be influenced by the promise of benefit in exercising his discretion. The wrongful agreement need not be made explicitly or in writing. A statement intending the conclusion of such a wrongful agreement can be made by an action implying intention. It is enough for the »official entitled to decide at his own discretion« to imply through his behavior that the benefit will be a factor in his decision. It does not matter whether or not this willingness is actually put into effect, i.e., it is immaterial whether or not the public official actually does succumb to influence when he makes his decision.[1]) The preemptive purpose of section 332 StGB intervenes at an earlier stage. This law is intended to prevent an erosion of public trust in the integrity of public officials. Therefore, it does not matter whether the public official actually did go so far as to perform an act in violation of his duty. The public official therefore also does not protect his *inner* conviction that he ordered supplies solely according to objective criteria and was not influenced by the benefit granted.

Pursuant to section 332 StGB, approval by the employer is no justification. Approval is only relevant in connection with section 331 StGB.

(1) The first case concerns the financing by a company of two conference trips for a senior physician who was responsible for the selection of certain medical products. The court contended that she had known that the invitation was extended to her only to induce her to continue placing orders at the same volume. The court argued that she had acquiesced in the company's expectations through her attendance at the congresses and implicitly expressed her consent to »take the gifts into account when deciding« what to order«. That in itself was in violation of her duty, said the courts, as the benefit itself need not be the deciding factor; it was enough for the public official to allow the benefit to have a bearing on her decision-making. That this was indeed the case, could be affirmed on the basis of knowledge of human nature, in view of the good contacts built up with the company staff over the years. The court refused to accept the objection that competitors made the same offers and also financed all-expenses-paid congress trips, saying: »It does not matter from whom the official accepts benefits. Section 323 StGB states that benefits should be accepted from nobody«.

In fixing the sentence (a fine amounting to 90 daily rates), the court took into account in the defendant's favor the purpose of the trip (professional education and improvement of medical care for patients) and the fact that the bestowal of considerations was a »widespread practice« in the medical and pharmaceutical industry and that physicians did not have »the same highly developed awareness of the obligations arising out of their status as public officials that other public sector employees have«.

(2) The second case concerns the medical director of a hospital. This man was in charge of selecting all the medical and pharmaceutical products used in his department. The annual departmental Christmas party was paid for over the years by a number of healthcare companies, who contributed different sums ranging from approximately DM 1500 to DM 5000. The defendant was aware that the purpose of this was to enhance his willingness to maintain or create a business relationship. Again, the court found the man to be guilty of corruptibility pursuant to the relevant StGB section, contending that it was enough for the perpetrator to »indicate by his behavior that he would take the benefit into account when making decisions«. This conclusion however could not be drawn solely from »the fact that he accepted anything at all«. Rather, section 332 subsection 3 no. 2 StGB presupposes that the perpetrator »showed himself willing to be influenced by the benefit in exercising his

---

[1] cf. BGHSt 15, 242

discretion«. The court argued that this willingness could be inferred from the overall circumstances of the case, e.g., the amounts received, the intensity of the contacts, the chronological connection between gift and order placement, etc.

The court sentenced the medical director to a fine amounting to 70 daily rates, saying that it considered the »standard practice of accepting monetary and material gifts« and the resulting »thoughtlessness in accepting such gifts, symptomatic of the insidious erosion of a sense of wrongdoing« to be a mitigating circumstance.

(3) The Federal Court of Justice (BGH) also clearly stated in an appeal decision from 19 October 1999 (1 StR 264/69) that a senior district hospital physician's acceptance of dinner invitations from a medical device manufacturer constituted corruptibility. The senior physician in question was in charge of procurement. The court contended that the employees of the supplier company would »have to infer from the defendant's acceptance of the invitations that the defendant was interested in continuing the business relationship«, and in the actual case in question, an invitation to a meal in a gourmet restaurant was followed by a larger order the next day!

a) *Public official*: Section 11 subsection 1 no. 2 a StGB says that a medical department head is a public official if he has *civil servant status*, is the incumbent of »another public office« (section 11 subsection 1 no. 2 b StGB) or is otherwise appointed to engage in public administrative tasks in the employment of a public agency or other office. The term »other office« includes public-law corporations and public-law institutions having legal capacity. Therefore, *chiefs of staff* at *district hospitals* or *municipal hospitals* having these legal forms qualify as »public officials«.[1])

aa) For physicians who are *civil servants* or hold an office, there is no need to examine whether they discharge public administrative duties. They are *public officials in the formal sense*. As for the rest, however, it mainly depends on the *function* performed and the public relevance of the organization financing the hospital. The duties of the public administrative system include the preservation of citizens' health and the cure of disease. These fundamental functions of the State are subsumed under the term »provision for elementary requirements«. As such, medical and nursing staff in university hospitals, district hospitals, municipal hospitals and other specialist hospitals fall under the definition of »public official«.[2])

bb) It is therefore immaterial whether the municipal hospital has the *legal form* of an independent limited company (GmbH), is a dependent organization run by a local authority, or operates in the form of a public-law corporation. Public official status does not depend upon these various legal forms, but upon whether functions related to »provision for elementary requirements« are carried out.

Majority rule applies in hospitals with a mixed public and private financial basis. If, for example, a municipal hospital has the legal form of a GmbH and the local authority has full or majority ownership of the GmbH shares, the employees of the municipal hospital are seen as discharging *public* duties. The necessary act of appointment is the long-term employment contract with

---

[1] Karlsruhe Higher Regional Court, NJW 1983, 352
[2] Karlsruhe Higher Regional Court, NJW 1983, 352

the physician. In the case of hospitals financed by foundations or associations, what again counts is whether the majority of shares is publicly owned.

cc) It is more difficult to assess the situation in hospitals financed by the *major churches*. These hospitals are primarily organized according to private law, but nevertheless are involved in »provision for elementary requirements« by virtue of the institutional character of churches as public-law corporations. Therefore, their employees in hospitals also qualify as »public officials«. This view is not undisputed, however.[1])

dd) Physicians and other staff of hospitals that are 100% *privately* financed are not public officials as they do not discharge public duties. However, non-public officials have to watch out for the new regulation in section 299 StGB, which may also apply to »recipients of considerations« in the healthcare system, including physicians and other persons employed in a hospital (see under II).

ee) To recapitulate, therefore, the *functional* approach in respect of the duties performed and *not the legal form* of the organization financing the hospital is what determines whether an employee is a public official. The only *certain exceptions* to the provisions of section 331 are physicians employed at a 100% *privately owned hospital* or private practice.

b) *Discharge of duty:* This ingredient of an offence is very *broadly* defined in case law. An act falls under this definition if it by nature is interrelated with the office and does not »lie completely outside the public official's scope of duties«.[2]) In the Federal Court of Justice's view, it is an instance of discharge of duty when the deed the public official performs is one of his official duties and is performed by him in an official capacity. The only essential element is therefore that the deed is not a *purely private* act of the chief of staff, but that the testing of the equipment is a task entrusted to him and is part of the hospital's scope of duties.

The chief of staff therefore performs official acts when he is engaged in research, gives lectures, orders particular medical devices himself, has another hospital staff member procure them, is involved in their selection, engages in talks with the manufacturers, etc. It is immaterial whether his activity is merely preparatory or supportive, takes place before the decision or actually represents the final decision.

Discharge of duty pursuant to sections 331 subsection 1 StGB in this respect is *not a violation of duty*, but permissible, licensed behavior – in contrast to bribery and corruptibility, which represent a *violation of duty* in the discharge of duty.

Unlike earlier legislation (until 13 August 1997) acceptance of benefit no longer needs to be in relation to a *concrete* act, in view of past difficulty in supplying proofs.

c) However, the letter of the law states that the benefit must be offered, promised or granted »*for*« the discharge of duty. The little word »*for*« expresses a close connection between the benefit and the discharge of duty (of the official act intended or performed). The connection is easier to understand when one consi-

---

[1] A Bruns, Arztrecht 1998,

[2] BGHSt 31, 264, 280

ders that the so-called criminal offenses by a public official want to avoid an »impression of venality«. What matters is that the benefit is granted »in return for« something that the public official does »in an official capacity«.

aa) This element known as »Beziehungsverhältnis«, also as »Äquivalenzverhältnis« (commutation, reciprocity, return in kind) in the sense of »do, ut des« and more commonly as »wrongful agreement« is a traditional core element of German anti-bribery legislation and was not made obsolete by the 1997 amendment. It is still a *sine qua non for an offense*. Therefore, the acceptance of a benefit by the chief of staff or other recipient of a consideration does not count if the consideration (the benefit) is granted merely *in consideration* of, *because* of, or on the *occasion* of an official act.[1]) The letter of the law explicitly refers to a benefit »*for*« the discharge of a duty and not »on the occasion of« or »in connection with«.[2]) The word »for« expresses the – explicitly or tacitly concluded – *wrongful agreement* consisting in the consensus between the perpetrator and granter (physician and manufacturer) that the public official, in the discharge of duty, »has performed or will perform some kind of official activity« as a »quid pro quo« for the consideration.[3])

According to the amended law, cases do not revolve around a (specified) official act. Therefore, according to widespread opinion, section 331 subsection 1 StGB also covers »unspecific« considerations or gifts for »enhancing the climate« or to procure the physician's »goodwill« or »favor«,[4]) but it very much depends on the individual case (e.g., the value of the consideration). Therefore, in this gray area of the constituent facts of an offense, by no means every consideration can be interpreted as »buying affection« and building up a dependency consistent with the offense of acceptance of benefit, especially as the subjective goal plays a significant role. As already stated, a connection in the sense of »do, ut des« – of which both parties are aware – must exist between the performed or imminent discharge of duty and the granting of the benefit, generating an »impression of venality«. Therefore, the motives of the partners are often decisive in determining whether a behavior was proper or improper.

bb) Möhrenschlager[5]) is in favor of reversing this broadening of the definition of an offense – which is hardly compatible with the principle of clarity and definiteness in the wording of elements of offences[6]) – versus the prior legis-

---

[1] The Federal Ministry for Education, Science, Research and Technology incorrectly commented on 10/5/97: »The new section 331 StGB constitutes an extension of the penal armentarium in respect of the public official in the case of a general relationship between acceptance of the benefit and discharge of duty, i.e., if the consideration is accepted merely in consideration of, because of or on the occasion of an unauthorized official act. Previously, the public official was only liable to disciplinary proceedings in such cases. According to the revised law, punishment is additionally governed by penal law«.

[2] Korte, NStZ 1998, 515

[3] Tröndle/Fischer, StGB, 49th edn., 1999, §331 lit. ref. 18

[4] Tröndle/Fischer, op. cit., lit. ref. 18

[5] Presentation to the »Medical and Legal« task force on 11/13/98 in Würzburg

[6] cf. Lüderssen, JZ 1997, 112, 119; König JR 1997, 397, 399; Tröndle/Fischer, § 331 lit. ref. 19

lation and says prosecution is not warranted if the consideration is not intended for the discharge of a duty of an *individual* public official but is for bestowal upon the public-law institution as such (hospital, institute, university). Möhrenschlager contends that this is the real intended purpose of third-party research[1]) and of legitimate sponsoring. Möhrenschlager therefore holds that compliance with the relevant rules and regulations such as the »Medical Devices« code[2]) rules out criminality because there is no connection with sales transactions and the consideration benefits the hospital as a facility engaged in »provision for elementary requirements«, not the individual interests of individual physicians. However, any industrial concern will only sponsor »a thing« if the measure has some kind of positive impact on business. The background will always be sales generated or expected – a legitimate, indeed natural motive on the company's side.

It is obvious that amendment of the law has taken away the former clarity of the definition of the constituent elements of section 331 subsection 1 StGB, and now we suddenly have a situation where cases such as third-party research are liable to fall under the prohibition of acceptance of benefit. It is essential that such cases be kept out of the realms of criminal law by »judicious interpretation«, in particular by taking legislative considerations into account. It is to be hoped that case law follows this restrictive approach which is reasonable and indicated as far as the intended goal of the legislation is concerned.

d) *Benefit:* This constituent part of an offense is interpreted very broadly in case law.

    aa) According to BGH case law, a *benefit* within the meaning of sections 331 StGB is »any consideration to which the public official has no legal claim and which objectively improves his economic, legal or personal situation«. The BGH rightly concludes that no »benefit« within the meaning of sections 331 ff StGB exists where there are contractual agreements. This is often the case, for example, in postmarketing studies, basic research, conferences, clinical trials, presentations at scientific congresses and similar events, where the doctors involved are entitled to the agreed financial compensation or payment for work performed (study, presentation and the like).

    bb) However, this argumentation contrasts with a BGH judgment according to which a benefit »may already be inherent in the *conclusion* of a contract resulting in considerations being provided to the public official, even if the considerations are only the appropriate financial compensation for the services owed by him on the basis of the contract«[3]). Otherwise, corruption could always be denied simply by referring to the existence of a contractual relationship between the public official and provider of the considerations (company)[4]). It is hardly necessary to point out that this case law is *extremely dangerous* for all cases of contractual agreement. Alone the *suspicion* of a crimi-

---

[1] See also Lüderssen, JZ 1997, 112
[2] NJW 1997, vol 24, p XX
[3] BGHSt 31, 280
[4] BGHSt 31, 279 .

nal act provides grounds for the launch of a preliminary investigation by the state prosecutor (section 152 subsection 2 StPO). Therefore, research projects such as screenings, postmarketing studies, lecture fees etc. must by all means be examined in the light of section 331 StGB. However, in the presence of appropriate payment and a genuine service performed, i.e., if the consideration provided and official act are equivalent, there would generally be no grounds for affirming a benefit within the meaning of section 331 subsection 1 StGB.

cc) According to invariable practice in BGH cases, in continuation of established case law under the Supreme Court of the German Reich, the *definition of benefit* in force until August 1997 implied that the consideration provided had to make the *public official* himself better off in some way and be to his »benefit«. »Considerations to the sole betterment of a third party – where the public official derives no personal advantage whatsoever – do not meet these requirements«.[1]) Because of this egoistic attitude, case law in the past overstrained the definition of benefit and stretched it to encompass not just *economic* betterment in the form of increased *assets* (material benefit), but also *intangible* benefits. In the case of the latter, the recipient does not receive a material asset and is not enriched, but the public official benefits instead from »satisfaction of *ambition, vanity*, or the *need for recognition*«. »*Career opportunities*« are also considered to be intangible benefits, but an »objectively measurable« added value must be demonstrable.[2])

The *literature* rightly presented *major objections* to this extensive interpretation of the law, which features in numerous precedents of the highest courts of the land, but always only by-the-way or as an abstract guiding principle with no implications for the case in hand. However, the controversy about the inclusion of third-party benefit in the definition of what constitutes an offense pursuant to sections 331 ff StGB barely has any practical significance now, as the *revised* wording clarifies that the law covers *not just egoistic* behavior on the part of the public official but also includes *considerations rendered to any third party*. Let us be clear that a benefit within the meaning of sections 331 ff StGB exists not only if there is an improvement in the public official's situation, but also if a benefit accrues to any third party – be that the patient, hospital, staff, or company. Some third party invariably benefits from considerations that help a hospital.

ee) For example, postmarketing studies and basic research benefit hospitals and patients in the form of the lasting effects of better healthcare,[3]) which go beyond the mere fulfillment of contractual obligations to the manufacturing company. The company also derives benefits when postmarketing studies

---

[1] BGHSt 35, 133

[2] cf. BGHSt 14, 123, 128; BGH, NJW 1985, 2652 with comments Marchelli, NStZ 1985, 500; Griebl, Der Vorteilsbegriff bei den Bestechungsdelikten, 1993, p. 27; Jescheck, in: LK/StGB, 11th edition, § 331, lit. ref. 9; Lackner/Kühl, StGB, 22nd Edition 1997, § 331, lit. ref. 5; Tröndle, StGB, 48th Edition, § 331 lit. ref. 11; Wagner, JZ 1987, 594, 602; Dahm, MedR 1992, 602;

[3] Lüderssen, JZ 1997, 115

and basic research are conducted using the hospitals' already existing technical facilities.

The »benefit« is also undisputed in cases where the money is used to purchase other – otherwise unaffordable – equipment from the same manufacturer or to *finance medical devices* from other manufacturers. The benefit for the organization financing the hospital and for the chief of staff lies in this case in the *prospective improvement of treatment and liquidation options*. The same applies in the case of the setting up of *assistantships and internships*, whether in the chief of staff's private liquidation area or on other wards. Because of the amendment to the law, all these cases are instances of a »*third-party benefit*«.

If the company money is used to pay projects remote from hospital life, such as *travel and accommodation expenses* for attending congresses, conferences, or symposia, or if it is used to finance the attendance of family members, these are cases where the recipient or third parties derive a mixture of direct private benefits and indirect benefits. As education at congresses and conferences is part of the professional duty of every physician (and all medical staff), the financial support provided by the manufacturing company, which this circle of people receive, improves their legal, economic and personal situation.

To sum up: all the many forms of industry sponsoring fall under the broad literal definition of »benefit« in case law pursuant to sections 331, 333 StGB.

ff)   Therefore, legal authors are right to assert that the definition of »benefit« as an ingredient of the offense should be interpreted more closely with regard to the sense and purpose of the provisions according to sections 331 ff StGB. Dauster contends that the provision of research funding to a research facility is *not* a personal or »third-party benefit« according to the definition of the offence. He argues that if the »considerations provided by third parties to a university research facility« have an *objectively quantifiable* impact – i.e., are measurable in monetary terms – only in the *official research area* of the university-based public official, the basic right of freedom of science calls for a restrictive interpretation of the definition of benefit pursuant to section 331 subsection 1 StGB. »*Freedom of science* means the right to sponsorship and the right to receive such considerations«. Therefore, Dauster says, there is a »constitutionally legitimated need to differentiate between the self-interest and private interest of receiving the consideration on the one hand and the interest of the state and research in transfer of the consideration on the other hand ... . The acceptance of considerations from third parties for the purpose of scientific research at universities is *not* acceptance of benefit within the meaning of section 331 I StGB«. The evasion in unquantifiable ambition or equally intangible recognition ignores these interpretations, however.[1])

In the same way, clinical trials of medical devices and medicinal products pursuant to section 40 ff of the German Drug Law (AMG) or Section 17 ff of the German Medical Devices Directive (MPG) should not be considered as

---

[1] Dauster, op. cit., p. 67

meeting the definition of an offense under section 331 (no »benefit«, no »wrongful agreement«), as these laws *oblige* the manufacturer to conduct clinical tests on pain of penalty. Therefore, in view of the obligations pursuant to AMG/MPG, conclusion of a research contract for a clinical trial cannot be interpreted as a »benefit« in the criminal sense if the funds provided for this purpose do *not constitute uncompensated considerations* and the mutual services rendered are in proportion to each other, i.e. the financial compensation provided is not inappropriate.[1]) In my opinion, the same must apply to *research funded by third parties*, provided that the considerations go to finance »genuine« research projects in the university area [see section 35, Third Level Education Framework Act (HochschulrahmenG)]. The freedom of research and teaching in accordance with article 5 III 1 of the Basic Law is exceeded only in the case of inappropriately high levels of payment or the associated goal of obtaining preferential treatment in the procurement of products, in which case »self-interest« is predominant and the legitimation for restrictive interpretation of the »benefit« offense no longer applies.

d) The *subjective* element of section 331 subsection 1 StGB presumes *intent*. This means the public official must know his position and be aware that the act is relevant to his public office and grants him or a third party a legally unjustified benefit as quid pro quo for discharge of his duties.

To make sure there is no misunderstanding: the physician (or other staff member) of the hospital needs not know the *legal definition* of a public official or the other elements of the offense, e.g., the definition of benefit. It is enough for them to know the facts on which the legal appraisal is based, i.e. that the physician is engaged in »provision of elementary requirements« in the interest of patients and public health and either he or a third party will derive some betterment from the company's measures. However, a so-called »intent-excluding factual mistake« often seems likely in cases in which the literature denies the presence of a »benefit« or »wrongful agreement« (e.g., in clinical trials, research assignments, and third-party funding within the meaning of the Third Level Education Framework Act). By contrast, the belief that there is nothing wrong in having a sponsor and accepting considerations from a sponsor – a belief that is widespread and understandable in view of decades of »practice« – is an »error as to the prohibitive nature of an act«, which excludes guilt only in the case of unavoidability.

The courts interpret doctors' frequent lack of a sense of wrongdoing as an avoidable »error as to the prohibitive nature of an act«. One such error is the assumption that, because the hospital administration knew how the educational trips were being financed, it was legitimate to accept the benefits. When a physician knows all the facts and merely draws a legally false conclusion, this »error as to the prohibitive nature of an act« is avoidable; the physician could easily have found out (by asking a lawyer, for example), that the employer's approval does not constitute justification in connection with section 332.[2])

---

[1] Tröndle/Fischer, §331 lit. ref. 21a; Pfeiffer NJW 1997, p. 783f.
[2] AG Tuttlingen, case no. 5 Cs 411 Js 91480/96, ruling of 2/8/1999

In view of the excessively broad interpretation in court practice of what constitutes an offense pursuant to section 331 subsection 1 StGB, the objective and subjective elements amount to an offense in most cases. The grounds for justification pursuant to section 331 subsection 3 StGB are therefore of eminent practical relevance.[1]) According to the justification clause, public officials are not liable to prosecution »if the competent authorities, acting on the powers vested in them, approved the acceptance of a benefit by the recipient beforehand or did so upon prompt notification by the recipient«. Acceptance of benefits *solicited* by the public official is not approvable in the context of section 331 *subsection 1*. The issue as to whether a benefit was »*solicited*« could be problematic in connection with research projects where the *initiative is launched by the hospital*. If a physician approaches a company to propose the conduct of a study and asks for support, this could well constitute »solicitation« pursuant to section 331 StGB. Approval by the administration would in this case *not constitute justification*, but it greatly depends upon the circumstances of the individual case. »Solicitation« is a demand, i.e., more than a request or query or »suggestion«, which is used to seek a benefit for the discharge of duty.

If the acceptance of benefit was approved and the approval is effective, the deed is also justified (for company members) according to section 333 subsection 1 StGB. I would therefore strongly *advise public officials (physicians) and company members* to apply the principle of transparency and, in all the various cases of industry sponsoring discussed in the foregoing, to ensure that the »competent authorities, acting on the powers vested in them«, *approve* the consideration or acceptance of benefit.

If in doubt, one should always *ask for permission* and obtain it *in writing* for documentation purposes (evidence). *General permission* can be obtained *for specific areas*. Once permission has been obtained, there can no longer be the least suspicion of wrongdoing on the part of the recipient or the company and its staff and the actions of both parties are confined in a safe, legally admissible area, free from the odium of criminal law and possible procedural consequences (search of buildings, confiscation).

Accordingly, the federal government specified in a directive addressed to the *federal administration* dated June 17, 1998 that »the *prior agreement of top-level authority*« be obtained for *any kind of sponsoring* of activities, events and facilities of the administration. Going by the wording, the directive could also refer to *third-party funding of research facilities*.

The identity of the »competent authority« may differ from case to case. It is clear however that the »competent authority« for the granting of permissions to subordinates or to the purchasing department is not the »medical director« and not the »chief of staff« but the organization financing the hospital, i.e. somebody in the *personnel department*, possibly the administrative director himself. Responsibility is defined in the statutes of the respective organization financing the hospital, which can allocate responsibility as it sees fit.

A *false* assumption on the part of a physician that the necessary permission had been granted or that an invalid approval was effective, is a factual mistake that rules

---

[1] BGHSt 31, 264, 285

out *intent*.[1]) In the context of section 331 subsection 1 StGB, all that counts is what the recipient of the benefit (physician) believes to be true.[2])

3. Donations, gifts, clinical trials, postmarketing studies, speakers' fees, consulting fees, travel expenses, other expenses, financial support for education, etc., are all still legal if the recipient clears them with his employer. When making a notification to the competent authority, it is important to state the true facts, in particular the circumstance that the company providing the considerations is a medical devices manufacturer, and that these devices may already be in use at the hospital or are intended for use.

II.

As already stated under I. 2 a, the provisions outlined above do *not apply to fully privately owned facilities*. However, sections 299 and 300 StGB introduced in connection with the penal law reform of August 1997 may apply. These provide for the prosecution of those who »offer, promise or grant a benefit to an employee or designee of a business operation for that person or a third party in return for giving him or another unfair preferential treatment in the procurement of goods or services«.

1. The elements of the offense are as follows:

a) A business operation is any enterprise set up on a long-term perspective that carries out its characteristic tasks outside the private sphere by participating in business life through the exchange of outputs in return for other outputs.[3]) This definition includes any and all activity performed in trade and commerce with the goal of generating revenue. Business operations may therefore also be enterprises that exclusively pursue nonprofit, social or cultural goals.[4]) According to this definition, *hospitals* also fall under the category of »business operations« and consequently, the legal literature explicitly includes physicians' practices in the category.[1])

b) As the promotion of medical activity belongs to the area of »business operations« and the definitions of »benefit« and »wrongful agreement« agree with those pursuant to section 331 StGB, what I have said earlier applies.

c) Another essential element is unfair *preferential treatment* of the granter of the benefit (i.e., the industrial company) over the latter's competitors, resulting in impairment of free competition.[6]) The preferential treatment must be in relation to the procurement (ordering, delivery, acceptance, payment) of goods or industrial outputs and must be a means of promoting the company's own sales at the competition's expense.[7])

---

[1] BHSt 31, 264, 285
[2] Lackner/Kühl, § 331 lit. ref. 16
[3] BGHSt 2, 396, 403; 10, 358, 365, 366
[4] Pfeiffer, FS for von Gamm, 1990, p. 129, 134
[5] Fuhrmann, in: Erbs/Kohlhaas, comment 2d on §12 UWG
[6] Fuhrmann, op. cit., comment 2f
[7] Fuhrmann, op. cit, comment 2h, bb; RGSt 58, 429, 431

The preferential treatment is unfair if it is based on improper motives and »offends against morality«[1]) with the objective of eliminating the competition in this manner. Secrecy and objective harming of one's own or another business operation are not essential ingredients of the offense.[2]) Wrongful agreement linking the consideration (benefit) and counter-performance (preferential treatment in a concrete decision) is a characteristic of unfair preferential treatment. A consideration granted to create »a favorable disposition« or to maintain »general goodwill« unrelated to a *specific* action is *not* enough.[3])

d) The subjective element presupposes *intent*. Contingent intent suffices. The perpetrator must therefore know or at least be aware of the possibility of offering, promising or granting a benefit to an employee in the course of business, and must know that this benefit is intended and qualified as a quid pro quo for an act of unfair preferential treatment.

2. The essential constituents of an offense pursuant to the new section 299 StGB may *not be at all rare* in the case constellation studied here. As the offense was previously concealed in the law against unfair competition (section 12 of the Unfair Competition Act, UWG) and was contingent upon a demand for prosecution, it was *practically never prosecuted*. That will change in future now that the offense has been adopted in the penal code and now has the status of a »relevant offense requiring an application for prosecution«. This means that even without an *application for prosecution* by the competitor, the state prosecutor may investigate proceedings on his own initiative by virtue of his office, simply by affirming that this course of action serves a »special public interest« (section 301 StGB). As the definition of a »special public interest« is not revisable, it is enough for the state prosecutor to simply claim that a special public interest is involved, without having to substantiate this claim in detail.

3. Approval pursuant to section 331 subsection 3 StGB does *not* rule out the applicability of section 299 StGB. The medical community must therefore exercise caution as far as the laws on unfair competition are concerned. »Unfair« practices must not be allowed to prevail.

---

[1] BGH GRUR 1977, 619, 620
[2] Tröndle/Fischer, §299 lit. ref. 13
[3] Tröndle/Fischer, §299, lit. ref. 12

IX.a Poster: Hemophilia

Experience with Recombinant Factor IX (Benefix) in Pediatrics

N. NOHE, M. PRAUN, K. KURNIK

Introduction

Benefix is a lyophilized stable recombinant factor IX formulation containing no pre-servatives, blood or plasma products. With regard to its structural, functional, and clinical qualities, recombinant factor IX has proved to be comparable to monoclo-nal plasma-derived factor IX. The only difference found was a 72% lower recovery rate for recombinant factor IX compared to plasma-derived factor IX; this is most probably caused by minor differences in the post-translational modification [1]. In a canine model study, recombinant factor IX proved to be as effective as highly puri-fied plasma-derived factor IX in normalizing hemostasis. Canine pharmacokinetic studies showed a dose-proportional profile, and experiments in a model of throm-bogenicity indicated a low thrombogenic potential for recombinant factor IX [2]. In between pharmacokinetics, the safety and efficacy of recombinant factor IX have been evaluated in both previously treated and previously untreated hemophilia B patients. In a study including 56 previously untreated patients, 80% of 1070 bleeding episodes resolved after a single recombinant factor IX infusion. In 87% of a total of 1514 infusions, the clinical response was rated as excellent or good. Recombinant factor IX has also been successfully used in a surgical setting. In a total of 13 surgi-cal procedures, 97% of the clinical responses following a bolus or continuous infu-sion of recombinant factor IX were rated excellent or good [3].

In pharmacokinetic studies, the recovery of recombinant factor IX was shown to be 28% lower than the recovery of plasma-derived factor IX [1, 3, 4]. In 56 previously untreated patients following a single dose of 50 IU recombinant factor IX per kg body weight (b.w.), a recovery of 0.7 (range, 0.3–1.4) IU/dl for 1 IU/kg b.w. infused was measured. These data were confirmed in a crossover study including 11 patients in whom a recovery of 0.84±0.30 IU/dl for Benefix and of 1.17±0.26 IU/dl for plasma-derived factor IX was observed [4]. According to these data, the dose re-quirement for recombinant factor IX needs to be about 30% higher. The half-life of recombinant factor IX of 18.1±5.1 h was found to be comparable to that of plasma-derived factor IX (17.7±5.3 h) [4].

Patients

We treated five previously untreated patients aged 4–15 years with recombinant factor IX. One out of the five children suffered from moderate and four of the five

I. Scharrer/W. Schramm (Ed.)
30th Hemophilia Symposium Hamburg 1999
© Springer-Verlag Berlin Heidelberg 2001

children from severe hemophilia B. One child received treatment on demand, and four received prophylactic treatment.

Recovery/Half-Life

The recovery was determined in four out of the five children. The mean recovery of recombinant factor IX was 1.05% (range, 1.0%–1.1%), corresponding to a 7.1% lower recovery compared to plasma-derived factor IX, with a recovery of 1.13% (range, 0.9%–1.5%). Thus we were not able to confirm published data reporting a 28% lower recovery rate for recombinant factor IX in our patients (see Table 1).

The half-life was measured in one patient (patient 4). The half-life of recombinant factor IX was 14.5 h compared to 17.0 h under plasma-derived factor IX, corresponding to a 14.7% reduction in half-life for recombinant factor IX.

Table 1. Recovery of plasma-derived compared to recombinant factor IX

		Patient 1	Patient 2	Patient 3	Patient 4
Plasma-derived factor IX	Before	8%	13%	21%	57%
	30 min after	17 IU/kg b.w.: 37%	30 IU/kg b.w.: 39%	27 IU/kg b.w.: 47%	67 IU/kg b.w.: 142%
	Recovery	1.5%	0.9%	1.0%	1.1%
Recombinant factor IX	Before	21%	3%	25%	5%
	30 min after	42 IU/kg b.w.: 70%	30 IU/kg b.w.: 29%	57 IU/kg b.w.: 82%	30 IU/kg b.w.: 37%
	Recovery	1.1%	1.1%	1.0%	1.0%

Clinical Response/Factor IX Requirement

No changes in bleeding frequency or bleeding intensity were observed in two out of the five patients (patients 4, 5). It should be mentioned, however, that changing to recombinant factor IX, the substitution dose was increased from 36 IU/kg b.w. to 45 IU/kg b.w. twice weekly in patient 4.

In three out of five patients, an increase in both bleeding frequency and bleeding intensity occurred following the change to recombinant factor IX. Substitution doses in these patients had to be increased from 20 IU/kg b.w. to 33 IU/kg b.w. and finally to 44 IU/kg b.w. twice weekly (patient 1) and from 20 IU/kg b.w. to 30 IU/kg b.w. twice weekly (patient 3), respectively. The factor IX required by the patient receiving treatment on demand (patient 2) increased from 83–200 IU/kg b.w. per month to 272–333 IU/kg b.w. per month (see Fig. 1).

Conclusion

In contrast to the literature, the recovery of recombinant factor IX in our patients was found to be only 7.1% less than that of plasma-derived factor IX. With recom-

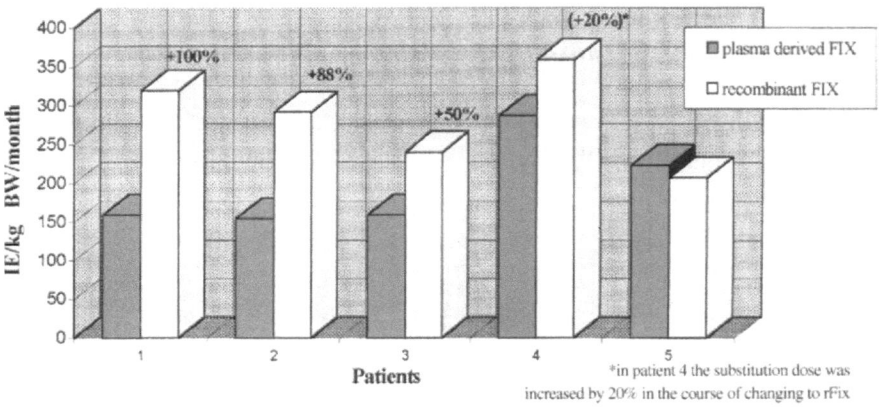

Fig. 1. Dose requirements for plasma-derived compared to recombinant factor IX

binant factor IX, three out of five children had a rise in bleeding frequency and intensity requiring a dose increase of 50% to 100% to achieve effective prophylaxis and therapy. As no half-life data for Benefix are available in these three children, we are not able to give any explanation for this observation.

In two out of five children, no change in clinical course or dose requirement was observed under recombinant factor IX. However, one of these two children received a 20% higher treatment dose of recombinant factor IX than of plasma-derived factor IX from the beginning.

References

1. White GC, Beebe A, Nilesen B (1997) Recombinant Factor IX, Thromb Haemost 78(1): 261–5
2. Schaub R, Garzone P, Bouchard P, Rup B, Keith J, Brinkhous K, Larsen G (1998) Preclinical studies of recombinant factor IX. Semin Hematol 35(2 Suppl 2): 28–32
3. White G, Shapiro A, Ragni M, Garzone P, Goodfellow J, Tubridy K, Courter S (1998) Clinical evaluation of recombinant factor IX. Semin Hematol 35 (2 Suppl 2): 33–8
4. Genetics Institute, Inc. Cambridge, MA: Benefix™. Coagulation Factor IX (recombinant)

Articular Cartilage Is More Susceptible
to Blood-Induced Damage in Young Than in Old Age

G. Roosendaal, J.M. Tekoppele, M.E. Vianen, H.M. van den Berg,
F.P.J.G. Lafeber, J.W.J. Bijlsma

Introduction

It has been demonstrated that cartilage is damaged upon intra-articular hemorrhage (patients with hemophilic arthropathy) [1, 7]. The present study investigates
differences in the susceptibility of young and old cartilage to blood-induced joint
damage in a canine in vivo model.

Methods

The right knees of six young (2.2±0.1 years) and six adult (7.4±0.3 years) dogs
(beagles) were intra-articularly injected twice in 4 days with autologous blood.
Dogs were killed 4 or 16 days after the first injection, and cartilage matrix proteoglycan content and synthesis were determined as described previously [8, 9].

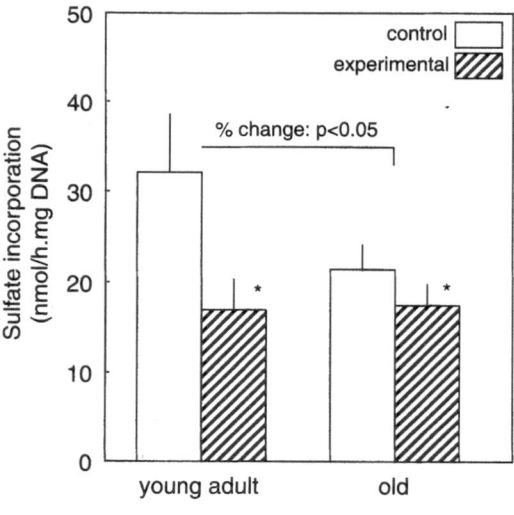

Fig. 1. »Short-term« effects observed 4 days after the first of two injections in 4 days of autologous blood into the knee joint cavity. The sulfate incorporation rate is shown as a measure of proteoglycan synthesis. *Open bars* represent contralateral control knees, and *hatched bars* blood-injected knees. *Asterisks* indicate statistically significant differences between experimental joints and contralateral control joints ($p \leq 0.01$ and $p \leq 0.03$ for young adult and old animals, respectively). The p values indicate statistical significance between percentage change in experimental joints compared to contralateral control joints for cartilage of young adult and old animals (–45% and –18%, respectively)

I. Scharrer/W. Schramm (Ed.)
30th Hemophilia Symposium Hamburg 1999
© Springer-Verlag Berlin Heidelberg 2001

Fig. 2. »Short-term« effects observed 4 days after the first of two injections in 4 days of autologous blood into the knee joint cavity. Glycosaminoglycan (*GAG*) content is shown as a measure of cartilage matrix proteoglycan content. *Open bars* represent contralateral control knees, and *hatched bars* blood-injected knees. *Asterisks* indicate statistically significant differences between experimental joints and contralateral control joints ($p \leq 0.03$ and $p \leq 0.003$ for young adult and old animals, respectively). No statistically significant difference was found between percentage change in experimental joints compared to contralateral control joints for cartilage of young adult and old animals (–13% and –14%, respectively)

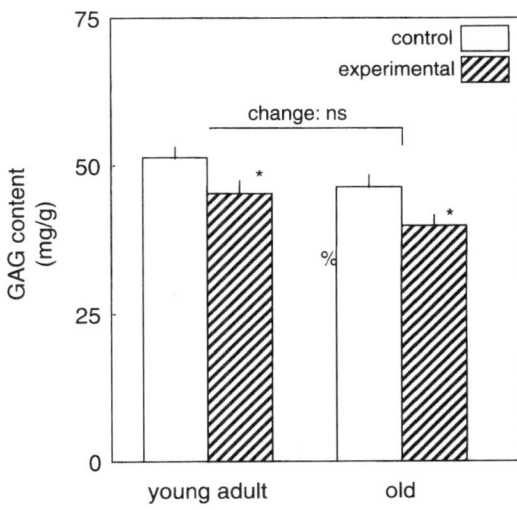

Fig. 3. »Long-term« effects observed 16 days after the first of two injections in 4 days of autologous blood into the knee joint cavity (in vivo recovery). Sulfate incorporation rate is shown as a measure of proteoglycan synthesis. *Open bars* represent contralateral control knees, and *hatched bars* blood-injected knees. *Asterisks* indicate statistically significant differences between experimental joints and contralateral control joints ($p \leq 0.05$ and $p \leq 0.01$ for young adult and old animals, respectively). No statistically significant difference was found between percentage change in experimental joints compared to contralateral control joints for cartilage of young adult and old animals (+27% and +38%, respectively)

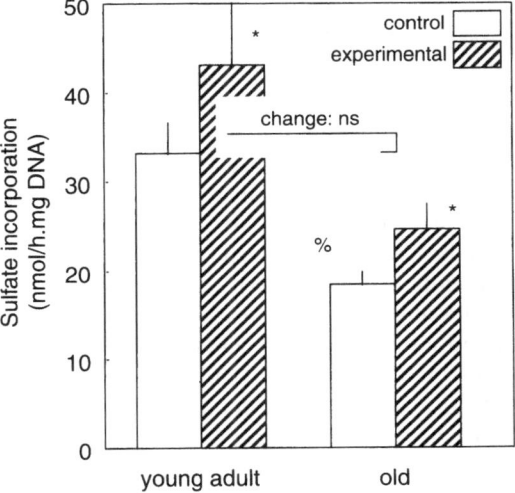

Discussion

Joint damage resulting in disability is a major problem in patients with hemophilia. It has been demonstrated that a limited number of bleeding episodes in joints, and maybe even a single episode, result in long-lasting changes in articular cartilage,

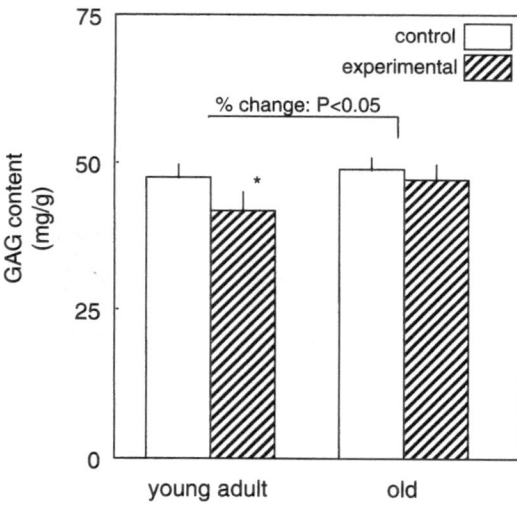

Fig. 4. »Long-term« effects observed 16 days after the first of two injections in 4 days of autologous blood into the knee joint cavity. Glycosaminoglycan (*GAG*) content is shown as a measure of cartilage matrix proteoglycan content. *Open bars* represent contralateral control knees, and *hatched bars* blood-injected knees. The *asterisk* indicates a significant difference in the glycosaminoglycan content of the cartilage obtained from experimental joints and contralateral control joints of young adult animals ($p \leq 0.005$). No statistical difference was found between the experimental joints and contralateral control joints of old animals. The p value indicates the statistical significance between the magnitude of changes in the GAG content in cartilage obtained from joints of young adult and old animals (–12% and –4%, respectively)

independent of synovial changes. These cartilage changes as observed both in vitro [9, 10] and in vivo [8] are predictive of irreversible joint damage in time. These data warrant more intensive prophylactic treatment of patients with hemophilia to completely prevent joint bleeding.

There is the general impression among physicians who treat patients with hemophilia that joints deteriorate more quickly in children than in adult patients. A retrospective study showed that young patients with hemophilia had more rapid progression of joint damage than patients older than 20 years, even though the clinical status was comparable, including the number of bleeding episodes in joints and the treatment protocol [4]. As a prospective clinical study takes many years, the presently described approach was chosen first.

Results showed that cartilage from young adult beagles is more susceptible to blood-induced impairment of cartilage matrix turnover, predicting damage in time, than cartilage from old animals. The inhibition of proteoglycan synthesis was significantly greater in young adult animals than in old animals. This cannot be attributed to changes in the cellularity of the cartilage, since no significant differences in DNA content between blood-injected and control joints were observed (data not shown). Interestingly, control proteoglycan synthesis was significantly lower in cartilage from old animals than in cartilage from young adult animals. This has been reported also for human cartilage [3, 4, 6] and was attributed to aging of chondrocytes and to interactions with an aged matrix. An in vivo recovery period resulted in an increase in proteoglycan synthesis. This phenomenon can be considered as a »rebound« effect of proteoglycan synthesis. A rebound such as this has been reported for articular cartilage from osteoarthritic joints, both in animal models and in human in vitro experiments, and has been described as an attempt to repair the osteoarthritic features [5]. In the present study, this rebound was stronger in cartilage obtained from old dogs than in that from young adult animals. During the recovery period, the proteoglycan content of cartilage from old animals normalized. This contrasted to the cartilage of young adult animals, which still showed a significantly diminished proteoglycan content, not statistically different from the change observed immediately after the injections of blood. This difference in the integrity of young adult and old cartilage (with respect to proteoglycans) after a short exposure to intra-articular blood, as assessed after 12 days of recovery, was not accompanied by a difference in collagen damage (data not shown).

The present study demonstrates that the cartilage of young adult dogs is more susceptible to blood-induced impairment of cartilage matrix turnover than is the cartilage of old dogs. Whether these findings can be extrapolated to young and old patients with hemophilia is uncertain. The present results nevertheless underscore clinical experience that young hemophilia patients with recurrent bleeding show a faster progression of joint damage than older patients. Since iron accumulation in joints is a major cause of the destructive process, it is interesting to note that, when iron injections were given to rabbits, iron only accumulated in cartilage in immature rabbits, with the subsequent destructive effects on the cartilage. No effect was observed in mature rabbits [2]. Based on these findings, our present results, and clinical data, young adult cartilage seems to be more susceptible to blood-induced damage than old cartilage. Thus, awaiting further prospective clinical studies, the prophylactic regimen of clotting factor substitution should be reconsidered, with earlier and higher levels at a younger age and possibly lower levels and only treatment on demand in older patients.

References

1. Arnold WD, Hilgartner MW. Hemophilic arthropathy. Current concepts of pathogenesis and management. J Bone Joint Surg [Am] 1977; 59: 287–305.
2. Brighton CT, Bigly EC, Smolensky BI. Iron induced arthritis in immature rabbits. Arthritis Rheum1970; 13: 849–57.
3. De Groot J, Verzijl N, Bank RA, Lafeber FPJG, Bijlsma JWJ Te Koppele JM. Age-related decrease in proteoglycan synthesis of human articular chondrocytes: the role of non-enzymatic glycation. Arthritis Rheum 1999; 42: 1003–1009.
4. Fischer K, van den Berg HM, Mauser-Bunschoten EP, Roosendaal G. Changing treatment strategies for severe hemophilia A; Effects on clinical outcome and costs. Blood 1997; 90 (suppl): 35 A (abs 142).
5. Lafeber FPJG, van Roy JLAM, Wilbrink B, Huber-Bruning O and Bijlsma JWJ. Human osteoarthritic cartilage is synthetically more active but in culture less vital than normal cartilage. J Rheumatol 1992; 19: 123–29.
6. Maroudas A, Schneiderman R, Weinberg C, Grushko. Choice of specimens in comparative studies involving human femoral head cartilage. In: Maroudas A, Kuettner K editors. Methods in cartilage research. London: Academic Press; 1990: 2–25.
7. Roosendaal G, van den Berg HM, Lafeber FPJG, Bijlsma JWJ. Pathologie der Synovitis und haemophilen Arthropathie. Der Orthopäde 1999; 28: 323–328.
8. Roosendaal G, TeKoppele GM, Vianen ME, van den Berg HM, Lafeber FPJG and Bijlsma JWJ. Blood-induced joint damage: a canine in vivo study. Arthritis Rheum 1999; 42: 1033–1039.

9. Roosendaal G, Vianen ME, Marx JJM, van den Berg HM, Lafeber FPJG and Bijlsma JWJ. Blood-induced joint damage: a human in vitro study. Arthritis Rheum 1999; 42: 1025–1032.
10. Roosendaal G, Vianen ME, van den Berg HM, Lafeber FPJG, Bijlsma JWJ. Cartilage damage as a result of hemarthrosis in a human in vitro model. J Rheumatol 1997; 24: 1350–54.
11. Verbruggen G, Malfait AM, Cornelissen M, Broddelez C, Veys EM. Human chondrocytes cultured in suspension culture in agarose. Reliability of the system to predict 'structure modifying' capacity of osteoarthritic drugs. Clin Rheumatol 1996; 15: 534.

Chronic Liver Disease in Hemophilia Patients

Z. VORLOVÁ, M. MATÝŠKOVÁ, I. MARTINKOVÁ

Introduction

Chronic liver disease is an important complication when treating hemophilia patients with factor VIII and IX concentrates. Hepatitis B (HBV) and C (HCV) virus infection is the major cause of chronic liver disease [5]. Chronic HCV infection is characterized by persistently or intermittently raised liver transaminases [4, 6].

Affected patients are asymptomatic or may develop cirrhosis. Liver biopsy studies in these patients showed evidence of cirrhosis in around 25% [1] of patients. It has been demonstrated that liver disease only develops after prolonged infection. Human immunodeficiency virus (HIV) coinfection is associated with more severe hepatic failure [3]. In patients with cirrhosis, there is a clearly increased risk of hepatocellular carcinoma. The main cause of HCV infection was treatment with non-virus-inactivated concentrates [2].

The Czech hemophiliac population was mainly treated with cryoprotein prepared from small pools of plasma. The concentrates began to be used in 1992, when virus-inactivated concentrates were produced. Our aim was to assess the extent of liver disease in Czech hemophilia patients. In comparison with published studies, the incidence of liver disease in the Czech hemophilia population has been low, although clinical hepatitis occurred in 60% of our patients during their lifetime. The aim of this study was to find an explication for the low incidence of liver disease. Our first systematic laboratory investigation was started in 1975 and has followed this population during the following 24 years. In order to obtain more representative results, 292 hemophilia patients were examined in 1999.

Methods

A total of 292 adult patients with hemophilia (hemophilia A and hemophilia B) were followed up in three regional hemophilia centers: in South Moravia (116 patients), West Bohemia (72 patients), and Central Bohemia (104 patients) (Table 1). They were referred to as Group I, II, and III, respectively. The data obtained from each group are reviewed separately. In group III, 51 patients (10 hemophilia B and 41 hemophilia A) were enrolled in the study in 1975 and were followed up for the following 24 years. Special attention was paid to the clinical status and to laboratory

I. Scharrer/W. Schramm (Ed.)
30th Hemophilia Symposium Hamburg 1999
© Springer-Verlag Berlin Heidelberg 2001

Table 1. Characteristics of study groups (year 1999)

Hemophilia patients	Group I (n=116) (%)	Group II (n=72) (%)	Group III (n=104) (%)
Severe <1%	38	43	45
Moderate 2%–5%	24	26	40
Mild >5%	38	30	15

parameters, i.e., aminotransferases, hepatitis B surface antigen (HBsAg), and anti-HB.

In 1999, other parameters were added: HIV, HBsAg, anti-HBs, anti-HCV, HCV genotype, anti-HAV, and parvovirus B19.

Results

The 51 patients in group III were examined in 1975 to establish the extent of liver disease. The youngest patient was 16 and the oldest 49 years old. No hepatomegaly or splenomegaly was demonstrated. Alanine aminotransferase (ALT) was normal in 40% of patients; in 36% of patients, it was increased to a value less than twice the upper normal limit, and in 24% it was higher than twice the normal upper limit. Aspartate aminotransferase (AST) and GGT were elevated in 12% of patients (Table 2). In 1975, HBsAg was positive in 1% and anti-HBs were demonstrated in 65% of patients. Chronic hepatitis was suspected in three patients, and the initial stage of cirrhosis in one patient. None of the other patients had any clinical symptoms of illness.

Thirteen years later, the clinical status of these patients had not changed significantly, and no progressive liver disease had developed. As was later demonstrated, 80% of these patients were infected by HCV, which was demonstrated by anti-HCV positivity. Patients in groups I and II were not studied longitudinally. Table 3 contains laboratory data from 1999.

Of these 292 patients, 60% were found to be HCV positive, and 55% were confirmed using the polymerase chain reaction (PCR) method. HBsAg was found to be positive only in 1% of patients, and the antibody was found to be positive in 60% of patients. Aminotransferases were elevated in 24%–64% of patients (Table 4).

Table 2. Alanine aminotransferase (sALT), aspartate aminotransferase (sAST), and sGMT in 51 patients with hemophilia (year 1975)

Aminotransferase values	Patients (%)		
	sALT	sAST	sGMT
Normal	40	44	72
Up to twice the upper limit	36	44	16
More than twice the upper limit	24	12	12

Table 3. Virology in 292 hemophilia patients

| | Patient group (positivity in %) | | |
	I	II	III
HBAg	1	0	0.5
HBAb	37	51	72
HCV	39	53	85
HCV PCR	28	44	50
HAV	18.6	–	21
Parvo B19	95	–	89

HBAg, hepatitis B antigen; HBAb, hepatitis B antigen; HCV, hepatitis C virus; PCR, polymerase chain reaction; HAV, hemoabsorption vius.

Table 4. Laboratory parameters in 292 hemophilia patients in 1999

| ALT values | Patient groups (%) | | |
	I	II	III
Normal	66	57	44
Up to twice the upper limit	17	13	33
More than twice the upper limit	16	21	19

During these 23 years, one patient died of hepatoma and one due to bleeding from esophageal varices. Three patients developed progressive liver disease. Interferon therapy was used in exceptional cases. In all the groups, patients were mainly treated with cryoprotein up until 1991. Cryoprotein was prepared from small pools of plasma (eight to 12 plasma units). Treatment by concentrates was not introduced until 1992.

Conclusion

Longitudinal 24-year follow-up of severe hemophilia patients demonstrated only mild liver disease and no higher incidence of cirrhosis than found in the control population.

The low incidence of severe liver disease in hemophilia patients in our study may correlate with a relatively short use of concentrates of factor VIII and IX and with a low incidence of HIV positivity (2%) in these patients.

The high frequency of evidence of HCV infection (anti-HCV and HCV antigen PCR) in our hemophilia patients prompted us to find other factors that are involved in the development of hepatic failure.

Summary

Chronic liver disease is an important complication of treatment with factor VIII and IX concentrates in hemophilia patients. The concentrates are prepared from a plasma pool comprising thousands of donor units. Liver biopsies of such patients confirm cirrhosis in 10%–20% of cases. Aledort et al. reported a 7% incidence of severe chronic active hepatitis and a 15% incidence of cirrhosis. All patients were treated using commercial factor VIII and IX concentrates.

In the Czech Republic, patients with hemophilia were preferentially treated using cryoprotein prepared from small pools of plasma donors until 1989. In 1975, a group of 60 patients with severe hemophilia were studied. 9 patients suffered from hemophilia B and 51 from hemophilia A. The median age was 32 years (range, 16–49). A total of 26% of patients demonstrated an elevated level of aminotransferases. The levels of the antibodies against HBV were positive in 36% of patients, and the antigen was negative in all of them. When the same group of patients was followed up 13 years later, 45% of patients demonstrated elevated aminotransferases (up to twofold the upper normal limit) without clinical illness. Anti-HCV was positive in 64% and anti-HBV in 40% of patients. Four patients were HIV positive. During the subsequent 10 years, the treatment changed. Only commercial factor VIII and IX concentrates were used, and the total amount of infused units was doubled.

One patient died at age 52 of hepatoma, and another died due to cirrhosis with bleeding from esophageal varices. The low incidence of clinical symptoms of hepatitis and no development of symptoms of chronic hepatitis during more than 20 years in a cohort of 60 patients is compared with the present hepatic status in a large number of hemophiliacs from two other hemophilia centers.

References

Aledort LM, Levine PH, Hilgartner M, Blatt P, Spero JA, Goldberg JD, Bianci L, Desmet V, Scheuer P, Popper H, Berk PD (1985) A study of liver biopsies and liver disease among hemophiliacs. Blood 66:367

Blanchette VS, Vorstman E, Allyson S,Wang E, Petric M, Jett BW, Alter HJ (1991) Hepatitis C infection in chidren with Hemophilia A and B. Blood 78 :285–289.

Ahmed MM, Mutineer DJ, Elias E, Linin J, Carrido M, Hubscher S, Jarvis L, Simmonds P, Wilde JT (1996) A combined management protocol for patients with coagulation disorders infected with hepatitis C virus. British Journal of Haematology 95: 383–388

Dashiki GM (1998) Therapy for chronic hepatitis B and C infection in haemophilia. Haemophilia 4: 577–586.

Fukuda Y, Nakano I, Katano Y, Toyoda H, Imoto M, Takamatsu J, Saito H, Hayakawa T (1998) Assessment and treatment of liver disease in Japanese hemophilia patients. Haemophilia 4: 595–600.

Hanley JP, Jarvis LM, Andrews J, Dennis R, Lee R, Simmonds P, Piris J, Hayes P, Ludlam ChA (1996) Investigation of chronic hepatitis C infection in individuals with hemophilia: Assessment of invasive and non–invasive methods. British Journal of Haematology 94: 159–165.

Lee ChA (1997) Investigation of chronic hepatitis C infection in individuals with haemophilia British Journal of haematology.98:424

Human Immunodeficiency Virus-Negative »High-Risk Patients« with Hemophilia or Severe von Willebrand Disease Type 3: Coincidence or Genetics?

R. Schneppenheim, S. Krey, G. Auerswald, R. Ganschow, H. Holzhüter, H.J. Klose, W. Kreuz, A. Kurme, R. Linde, E. Maass, M. Rendtorff, J. Weisser

Introduction

Patients with inherited hemorrhagic disorders who were treated with plasma-derived factor concentrates in fairly high dosages before 1985 carried a high risk of infection with human immunodeficiency virus (HIV). However, a significant number of them remained HIV negative. In addition to differences in viral load or coincidence, a certain genetic predisposition has been discussed. Subsequent to the detection of a new essential co-receptor for the infection of monocytic cells or macrophages, the chemokine receptor CCR5, high-risk probands in cohorts of homosexuals were identified who were HIV negative in spite of repeated exposition to HIV. In some of them, a homozygous 32bp deletion of the CCR5 gene (CCR5del32) was found [1]. CCR5del32-heterozygous HIV-infected individuals seemed to have a prolonged course of HIV infection before developing acquired immunodeficiency syndrome (AIDS) [2].

Patients

We analyzed 50 patients with hemorrhagic disorders in a multicenter study. 30 of them had hemophilia A, 3 had hemophilia B, 16 had severe von Willebrand disease (vWD) type 3, and 1 had severe factor X deficiency. 21 of the 30 patients with hemophilia A, all 3 of the patients with hemophilia B, and 3 of the 16 patients with vWD were HIV positive. The patient with factor X deficiency was HIV negative.

Methods

A 174-bp fragment of the CCR5 gene harboring the region of the 32bp deletion was amplified by polymerase chain reaction (PCR) of DNA derived from patients' peripheral leukocytes. The deletion is easily detected by polyacrylamide electrophoresis and silver staining [3] due to the higher mobility of the shorter PCR product (Fig. 1).

I. Scharrer/W. Schramm (Ed.)
30th Hemophilia Symposium Hamburg 1999
© Springer-Verlag Berlin Heidelberg 2001

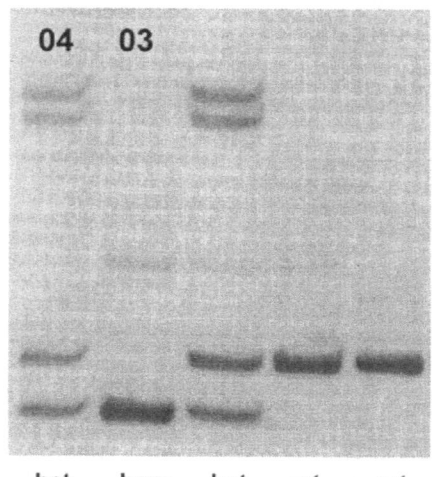

het   hom   het   wt   wt

Fig. 1. Polyacrylamide gel electrophoresis of polymerase chain reaction (PCR) products of the CCR5 gene. A CCR5del32 homozygote (*hom*), two heterozygotes (*het*), and two patients with wild-type sequence (*wt*) are shown. Numbers 03 and 04 are the same patients as in Fig. 2

Results

In line with the frequency of 20% in the normal population, heterozygosity for CCR5del32 was found in 4 out of 27 HIV-positive patients and in 4 out of 23 HIV-negative patients. However, among the 23 noninfected patients, we also identified 3 homozygotes for CCR5del32 (13%), although the expected frequency was only 1% ($p<0,02$). Interestingly, there were 2 brothers with severe hemophilia A who received comparable quantities of factor VIII concentrates from the same batches, one of them was HIV negative and the other HIV positive. The HIV-negative brother was homozygous for CCRdel32, while the HIV-positive brother was only heterozygous for CCR5del32 (Fig. 2).

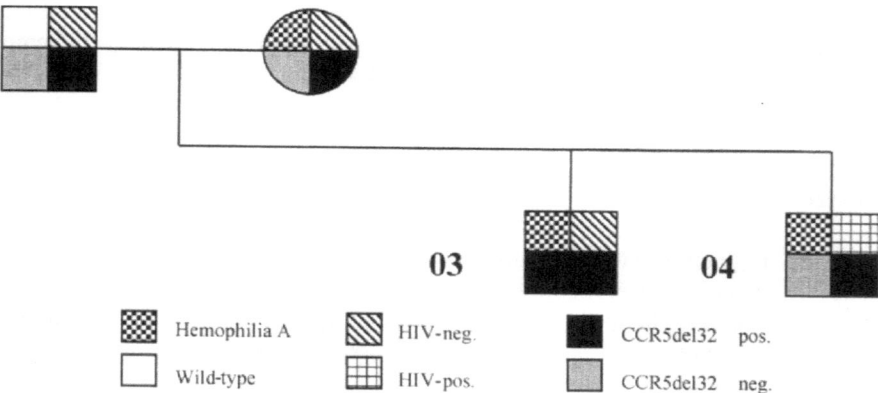

Fig. 2. Segregation of CCR5del32 in a family with hemophilia A. The patient who is CCR5del32 homozygous is HIV negative; his heterozygous brother is HIV positive. Both patients received comparable quantities of plasma-derived factor concentrates from the same batches

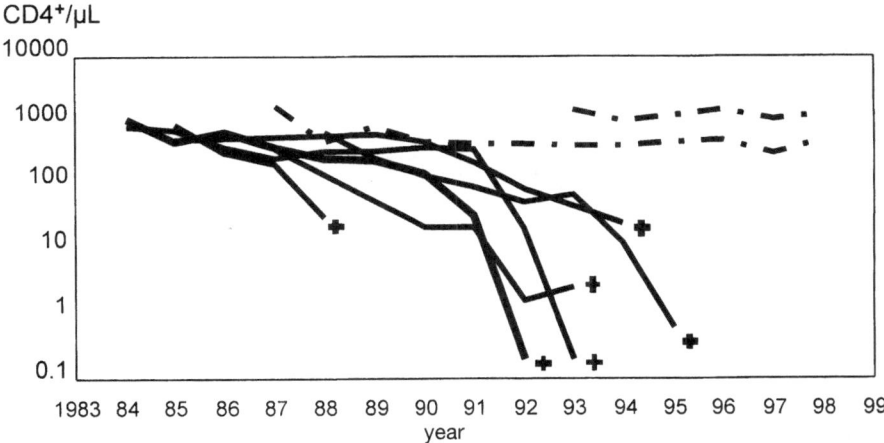

Fig. 3. Course of HIV infection in CCRdel32 heterozygous patients (*broken lines*) and in those without CCR5del32 (*solid lines*). The patients did not receive antiretroviral polychemotherapy or were noncompliant

Patients without the deletion who did not receive adequate antiretroviral poly-chemotherapy showed a more rapid and fatal course of their HIV infection (Fig. 3).

Discussion

In view of the situation in high-risk homosexual groups, homozygosity for CCR5del32 seems to be correlated with relative resistance against HIV infection; this was also true of our patients with hemorrhagic disorders. Thus genetically determined properties of individual patients contribute to the predisposition to HIV infection.

Heterozygosity for CCR5del32 is not sufficient to protect against HIV infection. However, according to our data, it seems to correlate with a slower course of HIV infection towards AIDS among patients who did not receive adequate antiretroviral therapy.

References

1. Liu R, Paxton WA, Choe S, Ceradini D, Martin SR, Horuk R, MacDonald ME, Stuhlmann H, Koup RA, Landau NR (1996) Homozygous defect in HIV-1 co-receptor accounts for resistance of some multiply exposed individuals to HIV infection. Cell 86: 367–377
2. Dean M, Carrington M, Winkler C, Huttley GA, Smith MW, Allikmets R, Goedert JJ, Buchbinder SP, Vittinghoff E, Gomperts E, Donfield S, Vlahow D, Kaslow R, Saah A, Rinaldo C, Detels R, O'Brian SJ (1996) Genetic restriction of HIV-1 infection and progression to AIDS by a deletion allele of the CCR5 structural gene. Science 273: 1856–1862

Quality Management and Economic Aspects in Hemotherapy in the Federal Republic of Germany: Description of a Retrospective Cross-Sectional Multicenter Trial

J. Hoffmann, L. Frey, C. Wittmann, C. Domsch, K. Thürmel, K. Berger, M. Spannagl, W. Schramm

The transfusion of blood components and the utilization of human blood-derived products for the treatment of patients and for preventive medicine are associated with medical consequences for the patients (e.g., risk of transmission of infectious diseases, immunosuppression, graft versus host reactions). As all of these components or products depend on the amount of donated human blood or plasma, the resources are limited. Furthermore, hemotherapy has an considerable economic impact. In the Federal Republic of Germany, more than 1 billion euros have been spent per year for blood products over the past decade.

Economic aspects have become more important in the modern healthcare system in an attempt to limit expenses for healthcare. Rationing of healthcare is an impending issue in the face of limited resources. Careful economic planning should mean that rationing of health care can be avoided. Rationing is focused on the limitation of resources, while rational decision-making involves guaranteeing and improving the productivity of the entire healthcare system. Utilization of resources therefore has to be evaluated and assessed.

Guidelines and recommendations for the use of blood products have been established. Over the past 10 years, these guidelines have been adapted to more restrictive transfusion criteria. In addition, the risks associated with transfusion and the growing economic constraints propagate a rationale for the definition of clear indications for transfusion and for quality management measures.

The use of human blood and blood-associated products was regulated by legislation in the EU for the first time in 1989 [1]. Members of the EU were encouraged to support voluntary blood donation on a complementary basis to achieve self-sufficiency in the production of blood products within the EU [2]. In 1994 and 1995, general agreements were reached on the processing of blood and blood components in the EU, resulting in improved safety of blood products [3, 4]. General recommendations for the development of national transfusion policies and guidelines on the clinical use of blood have also been developed by the World Health Organization (WHO), proposing the establishment of a National Committee on the Clinical Use of Blood in each country [5].

In the SANGUIS (safe and good use of blood) study, it has been demonstrated that there are still substantial differences within a country and between countries in the clinical use of red blood cells in the member states of the EU [6]. Thus there might be a lack of valid guidelines or insufficient implementation of guidelines in certain areas or hospitals.

I. Scharrer/W. Schramm (Ed.)
30th Hemophilia Symposium Hamburg 1999
© Springer-Verlag Berlin Heidelberg 2001

Table 1. Extract from the standardized protocol

Patient characteristics	Preoperation data	Operation data	Postoperation data (day 0)	Postoperation data (day 1 onward)
Sex	Use of anticoagulants:	Time of anesthesia	Administration of:	Administration of:
Day of birth	Cumarine	Time of surgery	Fresh frozen plasma	Fresh frozen plasma
Weight	Heparin	Administration of:	(auto/homo)	(auto/homo)
Height	Acetylsalicyl acid	Human albumin	Platelets	Autologous URBC
Day of surgery	Ticlopidine/clopidogrel	Fresh frozen plasma	Autologous URBC	Homologous URBC
Diagnosis (1, 2, 3, or 4)[a]	Use of erythropoietin	(auto/homo)	Homologous URBC	Laboratory data:
Associated diseases:	Iron supplementation	Platelets	Cell saver retransfusion	Coagulation parameters
Coronary heart disease	(i.v., s.c.)	Autologous URBC	Documented blood loss	Blood count
Liver disease	ABD:	Homologous URBC	Laboratory data:	Length of stay in:
Kidney disease	Hb value before first ABD	Documented blood loss	Coagulation parameters	ICU
	Hb value before second ABD	Use of a cell saver:	Blood count	Hospital
	Hb value before third ABD	Milliliters of saved blood		Survival
	Hb value before fourth ABD	Milliliters of retransfusion		Complications:
	ANH	Laboratory data:		Transfusion reaction
	Laboratory data:	Coagulation parameters		Infection
	Coagulation parameters	Blood count		Lung edema
	Blood count			Circulatory failure

ABD, autologous blood donation; auto, autologous; ANH, acute normovolemic hemodilution; Hb, hemoglobin; homo, homologous; i.v., intravenous; s.c., subcutaneous; URBC, units of packed red blood cells.

[a] 1, total hip replacement; 2, coronary artery bypass grafting; 3, hemicolectomy; 4, abdominal aortic aneurysm surgery.

Our aim was to investigate the actual utilization of blood products in the Federal Republic of Germany. The study was sponsored by the German Ministry of Health. In a multicenter retrospective, cross-sectional study, the clinical practice of transfusion in 30 hospitals was assessed and the compliance with current guidelines determined. Four surgical procedures that frequently require blood transfusions were selected, i.e., total hip replacement, coronary artery bypass grafting, hemicolectomy, and abdominal aortic aneurysm surgery.

Patients' records were analyzed using a standardized protocol, and all data regarding the transfusion of blood products, transfusion triggers, laboratory tests, complications, patient characteristics, medication, and preoperative health status were documented (Table 1). The use of preoperative blood donation programs and intraoperative blood saving was recorded. Furthermore, different outcome parameters (survival, length of stay in intensive care and in hospital) and the hematocrit value on the fifth postoperative day were also documented (Table 1).

We included 30 national hospitals of different categories (150–1500 beds) with different frequencies for a given surgical procedure per year.

Analysis of data primarily focused on decision-making for transfusion in the individual patient, the utilization of blood products, and the outcome of patients in the different hospitals. Economic evaluation of the utilization of resources together with the outcome parameters will allow to a sound cost-benefit analysis of the relevant transfusion practice to be established. Hence the agreement of clinical transfusion therapy with existing guidelines in the different hospitals can be assessed.

In conclusion, this study provides the necessary scientific basis for the implementation of guidelines on transfusion therapy and may allow an analysis of the economic impact of different transfusion practices.

References

1. Council Directive (89/381/EEC) of 14 June 1989 extending the scope of Directives 65/65/EEC and 75/319/EEC on the approximation of the provisions laid down by law, regulation or administrative action relating to proprietary medical products and laying down special provisions for medical products derived from human blood or human plasma. O.J.L 181 of 28.6.89. p. 44
2. Communication from the Commission to the Council, the European Parliament and the Economic and Social Committee on Blood Self-Sufficiency in the European Community. [COM(93) 198 final. Brussels, 25 May 1993. 13p.]
3. Communication from the Commission on Blood Safety and Self-sufficiency in the European Community. COM (94) 652 final. 21.12.1994. 23p.
4. Council Resolution of 2 June 1995 on blood safety and self-sufficiency in the Community (95/C 164/01). O.J. No C164.30.6.95. p. 1
5. WHO. Developing a national policy and guidelines on clinical use of blood – recommendations. Transfusion Today 1998; 37: 3–12. 7. Economic aspects in medicine.
6. Safe and good use of blood in surgery (SANGUIS) – Use of blood products and artificial colloids in 43 European hospitals. EUR 15398. G Sirchia et al. (eds). European Commission. 1994. 235p.

How Hemophiliacs View the Services Offered by »Bluter Betreuung Bayern e.V.«

Results of a Survey Carried Out for the Association's Tenth Anniversary

R. BACHHUBER, K.-H. FLEISCHER-KREIPL, W. SCHRAMM

Introduction

The survey aimed at reflecting upon and evaluating the advisory services offered by Bluter Betreuung Bayern e.V. (BBB), a service for hemophiliacs in Bavaria, Germany, and the form and content of the events it organizes. In addition, the survey was designed to establish how hemophiliacs view the BBB in general and what importance they attach to the advisory center.

Method

The questionnaire developed for the survey was sent out or handed out directly to hemophiliacs and their relatives.

Results

Of the approximately 400 questionnaires handed out, 39 (i.e., 10%) were filled in and returned. Of those who returned their questionnaires, 28 were male and 11 female, while 19 were hemophiliacs and 20 were relatives of hemophiliacs; they were aged between 14 and 67 years (median, 35 years).

A total of 50% of them had already made use of the services offered by the BBB in the field of social education and psychology, and all of them were »satisfied« or »very satisfied« with these services.

Only seven of the interviewees had not yet taken part in 1-day or weekend events organized by the BBB.

The manifold services offered by the BBB were widely approved of, and it seems that they meet the needs of the various subgroups, such as hemophilia patients, parents, hemophiliacs with human immunodeficiency virus (HIV), very well.

In order to evaluate the questions with open modalities, qualitatively categories were set up. While for parents the BBB serves mainly is a place where they can exchange information or meet and talk to others, for hemophiliacs it is more a place where they can feel safe and talk about their problems. Other important categories for hemophiliacs were: a link to medicine/to the hemophilia center, experts/competence, organizing events, the atmosphere of the events, providing support, indispensable representation/organization of hemophiliacs.

I. Scharrer/W. Schramm (Ed.)
30th Hemophilia Symposium Hamburg 1999
© Springer-Verlag Berlin Heidelberg 2001

Conclusion

On the one hand, the results of a survey such as this, which assumes that those affected are most familiar with their situation and needs, reflect what is already known; however, particularly when questions with open modalities are asked, such surveys help to gain a clearer idea of the needs of the different subgroups. Moreover, quality optimization strategies such as this help to foster the link between the counseling unit and its clients. Clients feel that they are taken seriously and that they are the main focus of all the unit's efforts. The BBB's work is obviously highly appreciated by its clients.

Alpha Tocopherol – A Medication with Few Side Effects for Treating Pain in Patients with Hemarthrosis

W. Kalnins, K. Vermöhlen, T. Wallny, W. Effenberger

Introduction

The effectiveness of vitamin E (alpha tocopherol) has been verified in patients with juvenile rheumatoid arthritis, with degenerative diseases (by W. Hunold and others), and with activated arthroses (by H. and M. Bartsch, among others). Since hemophilic arthropathy has much in common with the beforementioned diseases in terms of its course and pathophysiology, the question arose as to whether this substance might also have an effect in this patient group.

Patients and Methods

A total of 32 patients (2 female and 30 male patients, of which 25 had severe, 3 moderately severe, and 4 mild von Willebrand disease) took part in the double-blind, randomized, placebo-controlled study. Only patients with complaints in at least two joints and who received nonsteroidal antirheumatic (NSAR) medication at least occasionally were admitted.

These 32 patients received 2x600 mg vitamin E or placebo daily over a period of 10 weeks. The extent of movement of the patients' joints, the distance that could be walked without pain, the intensity of the pain, and improvements in activities of daily life (ADL) were measured. The patients were also asked about side effects such as increased frequency of bleeding or changes in the consumption of clotting concentrate.

It was also established whether NSAR treatment could be reduced or discontinued.

The study was carried out on patients at the Eifelhöhen Clinic in Marmagen and the Orthopedic Service of the Hemophilic Outpatients' Clinic at the Institute for Experimental Hematology and Blood Transfusion, University of Bonn. MOWIVIT capsules (Rodisma-Med Pharma) were used as medication. Each capsule contained 400 mg d-alpha tocopherol from natural vegetable oils. This corresponds to 600 I.U. vitamin E.

Note: When using synthetic vitamin E, which is often contained in other preparations, the dosage should be increased by 50%.

I. Scharrer/W. Schramm (Ed.)
30th Hemophilia Symposium Hamburg 1999
© Springer-Verlag Berlin Heidelberg 2001

Results

30 of 32 patients completed the study. 1 patient discontinued medication because he simultaneously took part in a study for a protease inhibitor and complained about an increased bleeding tendency, which we attributed to the protease inhibitor. 1 patient stopped seeing the doctor.

Vitamin E Group (*n*=20)

10 of 20 patients reported a reduction in pain, 9 of 20 patients said they had less trouble getting started in the mornings, and 8 of 20 patients reported improvements in ADL, e.g., climbing stairs. 9 of 20 patients were unable to establish a reduction in pain, fewer problems in getting started in the mornings, or an improvement in ADL.

6 of 10 ten patients in the group that reported a reduction in pain after taking vitamin E regularly took NSAR at the beginning of the study. 2 of these 6 patients were able to do without NSAR completely during the study period, while the other 4 were able to reduce the dosage of the NSAR medication by at least half, which, considering the hepatotoxic side effects of NSAR medicaments, is a positive result. In the group of 9 patients who did not report any reduction in pain while taking vitamin E, the consumption of NSAR remained unchanged.

A clear, objectifiable improvement in the extent of movement of the joints could not be ascertained; however, in view of the considerable joint changes that already existed, this would have been unlikely.

Placebo Group (*n*=12)

Of the 12 patients in this group, 10 completed the study. 2 patients reported a reduction in pain, 1 patient reported less trouble getting started in the mornings, and none of the patients reported improvements in ADL. 8 patients were unable to report any effect.

Discussion

Vitamin E is able to neutralize toxic, membrane-damaging oxygen radicals. In joint inflammation, increased numbers of cytotoxic radicals are formed in the joint in addition to cytokines and prostaglandins. Oxygen radicals destroy mesenchymal and cartilage cells by oxidation. The concentration of vitamin E in the synovial fluid of inflamed joints is lower than in healthy joints. Of the patients with hemophilic arthropathy, half of the group experienced a positive effect from taking vitamin E and, importantly, the dosage of NSAR and thus also its side effects could be reduced. This study shows that there is also an additional analgesic effect. Side effects from vitamin E have not yet been described in these dose rates.

Addendum: The antioxidative effect can probably be improved even further by a combination of vitamin E with vitamin C (EVINA 200 I.U. vitamin E plus 500 mg vitamin C). A hepatoprotective effect has even been discussed in connection with this vitamin combination. More than 30 patients at the Hemophilic Outpatients' Clinic in Bonn regularly take vitamin E preparations.

Neurosensorial Sequelae in Hemophilia

D. Mihailov, P. Tepeneu, K. Schramm, C. Petrescu, D. Lighezan, M. Pop, M. Serban

Introduction

Without adequate therapy, hemorrhage within the nervous system is the most frequent cause of mortality and morbidity and is also an important factor leading to sequelae in hemophiliacs of all ages. The neurological deterioration due to intrinsic bleeding within the central or peripheral nervous system is accompanied, with similar repercussions, by neurological adulteration due to an extrinsic compressive mechanism issued from juxtaneural hematomas.

Taking into account the therapeutic conditions in Romania (absence of the prophylactic therapy, inadequate doses and duration of therapy on demand, lack of factor concentrates in the majority of cases), we followed up patients with hemophilia or von Willebrand disease to assess the neurological manifestations due to nervous system bleeding (direct mechanism) and to nerve compression (indirect mechanism) and their long-term course in correlation with factors that depend on the patient (type of coagulopathy, severity, inhibitor status) and with factors that depend on the therapy (precocity and type of factor replacement therapy).

Patients and Method

The study was a retrospective study based on a group of 251 consecutive hemophilia and von Willebrand patients, registered and treated at the Timisoara Center of Hemophilia from 1989 to 1999.

A total of 76.10% of the patients had hemophilia A, 10.36% had hemophilia B, 1.19% had hemophilia C, and 12.35% had von Willebrand disease. Coagulopathy was severe in 53.0% of patients, moderate in 20.3%, and mild in 26.7%. On admittance, 0.4% of the patients were under the age of 1, 2.4% were aged 1–3 years, 9.9% were aged 3–6 years, 29.9% were aged 6–12 years, and 57% were older than 12 years.

The following parameters were recorded:
- Frequency and clinical symptoms
- Pathogenic mechanism
- Age of the patient at onset
- Evolution of neurological manifestations

I. Scharrer/W. Schramm (Ed.)
30th Hemophilia Symposium Hamburg 1999
© Springer-Verlag Berlin Heidelberg 2001

The study method consisted of the following:
- Physical examination (including neurological examination, ophthalmologic examination)
- Radiography (cranial, bone, abdomen)
- Echography (transfontanellar, abdomen)
- Computer tomography
- Examination of cerebrospinal fluid

Results

In our study group, neurological involvement was found in 52 patients (20.7%).

There were two different presumed pathogenic mechanisms of the neurological symptomatology (Table 1); it was due to either intrinsic bleeding within the nervous system (48% of patients) or to extrinsic compression of the hematoma located in the proximity of the nerve (52% of patients).

At the onset of neurological complications, 6.45% of the patients were younger than 1 month, 32.26% were between 1 month and 1 year, 16.13% were aged 1–3 years, 12.91% were aged 3–6 years, and 32.26% were older than 6 years.

All patients with neurosensorial sequelae had a severe form of coagulopathy.

Patients with inhibitors (16.17% in our study; 5.43% of them were low responders and 10.74% were high responders) were significantly less likely to recover full motor or sensory function than those without antibodies, and the time to full recovery in these patients was significantly longer.

A total of 18.80% of the patients with neurosensorial sequelae came from Timisoara.

Table 1. Pathogenic mechanism of the neurological symptomatology in patients with hemophilia or von Willebrand disease

Type	Patients (n)
Hemorrhage (direct action)	25
Cerebral	10
Extradural	2
Epidural	2
Subdural	3
Subarachnoidal	4
Ophthalmic	2
Otic	2
Compressive hematoma (indirect action)	27
Psoas	14
Arm	2
Forearm	3
Periorbital	5
Facial	3
Total	52

Table 2. Frequency and type of neurosensitive and neurosensorial sequelae

Sequelae	n	Frequency (proportion of patients) (%)	Frequency (proportion of total sequelae) (%)
Oligophrenia	4	1.60	11.77
First degree	(2)		
Second degree	(1)		
Third degree	(1)		
Epilepsy	8	3.18	23.53
Grand mal	(2)		
Petit mal	(6)		
Hydrocephalia	2	0.80	5.88
Progressive	(1)		
Stable	(1)		
Central paralysis	4	1.60	11.77
Hemiparesis	(1)		
Paraplegia	(1)		
Pyramidal syndrome	(1)		
Common oculomotor nerve	(1)		
Peripheral paralysis	8	3.18	23.53
Radial nerve	(1)		
Sciatic and femoral nerve	(3)		
Facial nerve	(2)		
Cubital nerve	(1)		
Lateral popliteal nerve	(1)		
Amyotrophic syndrome	2	0.80	5.88
Sensorial polyneuropathia	1	0.39	2.94
Deafness	1	0.39	2.94
Amblyopia	2	0.80	5.88
Hyperkinetic syndrome	2	0.80	5.88
Total	34	13.54	100

Twenty-two patients (42.30%) recovered fully from the neural damage; six of the patients (24%) with bleeding within the nervous system and 16 of the patients (59.25%) with juxtaneural bleeding had a complete remission of the symptoms. In 29 patients (55.77%), we observed long-term neurosensorial sequelae, 26 patients (89.65%) had one sequela, one (3.45%) patient had two sequelae, and two patients (6.90%) had three sequelae; 20 of them (68.96%) were hemophilia A, five (17.24%) hemophilia B, one (3.45%) hemophilia C, and three (10.35%) von Willebrand patients. One patient (1.93%) died due to a head trauma sustained in a car crash.

Neurosensorial sequelae were polymorphous (Table 2); epilepsy and peripheral paralysis occurred more commonly (23.53%), followed by oligophrenia and central paralysis (11.77%). We considered oligophrenia as a neurological sequelae only in patients who also had other neurological manifestations due to the hemorrhage or to the compressive hematoma (e.g., paralysis, epilepsy) at the same time.

Discussion and Conclusions

The medical literature from the last decade reflects how real the hemorrhagic risk is and the significant effect it has on the life and quality of life of hemophiliacs.

Despite the progress made in replacement therapy, the frequency of bleeding still remains high: 123 hemophilia A, hemophilia B, and von Willebrand patients who sustained head trauma between 1985 and 1992 in an American report [2], and 63 of 300 patients with 127 hemorrhagic episodes in an Latin American report [6].

The incidence of intracranial and extracranial bleeding in newborns with hemophilia is 3.58% [7] and is often associated with late neurological deficits; however, it is accepted that simple accidents during play are the most frequent cause of injury in children with coagulation disorders (>60%) [2].

Some cases draw attention to the often protean expression of the nervous system bleeding; this calls for sensitive nervous system imaging that can provide useful information for therapeutic decision-making. Immediate diagnosis and rapid medical management are mandatory if morbidity and mortality are to be minimized [2].

The majority of bleeding episodes in hemophilia patients occur within the musculoskeletal system, primarily in the joints, but approximately 30% occur within the muscles; recurrent iliopsoas muscle bleeding is common (14.2%). Neural involvement is found in almost 40% of cases [6].

In our study, the incidence of neurological complications was highest in children between the age of 1 month and 1 year and in those over 6 years (32.26%), and in most cases the mechanism of injury was a fall during play. One patient died due to a head trauma sustained in a car crash.

In conclusion, on account of the high frequency of neurological manifestations (20.7% in our study group) and the high rate of sequelae (55.77%), these complications warrant vigilant attention. They also call for hemophiliac families to be made aware of the need for rapid treatment of and for the diagnostic and the therapeutic attitude to be optimized in order to minimize the medical and symptomatic scale of handicaps due to late identification and treatment.

References

1. De Tezanos Pinto M, Fernandez J, Perez Bianco PR. Update of 156 episodes of central nervous system bleeding in hemophiliacs. Haemostasis 1992; 22 (5): 259–267
2. Dietrich AM, James CD, King DR, Ginn-Pease ME, Cecalupo AJ. Head trauma in children with congenital coagulation disorders. Journal of Pediatric Surgery 1994 Jan; 29(1): 28–32
3. Ray M, Ezhilarasan R, Marwaha RK, Marwaha N, Trehan A, Bapuraj JR. Facial nerve palsy in an infant with hemophilia A. Pediatr Hematol Oncol 1999 Jan-Feb; 16(1): 71–4
4. Guivarch M. Les hématomes du psoas iliaque. 29 observations. J Chir (Paris) 1997; 134(9–10): 382–9
5. Katz SG, Nelson IW, Atkins RM, Duthie RB. Peripheral nerve lesions in hemophilia. J Bone Joint Surg [Am] 1991 Aug; 73(7): 1016–9
6. Fernandez-Palazzi F, Hernandez SR, De Bosch NB. Hematomas within the iliopsoas muscles in hemophilic patients: the Latin American experience. Clin Orthop 1996 Jul; (328): 19–24

206 D. Mihailov et al.

7. Kulkarni R, Lusher JM. Intracranial and extracranial hemorrhages in newborns with hemophilia: a review of the literature. J Pediatr Hematol Oncol 1999 Jul-Aug; 21(4): 254–6
8. Leach M, Makris M, Hampton KK, Preston FE. Spinal epidural haematoma in haemophilia A with inhibitors – efficacy of recombinant factor VIIa concentrate. Haemophilia 1999 May; 5(3): 209–12
9. Friday RY, Pollack IF, Bowen A, Pollack A, Ragni M. Spontaneous spinal subdural hematoma in a young adult with hemophilia. J Okla State Med Assoc 1999 May; 92(5): 227–30
10. Schmitz A, Wallny T, Sommer T, Brackmann H-H, Schulze-Bertelsbeck D, Effenberger W, Kowalski S. Spinal epidural haematoma in haemophilia A. Haemophilia 1998 Jan; 4(1): 51–5
11. Chang C, Shen M. Mononeuropathy multiplex in hemophilia: an electrophysiologic assessment. Eur Neurol 1998 Jul; 40(1): 15–8
12. Ogawa K, Yoshida A, Ui M. Brachial plexus palsy presenting as an initial manifestation of hemophilia in a middle-aged man. J Shoulder Elbow Surg 1998 Sep-Oct; 7(5): 546–8
13. Zuckerman GB, Conway EE Jr. Neurologic complications of cancer, sickle cell disease, and hemophilia. Pediatr Ann 1998 Oct; 27(10): 640–50
14. Mizuguchi M, Kano H, Narita M, Chen RF, Bessho F. Weber syndrome caused by intracerebral hemorrhage in a hemophilic boy. Brain Dev 1993 Nov-Dec; 1

IX.b Poster: Thrombophilia

Effect of Vitamin Supplementation
in Venous Thrombosis Patients with Hyperhomocysteinemia

M. Krause, S. Ehrenforth, H.G. Koch, T. Vigh, A. Sewell,
I. Scharrer

Introduction

Venous thrombosis is a multifactorial disorder with an incidence of about 1–1.6 per 1000 population. In addition to the well-known risk factors for thrombosis (lack of AT or protein S/C, APC resistance or prothrombin mutation), other congenital and acquired disorders are also associated with an increased tendency to thromboembolic complications.

Hyperhomocysteinemia is an independent risk factor for both arterial and venous thrombosis [2]. The prevalence of hyperhomocysteinemia in the normal population is thought to be 5–10% compared to 18–25% in patients with venous thromboembolism [10]. The moderate form (30–100 mol/l) and the mild form (15–30 mol/l) of hyperhomocysteinemia occur in people with no disease who are heterozygous, with a prevalence of 0.4–1.5%, and in those with the thermolabile mutant of the MTHFR enzyme, which is the most common form of hyperhomocysteinemia with a prevalence of 5–20% [8]. The much more rare and more severe homozygous form of hyperhomocysteinemia occurs in 1:335,000 and is due to the absence of cystathionine-beta synthetase [1]. Meta-analysis studies show an odds ratio of 2.6 (95% CI; 1.8–3.8) for patients with venous thrombosis and hyperhomocysteinemia [3]. The relative risk of venous thrombosis rises 3.6-fold in patients in combination with an APC resistance [7].

It has also been shown [5] that patients with raised homocysteinemia run an increased risk of recurrent thrombosis compared to patients with normal homocysteine levels.

In addition to congenital causes of hypercysteinemia, lack of folic acid, vitamin B6 and vitamin B12 (all essential cofactors of homocysteine metabolism) also play a role. Supplementing folic acid, vitamin B6 and vitamin B12 can usually lead to a fall in homocysteine concentration in plasma, although folic acid alone or in combination with vitamin B12 is known to lead to a significant reduction in the homocysteine level (7% for vitamin B12, 25% for folic acid). It has not been possible to demonstrate a significant reduction using vitamin B6 alone [4,6] even though vitamin B6 is indispensable as cofactor in the transsulfuration in homocysteine metabolism [9]. As yet, no randomized placebo-controlled studies have been carried out to show the effect of vitamin supplements with regard to reduction or prevention of risk of recurrence of thrombosis.

I. Scharrer/W. Schramm (Ed.)
30th Hemophilia Symposium Hamburg 1999
© Springer-Verlag Berlin Heidelberg 2001

Patients and Methods

We examined the frequency of hyperhomocysteinemia in a group of 315 patients (193 women and 122 men) with venous thrombosis with a median age of initial onset of 38 years (range 15–70 years).

Enzyme immunoassay was used for estimation of homocysteine plasma levels, with a normal level for both men and women of 3.8–13.8 mol/l. In a randomized double-blind and placebo study, the patients with homocysteinemia were given vitamin supplements (with the combination: folic acid 2.5 mg, vitamin B6 25 mg and vitamin B12 250 g) or placebo, daily for 3–6 months. The homocysteine level, erythrocyte folic acid and serum vitamin B12 levels were measured before treatment or placebo, and again after 3 months and 6 months. The C677 T polymorphism of the MTHFR gene, the cystathionone-beta synthetase mutation (CBS), the APC resistance (APC-R; FV:R506Q) and the prothrombin G20210 A mutation (PT G20210 A) were also assessed. Patients were excluded who had illnesses directly associated with hyperhomocysteinemia. The objective of the study was to assess the effect of vitamin supplements on patients with venous thrombosis and hyperhomocysteinemia.

Results

Hypercysteinemia was present in 9.8% of patients with venous thrombosis (i.e. 31/315 patients: female 14/male 17). The median plasma homocysteine concentration was 18.5 1 mol/l (range 13.91–68.92 mol/l).

Of these 31 patients, 22 (11 men and 11 women) were given vitamin supplements as described (n=14, female 8/male 6) or placebo (n=8, female 3/male 5). Twenty-one patients had deep-vein thromboses, 6 (otherwise similar) had lung embolism, and 4 had recurrence; 1 patient had an arm vein thrombosis.

During the first 3 months 12/14 patients, and after 6 months 13/14 patients, showed a normalization of homocysteine plasma concentrations (tHcy females/males: 7.0/9.0 µmol/l) and in 1/14 patients a reduction of the initially raised level (tHcy 15.8 µmol/l). In the placebo group, 6/8 patients showed levels within the normal tHcy (mean female/male: 9.68/13.23) during the first 3 months (Fig. 1).

Serum vitamin B12 level was low in 5/22 patients before treatment: median 167 pg/ml (normal 220–1000 pg/ml), although 1/5 patients was homozygous and 3/5 were heterozygous for the C677T polymorphism of the MTHFR gene. One of the patients showed no change in vitamin B12 levels even though she was receiving B12 (Fig. 2).

Four of 14 patients showed initial low erythrocyte folic acid levels (normal 130–500 ng/ml) in the treatment group as well as 2/8 in the placebo group. Normal levels were achieved with vitamin supplements within the first 3 months (Fig. 3)

Of the 22 patients with hyperhomocysteinemia, 8 patients were homozygous and 7 were heterozygous for the thermolabile variant of MTHFR C677T, and 2 were

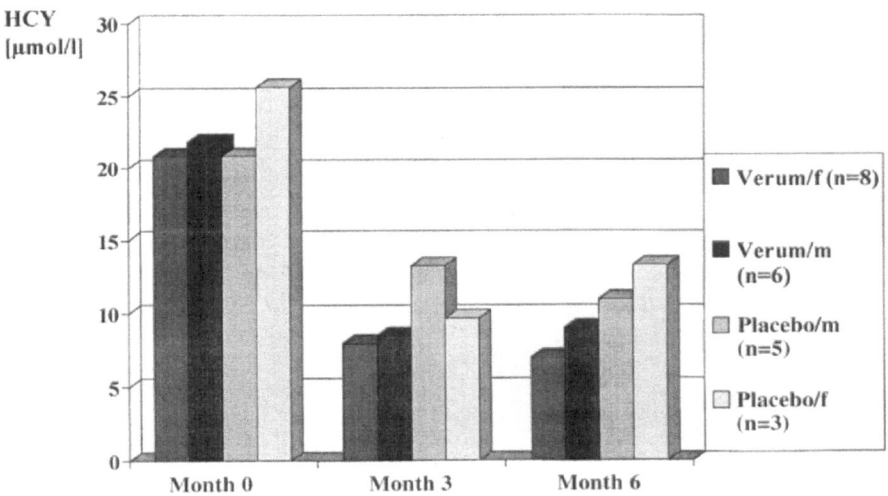

Fig. 1. Homocysteine plasma concentrations in the treatment- and placebo group

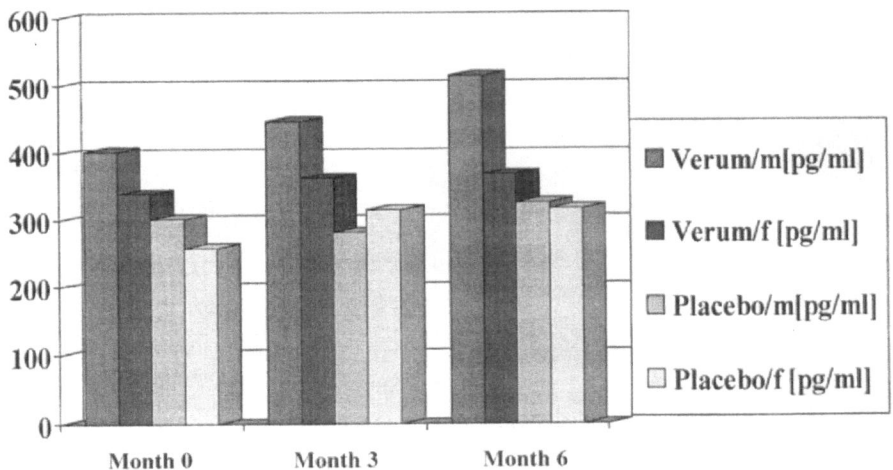

Fig. 2. Serum vitamin B_{12} levels in the treatment- and placebo group

heterozygous for the CBS mutation. A homozygote FV:R506Q mutation was present on 1 patient, and the reminder were homozygous for this gene. Two patients had heterozygous prothrombin G20210A. The combination of these defects are shown in Fig. 4.

No patient with hyperhomocysteinemia showed any further venous or arterial thromboembolic complications during the observation/treatment period.

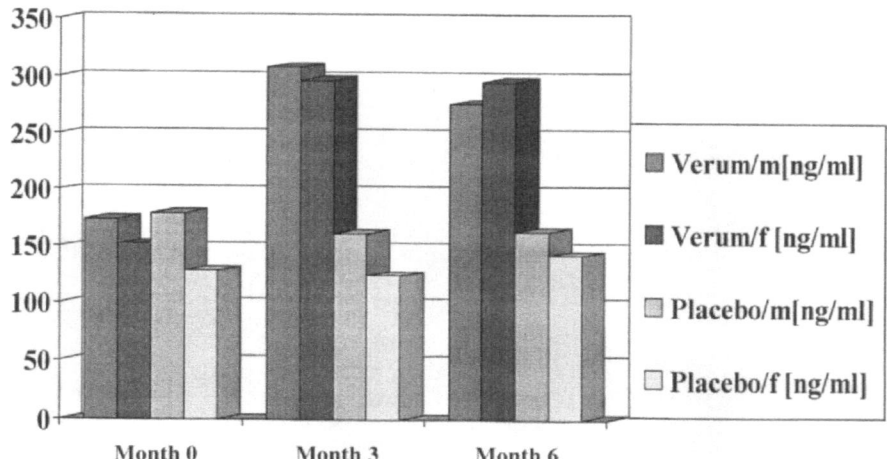

Fig. 3. Folic acid levels in the treatment- and placebo group

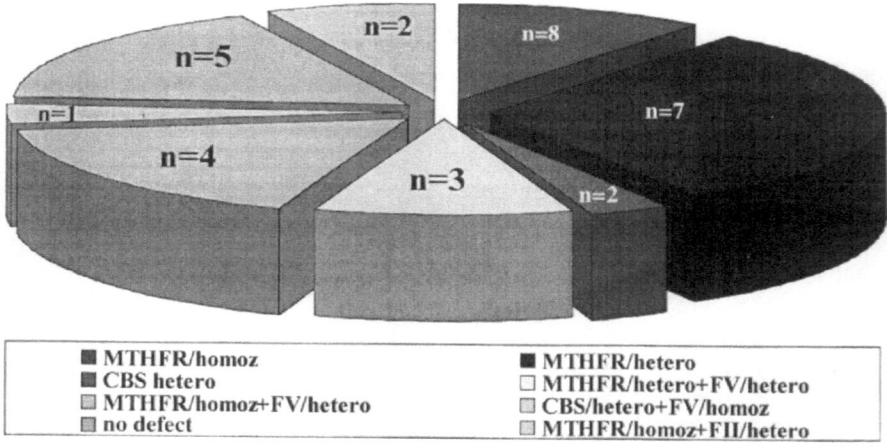

■ MTHFR/homoz	■ MTHFR/hetero
■ CBS hetero	☐ MTHFR/hetero+FV/hetero
☐ MTHFR/homoz+FV/hetero	☐ CBS/hetero+FV/homoz
▦ no defect	☐ MTHFR/homoz+FII/hetero

Fig. 4. Combined defects in patients with hyperhomocysteinemia

Discussion

In the group that we examined, it could be shown that supplementation with vitamins resulted in a reduction or normalization of the plasma homocystein level in all patients, regardless of whether or not a genetic disposition was present. An individual dietetic influence of vitamin substitution could not be excluded in the placebo group.

A combination of all three vitamins is needed to effectively lower the homo-cysteine level, raised by methionine breakdown. As homocystein metabolism needs the three essential cofactors, folic acid, vitamin B12 and vitamin B6, especially B6 which plays a critical role as cofactor in transsulfuration to cysteine, the combination of all three is vital for an adequate therapy of hyperhomocysteinemia [6]. The positive effect of the reduction of the plasma homocystein level has been shown in many studies, although the minimization of risk of further vascular effects is still unexplained. Prospective, randomized studies are needed to confirm the effect of vitamin supplements with regard to risks of thromboembolism, and the prevention of recurrent thrombosis.

Therapy and Prophylaxis of the Thromboembolic Syndrome in Pregnancy and Post Delivery

R. Klamroth, S. Gottstein, C. Heinrichs

Introduction

Thromboembolism is a dangerous complication during pregnancy and confinement. The risk for thromboembolism is increased six times for healthy females under these circumstances [3]. Fatal pulmonary embolism from deep vein thrombosis remains the main cause of death in females in labor [1].

Apart from well-known risk factors the physiologic increase of the thrombophilic potential contributes to the frequent occurrence of thromboembolism in pregnancy. In patients who had a thrombosis before and/or show a thrombophilic defect in hemostasis the risk for thromboembolism is even higher. After a previous thrombosis the risk of recurrence is 4% to 15% [2, 3].

Aim of the Study

We examined the effect of a risk-adapted therapy with low molecular weight heparin in woman during pregnancy and post partum for prophylaxis and treatment of thromboembolism. This therapy was preceded and monitored by laboratory controls of factors of hemostasis with known thrombophilic potential.

Patients

Twenty-four patients at the median age of 32 years (range 22–42) were treated; 1 patient was treated twice during two pregnancies. Sixteen women were pregnant for the first time, 5 had given birth once before, 2 twice before, and 1 three times previously.

The patients were referred to our thrombophilia center by the gynecological department of the Krankenhaus im Friedrichshain or by gynecologists in private practise.

The reasons for treatment before delivery were the following:
- Previous thromboembolism in 18 patients
- Acute thromboemboolism during pregnancy in 4 patients
- Primary thrombophilia in 2 patients

I. Scharrer/W. Schramm (Ed.)
30th Hemophilia Symposium Hamburg 1999
© Springer-Verlag Berlin Heidelberg 2001

Methods

The thrombophilia screening before treatment included the investigation of:
- Factor V mutation (Leiden)
- Prothrombin mutation
- Antithrombin activity and concentration
- Protein C activity
- Protein S activity
- Factor VIII activity
- Resistance against activated protein C (APCR)
- Fibrinogen concentration
- Lupus anticoagulant
- Anti-cardiolipin antibodies (IgG, IgM)
- Homocystein concentration
- Plasminogen-activator-inhibitor (PAI)

Follow-up examination were done on the factors known to be influenced by hormonal changes in pregnancy: protein S, factor VIII, fibrinogen, PAI, APCR.

Laboratory controls were continued until 6 weeks after delivery. All patients learned to perform subcutaneous self-injection.

The regimen for the prophylactic treatment was determined relating to individual risk factors. The injections were started from the 25th week of pregnancy at the latest. Reviparin was given twice daily and was monitored by measurement of antiXa-activity (Heptest) aiming at 2.5–4.5 ratio 4 h after injection.

Venous thrombosis during pregnancy was initially treated by the gynecologists with intravenous infusion of unfractionated heparin for 3–5 days adjusted to PTT; treatment was then continued with Reviparin twice daily aiming at Hep test 3.5–4.5 ratio.

All patients were treated until the 4th to 6th week after delivery; patients with thrombosis were treated until at least the 3rd month after delivery.

Results

The thrombophilia screening revealed:
- Heterozygote factor V mutation (Leiden) in nine patients
- Heterozygote prothrombin-mutation in two patients
- Protein S deficiency in three patients
- Protein C deficiency in one patient

Nine patients had none of the above listed thrombophilic defects. All of them showed pregnancy-related changes in protein S, fibrinogen, PAI or factor VIII. In five patients these changes were more pronounced and reached unphysiological levels, e.g., factor VIII activity elevated over four times of normal or protein S less than 50% of normal. These changes had normalized in all patients within 6 weeks after delivery.

The therapy with low-molecular-weight heparin was well tolerated. There were no complications concerning the technique of self-injection. Median period of therapy was 26 weeks (range 9–48 weeks).

No new thromboembolic complications, no bleeding complications, no premature deliveries or abortions, no clinical signs of osteoporosis and no heparin induced thrombocytopenia (HIT II) were seen.

None of the patients reported undesirable side-effects apart from superficial hematomas at the injection sites. All children were healthy after delivery.

Conclusions

Low-molecular-weight heparin is a well tolerated and efficacious substance for prophylactic and therapeutic treatment of thromboembolism during pregnancy and postnatal period. There are no obvious side effects in long-time use and subcutaneous application.

References

1. Koonin LM, Atrash HK, Lawson HW, Smith JC. Maternal mortality surveillance, United States, 1979–1986. MMWR CDC Surveill Summ. 1991; 40: 1–13
2. McColl MD, Ramsey JE, Tait RC, Walker ID, McCall F, Conkie JA, Carty MJ, Greer IA. Risk factors for pregnancy associated venous thromboembolism. Thromb Haemost 1997; 78: 1183–1188
3. Toglia MR, John GW. Venous thromboembolism during pregnancy. NEJM 1996; 335: 108–114

Is Factor V Leiden Associated with an Increased Risk for Fetal Loss?

P. Dulíček, L. Chrobák, I. Kalousek, L. Pešavová, M. Pecka,
P. Stránský

Introduction

Deep venous thrombosis is a serious but rare vascular complication during pregnancy and puerperium and pulmonary embolism is one of the most important causes of maternal mortality [10,15].

The physiological changes in hemostasis increase the risk of thromboembolism in pregnancy [16]. The risk is even higher in women with congenital thrombophilia [13, 6]. In 1993 Dahlbäck et al. [9] identified a new mechanism causing inherited thrombophilia, characterized by a poor anticoagulant response to activated protein C (APC resistance-APC-R). The molecular defect underlying this phenomenon was identified as an amino acid substitution at the cleavage site of factor V gene (1691 G to A) [2]. Point mutation in the FV gene is responsible for APC-R in more than 90% of cases [14]. APC-R without FV Leiden is called » acquired« APC-R and is usually found in the association with pregnancy [19], use of oral contraceptives [20] and in cancers [12]. This imbalance of the hemostatic equilibrium increases the life long risk of thrombosis five- to tenfold in heterozygous and 50- to 100-fold in homozygous [7]. In Caucasians, APC-R is the most common of the known inherited risk factors for venous thromboembolism (VTE) [8, 25]. Women with APC-R and FV Leiden have an eightfold increased risk of VTE in pregnancy [18].

A successful outcome of pregnancy requires an efficient uteroplacental vascular system. Congenital thrombophilia may lead to a hypercoagulable state. This state can cause placental infarctions. Placental infarctions can result in the following complications in pregnancy: abortion, intrauterine fetal growth retardation, premature delivery, preeclampsia, and intrauterine death [4]. Placental thrombosis was previously described not only in women with lupus anticoagulant, but also in women with antithrombin (AT), protein C and protein S deficiencies [23].

The reported early loss rate among recognized pregnancies is between 12% and 15% [24]. Approximately 5% of women have the experience of two or more consecutive abortions [3]. The recurrent fetal loss defined by at least three successive abortions affects 1–2% of women at the reproductive age [3].

The aim of our study was to assess the association of APC-R and FV Leiden with spontaneous abortion. A miscarriage was considered to be fetal loss before the 28th week of pregnancy, a stillbirth a termination of pregnancy after the 28th week. As mentioned above, the recurrent fetal loss was defined by at least three successive abortions.

I. Scharrer/W. Schramm (Ed.)
30th Hemophilia Symposium Hamburg 1999
© Springer-Verlag Berlin Heidelberg 2001

Materials and Methods

In 1996 we examined 500 blood donors (309 males, 191 females) to determine the prevalence of APC-R in the East Bohemian region. This prevalence has been found to be 1.6%. We assessed the association of APC-R and FV Leiden with spontaneous fetal loss in two cohorts of women.

A Retrospective Group

In this group we assessed the course of 255 pregnancies in 127 women with APC-R and FV Leiden (114 heterozygous, 13 homozygous) from 90 unrelated families. Diagnosis of APC-R and FV Leiden was made either in the laboratory work-up of women with personal history of thrombosis event or in the laboratory work-up of family members of individuals with personal history of thrombosis and with APC-R and FV Leiden. Characteristics of this group are shown in Table 1. All women with history of fetal loss were also tested for anticardiolipin antibodies (ACA), lupus anticoagulans (LA), protein C, protein S, and AT.

Table 1. Characteristics of females with APC-R and FV Leiden

No. of women	127
Mean age (years)	44
Age range (years)	21–70
No. of pregnancies	255
Mean age of pregnant women (years)	24
Age range of pregnant women (years)	18–37

A Control Group

In this group we evaluated the course of 171 pregnancies in 80 women without APC-R and FV Leiden. These women are relatives of individuals with history of thrombotic event and with diagnosis of APC-R and FV Leiden. Characteristics of this group are shown in Table 2. All women with the history of pregnancy loss were tested for ACA, LA, protein C, protein S, and AT.

Table 2. Characteristics of females without APC-R and FV Leiden

No. of women	80
Mean age (years)	42
Age range (years)	19–75
No. of pregnancies	171
Mean age of pregnant women (years)	24
Age range of pregnant women (years)	18–42

Methods

Blood samples were collected by venipuncture into plastic tubes containing either 1/10 volume of 3.8% sodium citrate for coagulation assays or 1/10 volume of 0.5 mol/l sodium EDTA for DNA extraction. After centrifugation (15 min at 2500 g) for prothrombin time (PT), activated partial thromboplastin time (aPTT) and AT assays or after double centrifugation (+10 min at 1500 g) for protein C, protein S, APC-R, and LA assays, citrated plasma was either analyzed immediately (PT, aPTT, LA) or stored at −70°C until analyzed (AT, protein C, protein S, APC-R). APC-R was determined by COATEST APC RESISTANCE kit (Chromogenix). Low response for APC-R was defined as SR<2.05 (SR = sensitivity ratio-clot time APTT+APC to aPTT without APC).

Protein C and protein S were determined by coagulation assays using STACLOT PROTEIN C and STACLOT PROTEIN S kits. AT was determined by Chromogenix assays using STA-STACHROM AT kit. All kits are from STAGO Diagnostics. To detect LA, the following assays were performed: PT, aPTT (PTT Automate, Stago D), aPTT with high sensitivity to LA (PTT-LA,STAGO D), TTIT (Tissue Thromboplastin Inhibition Time), dRVVT (diluted Russell's Viper Venom Time). A solid-phase immunoassay technique was used to quantify anticardiolipin levels. IgG level >10 U/ml and IgM level >7 U/ml were considered as positive results. PCR method was used for FV Leiden determination. Data were evaluated by software program NCSS 6.0.1. using Fisher's test for categorical variables.

Results

The Retrospective Group

Assessment of 255 pregnancies in 127 women with FV Leiden provided the results shown in Table 3. Stillbirths did not occur in any of these women. Protein C, protein S, and AT deficiencies were not found in any of 14 women with abortions. Antiphospholipid syndrome was diagnosed in one woman with recurrent abortions (positivity of LA and ACA). Frequency of women with abortion in this group is 11%. Frequency of abortions is 7%.

Table 3. The results in the retrospective group

No. of abortions	18
No. of women with abortions	14
Mean week of abortion	11
Week range of spontaneous abortion	6–26

The Control Group

The results from the cohort of women without FV Leiden are shown in Table 4. Stillbirths did not occur in any of these women. Protein C, protein S, and AT deficiencies were not found in any of 11 women with spontaneous abortions either.

Table 4. The results in the control group

No. of abortions	13
No. of women with abortions	11
Mean week of abortion	10
Week range of spontaneous abortion	6–18

Frequency of women with abortion in this group is 14%, and frequency of abortions is 8% (2–12%). Using Fisher's exact test we found no statistical difference between the frequency of women with abortions in the retrospective group and in the control group. We have not proven a statistical difference between frequency of abortions in women in these groups either.

Discussion

Since 1996 several reports have been published about the relationship between FV Leiden and fetal loss. These studies assessed either the association of FV Leiden with recurrent fetal loss or the association with miscarriages and stillbirths. EPCOT study (European Prospective Cohort on Thrombophilia) is the largest study which analyzed the risk of fetal loss in women with known thrombophilia. Researchers found that the odds ratios were 3.6 (95% CI 1.4–9.4) for stillbirths and 1.3 (95% CI 0.94–1.71) for miscarriages. The odds ratios were 2.0 (0.5–1.77) for stillbirths and 0.9 (0.5–1.5) for miscarriages in women-carriers of FV Leiden [21]. On the other hand, in Berkane's study, FV Leiden was not found to be a common risk for stillbirths [1]. The most recent prospective study performed in Sweden, comprising 2480 women with APC-R in early pregnancy, elucidated its obstetrics consequences. The presence of APC-R was unrelated to adverse pregnancy outcome apart from an eightfold increased risk of VTE [18].

Three recent case control studies documented a significantly increased prevalence of factor V Leiden mutation in women with recurrent fetal loss [5, 11, 22]. The increased prevalence was not found in the study done by Kotwal [17]. The discrepancies in these results may be explained by differences in selection criteria, including the ethnic origin of the study populations. Other potential causes for recurrent fetal loss, like chromosomal abnormalities, autoimmune disorders, endocrinologic diseases, infections and anatomic abnormalities should be eliminated as well. FV Leiden is a mild risk factor for thrombosis and is also a mild risk factor for recurrent pregnancy loss [3] but the majority of women who are carriers of FV Leiden will not experience a recurrent fetal loss.

Conclusion

Resistance to activated protein C and FV Leiden were not the risk factors for miscarriage and stillbirth in our study group. They have not been found to be the risk factors for recurrent fetal loss either.

References

1. Berkane A, Verdy E, Heim A et al. Does the Q^{506} mutation of factor V contribute to fetal loss or stillbirth? Thromb Haemost 1997; Suppl. 1: 759–60.
2. Bertina RM, Koeleman BPC, Koster T et al. Mutation in blood coagulation factor V associated with resistance to activated protein C. Nature 1994; 369: 64–7.
3. Brenner B. Inherited thrombophilia and pregnancy loss. Thromb Haemost 1999; 82: 634–40.
4. Brenner B, Mandel H, Lanir A et al. Activated protein C resistance can be associated with recurrent fetal loss. Br J Haematol 1997; 97: 551-4.
5. Brenner B, Sarig G, Weiner Z, Younis J, Blumenfeld Z, Lanir N. Thrombophilic polymorphism in women with fetal loss. Blood 1998; 92 [Suppl. 1]: 558a.
6. Conard J, Horellou MH, VanDreden P, Lecompte T, Samama M. Thrombosis and pregnancy in congenital deficiencies in AT III, protein C or protein S. Thromb Haemost 1990; 63: 319-20.
7. Dahlbäck B. Resistance to activated protein C, the Arg^{506} to Gln mutation in the factor V gene, and venous thrombosis. Thromb Haemost 1995; 73: 739–42.
8. Dahlbäck B. Inherited thrombophilia: resistance to activated protein C as a pathogenic factor of venous thromboembolism. Blood 1995; 85: 607–14.
9. Dahlbäck B, Carlsson M, Svensson PJ. Familial thrombophilia due to a previously unrecognized mechanism characterized by poor anticoagulant response to activated protein C; prediction of a cofactor to activated protein C. Proc Natl Acad Sci U.S.A 1993; 90: 1004–8.
10. Franks AL, Atrash HK, Lawson HW, Colberg KS. Obstetrical pulmonary embolism mortality. United States 1970–85. Am J Public Health 1990; 80: 720–2.
11. Grandone E, Margaglione M, Colaizzo D et al. Factor V Leiden is associated with repeated and recurrent unexplained fetal losses. Thromb Haemost 1997; 77: 822–4.
12. Green D, Maliekel K, Sushko E et al. Activated protein C resistance in cancer patients. Thromb Haemost 1997; Suppl 1: 316.
13. Hellgren M, Tengborn L, Abildgaard U. Pregnancy in women with congenital antithrombin III deficiency: Experience of treatment with heparin and antithrombin. Gynecol Obstet Invest 1982; 14: 127–41.
14. Hillarp A, Dahlbäck B. Activated protein C resistance. Vessels 1997; 3: 3–10.
15. Högberg U. Maternal mortality in Sweden. Thesis, Umea, Sweden 1985; 118.
16. Kjellberg U, Andersson NE, Rosen S, Tengborn L, Hellgren M. APC resistance and other haemostatic variables during pregnancy and puerperium. Thromb Haemost 1999; 81: 527-31.
17. Kotwal J, Saxena R, Mohanty S et al. APC resistance in recurrent fetal loss in the Indian population. Br J Haematol 1998; 103: 588.
18. Lindqvist PG, Svensson PJ, Maršál K, Grenner L, Luterkort M, Dahlbäck B. Activated protein C resistance (FV Q^{506}) and pregnancy. Thromb Haemost 1999; 81: 532–7.
19. Meinardi JR, Henkens CMA, Heringa et al. Acquired APC resistance related to oral contraceptives and pregnancy and its possible implications for clinical practice. Blood Coag Fibrinol 1997; 8: 152–4.
20. Olivieri O, Friso S, Manzato F et al. Resistance to activated protein C in healthy women taking oral contraceptives. Br J Haematol 1995; 91: 465–70.
21. Preston FE, Rosendaal FR, Walker ID et al. Increased fetal loss in women with heritable thrombophilia. Lancet 1996; 348: 913–16.
22. Ridker PM, Miletich JP, Buring JE et al. Factor V Leiden mutation as a risk factor for recurrent pregnancy loss. Ann Intern Med 1998; 128: 1000–3.
23. Sanson BJ, Friedrich PW, Simioni P et al. The risk of abortion and stillbirth in antithrombin-protein C and protein S deficient women. Thromb Haemost 1996; 75: 387–8.
24. Stirrat GM. Recurrent miscarriage I: definition and epidemiology. Lancet 1990; 336: 673–5.
25. Svensson PJ, Dahlbäck. Resistance to activated protein C as a basis for venous thrombosis. N Engl J Med 1994; 330: 517–22.

IX.c Poster: Molecular Biology

Congenital Deficiency of Vitamin K Dependent Coagulation Factors in Two Families: Evidence for a Defective Vitamin K-Epoxide-Reductase Complex

B. von Brederlow, A.H.E. Fregin, S. Rost, W. Wolz, W. Eberl,
S. Eber, E. Lenz, R. Schwaab, H.H. Brackmann, W. Effenberger,
U. Harbrecht, L.J. Schurgers, C. Vermeer, C.R. Müller,
J. Oldenburg

Introduction

Hereditary combined deficiency of the vitamin K-dependent coagulation factors II, VII, IX, X, Protein C and Protein S is a rare bleeding disorder that has been reported in only few families [1–11]. The phenotypic presentation of the disorder shows great variety. Levels of vitamin K-dependent proteins ranged from less than 1% to 50%. In some of the families the phenotype could be completely corrected by oral application of vitamin K [11, 12], whereas in other families even a high intravenous vitamin K dosage showed no effect [5, 7]. Notably, three families exhibited skeletal abnormalities [1, 9, 11], suggesting the involvement of vitamin K-dependent bone related proteins, such as osteocalcin and matrix Gla protein [13].

The phenotype is caused by a defect of the post-translational γ-carboxylation of selected glutamic acids in vitamin K-dependent proteins. γ-Carboxy-glutamic acids can bind calcium which is required for the attachment of these proteins to phospholipid membranes, the location of coagulation factor activation [14].

The carboxylase reaction is catalyzed by the γ-glutamyl carboxylase, an integral membrane enzyme located in the rough endoplasmatic reticulum. The corresponding gene is located on chromosome 2p1.2 [15] and contains 15 exons encoding a 758 amino acid polypeptide chain [16,17]. Vitamin K hydrochinone (KH_2) functions as a cofactor and is converted to vitamin K epoxide (KO) during carboxylation. To continue carboxylation, vitamin KO is regenerated to vitamin KH_2 by the vitamin K epoxide reductase (VKOR).

A hereditary deficiency of all vitamin K-dependent proteins may result from functional deficiency of either the γ-glutamyl carboxylase or the VKOR complex. So far, the molecular defect has been resolved in a single family, where a missense mutation in the gene coding for the γ-glutamyl carboxylase enzyme has been identified [1]. In a second family with additional signs of skeletal abnormalities evidence for a likely involvement of the VKOR complex has been reported [2].

Here we report another two families with recessively inherited combined deficiency of the vitamin K-dependent coagulation proteins. Molecular analysis of the γ-glutamyl carboxylase gene and determination of vitamin KO levels indicated that a dysfunction of a protein related to the VKOR complex is likely be causative for the disease.

I. Scharrer/W. Schramm (Ed.)
30th Hemophilia Symposium Hamburg 1999
© Springer-Verlag Berlin Heidelberg 2001

Materials and Methods

Coagulation Assays

Prothrombin, factor VII, IX and X were determined by one stage assays on a coagulometer Amax C160 (Sigma/Amelung) using commercial immunoadsorbed plasmas. Reagents were purchased from Dade/Behring (factors VII, IX, X) and Bio Merieux (Factor II). Protein C activity was measured on a Cobas Bio (Roche) with the Berichrom test from Dade/Behring.

Serum Vitamin K and KO

Blood was taken before and 5 h after oral substitution of 10 mg vitamin K (Konakion N Dragee, Hoffmann-La Roche) at the expected peak values for vitamin K and vitamin KO concentrations (C. Vermeer, personal communication). Encapsulated form was chosen to allow for easy application and standardized dosage. Blood was centrifuged and aliquoted portions of 1 ml serum were stored frozen at −70°C. Measurement of vitamin K and vitamin KO levels were performed by high performance liquid chromatography (HPLC) according to the method of Thijssen and Drittij-Reijnders [18].

Molecular Analysis of the γ-Glutamyl Carboxylase Gene

The 15 exons and their flanking regions of the γ-glutamyl carboxylase gene were screened for mutations using primers and PCR conditions indicated in Table 1. Both strands of the PCR templates were sequenced by the dideoxynucleotide chain termination method and the sequenase 2.0 DNA sequencing kit (US Biochemical).

Haplotypes of the γ-glutamyl carboxylase gene were constructed using two polymorphisms in exon 8 at nt8762 (Arg[CGA]325Gln[CAA]) and in exon 9 at nt9167 (Arg[CGT]406Arg[CGC]) that have been described by Wu et al [17]). Additionally, two novel polymorphic sites in the γ-glutamyl carboxylase gene that were detected in the families during sequence analysis were included. These polymorphic sites were located in exon 7 at nt7980 (Gly[GGC]379 Gly[GGA]) and in exon 9 at nt9191 (Pro[ACC]414 Pro[ACT]), respectively. All four polymorphic sites were investigated by PCR and direct sequence analysis.

Results

Clinical Presentation

Family A is of Lebanese origin. Pedigree analysis (Fig. 1A) revealed consanguinity of the parents (first-degree cousins). Eight children, seven female and one male, born between 1981 and 1997 are alive. Two children have died, one on day 3 after birth

Table 1. Primers and PCR conditions for sequencing of γ-glutamyl carboxylase gene

Exon No.	Annealing Temp. (°C)	Primer	Sequence 5'-3'
Exon I	65	E-I-F	GTT CAG ACG CGG CAG CTG TG
		E-I-R	CGG AGG GCG GGG TCC TAA G
Exon II	57	E-II-F	CCC CCG CAC ACA TAT TTT CT
		E-II-R	CCA AAT TGC TCC CAC CCA TA
Exon III	58	E-III-F	AGC TGA GGC CCA ATG ACC AA
		E-III-R	AGG CCA GTC AAT ATT TCC CA
Exon IV	54	E-IV-F	CTC TTA ATC CTC TCC CTA CA
		E-IV-R	TCC CCT TTG TCC CCC CTG AC
Exon V	54	E-V-F	CTC CCC CCT CCA ATG TTT AC
		E-V-R	TCC TCC CTC TGT CCT AAA AT
Exon VI	54	E-VI-F	TTT ATT CTT GCC TAT CTG TA
		E-VI-R	CTG CTT CTG CTG AAT AGG GA
Exon VII	56	E-VII-F	CTC CAG TGG GCT GGT GCT TG
		E-VII-R	TGT GGT TCC TGT TTC CTC CC
Exon VIII	55	E-VIII-F	GCC AAA CTC CTG AAA TAT GT
		E-VIII-R	GCC TTT GCT GTA CAC TCC AC
Exon IX	57	E-IX-F	CAG TGT GAG AAG CAT TGA GC
		E-IX-R	ACA AAA CCA GAC CCC AAA GC
Exon X	55	E-X-F	GGT GGG ACT AAT ATG GGG GT
		E-X-R	CTT GGT AAA AAG AAC TGT GCT
Exon XI	55	E-XI-F	CCT TAG GAA TGA TGA TGA AA
		E-XI-R	CAA AAA CAT TCC CTC TCC CC
Exon XII	59	E-XII-F	TGG GGT GGG ATG ATG AAC TC
		E-XII-R	TTA CTG GTG TGA GCT ACT GC
Exon XIII	52	E-XIII-F	ATT TAT CCA TTT CTT CTC CC
		E-XIII-R	CTA TCT CAG CCC AAA TGT TC
Exon XIV	59	E-XIV-F	AGG GGA TGA GAG TGA TCC ATC
		E-XIV-R	CCA GGG GAA AGT TAC CAA GC
Exon XV	59	E-XV-F	ACT TGG TCG GCT TTT TCC TG
		E-XV-R	CTA CAT CTG CAC CCA ACA TC

because of an intracerebral hemorrhage and one during the 1st year of life. Four children (A5, A6, A8, and A10) had experienced severe bleedings in the past. Two of them (A6 and A8) had been transfused with blood components. Patient A5 had received a ventriculoperitoneal shunt after the occurrence of an intracerebral bleed. In the last born boy, a hydrocephalus internus was diagnosed by ultrasonography as a result of an intracerebral bleeding at the beginning of the third trimester of gestation. A ventriculoperitoneal shunt has been implanted directly after birth. Today the boy is suffering from severe mental and physical retardation associated with blindness and epilepsy. No clinical abnormalities apart from those caused by the bleedings were present in any of the affected offspring.

Family B is of German origin. Pedigree analysis and family questionnaire showed no consanguinity. However, consanguinity cannot be ruled out since both mater-

Fig. 1A

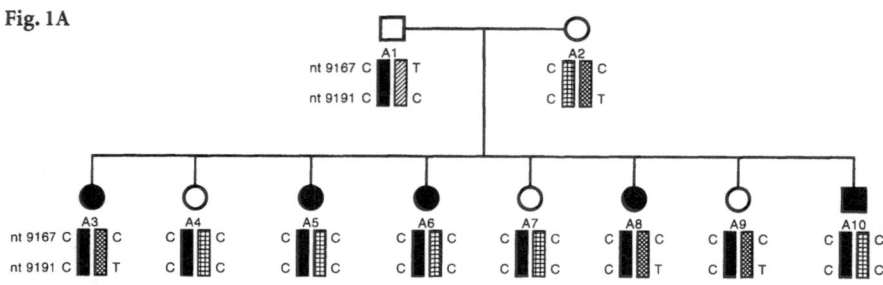

Fig. 1B

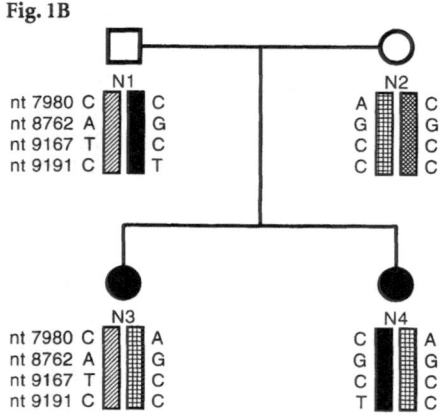

Fig. 1A+B. Haplotype analysis of the alleles of the γ-glutamyl-carboxylase gene in family A (fig. **A**) and family B (fig. **B**). The position of the polymorphisms are given by the nucleotide (*nt*) numbers according to Wu et al. [17]. The haplotypes are shown as *bars* and were constructed from the nucleotides that were found at the polymorphic sites by sequencing

nal and paternal grandparents originate from closely neighboring regions. The two female offspring were born in 1989 and 1993, respectively. After birth, the first born child (B3) developed a large cephal hematoma. At the age of 5 months a spastic paresis of the left body side was recognized. Further diagnosis revealed hydrocephalus internus caused by an intracerebral bleeding in the past. During the first years of life several episodes of epilepsy occurred. Mild mental and physical impairment is still present.

Levels of Vitamin K-Dependent Coagulation Factors

The levels of the vitamin K-dependent coagulation factors II, VII, IX, X and of Protein C are shown in Table 2. The affected individuals from family A (A3, A5, A6, A8, A10) and family B (B3, B4) showed a mild deficiency of these coagulation factors ranging from 20% to 60% of normal. Patients A3 and B4 appeared clinically asymptomatic and were diagnosed only by the laboratory values. In all other members of both families, especially in the parents, who are expected to be heterozygous carriers of the disease allele, normal levels of the vitamin K-dependent clotting factors were found. Pedigree data and consanguinity in at least one of the families suggest an autosomal recessive inheritance of the disorder.

Table 2. Vitamin K-dependent factor levels in affected (bold) and non-affected members of families A and B (family structure is shown in Figs. 1A and 1B)

(Normal Range)	A1	A2	A3	A4	A5	A6	A7	A8	A9	A10	B1	B2	B3	B4
II:C (70–130 U/dl)	114	127	63	103	40	59	88	42	105	79[a]	88	93	45	44
VII:C (70–130 U/dl)	97	102	47	76	20	55	98	45	79	62[a]	81	144	29	42
IX:C (70–130 U/dl)	125	120	66	142	52	99	91	40	111	51[a]	116	137	55	51
X:C (70–130 U/dl)	140	135	40	123	24	49	97	32	116	56[a]	111	140	33	30
PC:C (70–130 U/dl)	109	n.d.	56	112	61	80	101	43	n.d.	n.d.	91	113	60	55

[a]Measured several days after substitution of Vitamin K, basic coagulation factor levels were not available. n.d., not determined.

Table 3. Vitamin K-dependent factor levels in affected individuals 1 day after oral substitution of 5 mg (A5, A6, A8) and 1 mg (B3) Vitamin K, respectively

(Normal Range)	A5	A6	A8	B3
II:C (70–130 U/dl)	86	110	96	104
VII:C (70–130 U/dl)	77	107	101	90
IX:C (70–130 U/dl)	135	140	110	87
X:C (70–130 U/dl)	91	138	99	85
PC:C (70–130 U/dl)	n.d.	n.d.	n.d.	66

n.d., not determined

As shown in Table 3, the levels of all vitamin K-dependent proteins could be completely corrected by oral substitution of vitamin K. Measurement was carried out in family A after substitution of 5 mg vitamin K during 3 subsequent days and in family B after substitution of 1 mg vitamin K every other day.

Molecular Analysis of the γ-Glutamyl Carboxylase Gene

The phenotype of inherited combined deficiency of vitamin K-dependent proteins may be caused either by a defect in the γ-glutamyl carboxylase enzyme or a defect in the vitamin K epoxide reductase (VKOR) complex. We decided to start our investigation with the molecular analysis of γ-glutamyl carboxylase gene because the phenotype in both families presented here was similar to that of the family with the reported missense mutation in the γ-glutamyl carboxylase gene [1] with respect to phenotype correction by oral substitution of vitamin K. The only family with a suggested defect in the VKOR complex [2] showed only partial correction of the clotting factors by vitamin K substitution and also skeletal abnormalities.

All 15 exons with their flanking intron regions of the γ-glutamyl carboxylase gene were amplified by PCR and directly sequenced in at least one index patient of each family. No causative mutation could be found in the affected probands.

Since a genetic defect in the non-coding region of the γ-glutamyl carboxylase gene could not be excluded, haplotypes of the γ-glutamyl carboxylase gene were constructed to ascertain whether the phenotype in the families is segregating with one allele of the γ-glutamyl carboxylase gene.

For haplotype analysis, we investigated two known polymorphisms (exon 8 at nt8762 Arg[CGA]325Gln[CAA] and exon 9 at nt9167 Arg[CGT]406Arg[CGC]) that have been described previously by Wu et al [17], and two novel polymorphisms (exon 7 at nt7980 Gly[GGC]379 Gly[GGA] and exon 9 at nt9191 Pro[ACC]414 Pro[ACT]) that were detected in our study. As shown in Figs. 1A and 1B haplotype analysis excluded that the phenotype in both families co-segregates with the gene locus of the γ-glutamyl carboxylase.

Plasma Levels of Vitamin K and Vitamin KO

The finding of a normal γ-glutamyl carboxylase gene in both families points to a defect in a protein of the VKOR complex. To prove this hypothesis, affected and normal subjects of both families were supplemented with 10 mg vitamin K1. Blood was taken before and 5 h after oral drug intake at the expected maximum of plasma vitamin K and KO levels. The results are shown in Table 4. While vitamin KO is normally undetectable in serum, all tested individuals of both families with the disease phenotype showed highly increased vitamin KO levels ranging from 19.5 ng/ml to 59.7 ng/ml in family A and from 38.6 ng/ml to 66.2 ng/ml in family B. The vitamin K/KO ratio that includes the information on the vitamin K levels ranged between 2.4 and 4.3 in family A and 7.4 and 10.6 in family B. Vitamin KO could not be detected in the non-affected individuals of families A and B with the exception of individual B2 who exhibited a very low vitamin KO level (VK/VKO ratio 119.3). These findings indicate that a defect of the VKOR complex is likely to be causative for the deficiency of all vitamin K-dependent proteins in both families. These families therefore represent the second and the third kindreds in whom a defect in the VKOR complex explains a coagulation disorder.

Table 4. Serum concentrations of Vitamin K (VK) and Vitamin K epoxide (VKO) before and 5 h after oral substitution of a 10 mg vitamin K dragee. Affected individuals are in **bold**

	Basal serum concentrations (ng/ml)		Serum concentrations (ng/ml) 5 h after oral substitution of 10 mg vitamin K		
	VK	VKO[a]	VK	VKO	VK/VKO
A4	0.4	<0.05	201.8	<0.05	>1000
A5	**0.4**	**<0.05**	**84.6**	**19.5**	**4.3**
A6	**0.6**	**<0.05**	**219.6**	**52.6**	**4.2**
A7	0.4	<0.05	262.5	<0.05	>1000
A8	**n.d.**	**n.d.**	**147.0**	**59.7**	**2.5**
A9	n.d.	n.d.	607.3	<0.05	>1000
B1	0.5	<0.05	112.5	<0.05	>1000
B2	0.5	<0.05	310.3	2.6	119.3
B3	**0.7**	**<0.05**	**490.4**	**66.2**	**7.4**
B4	**0.4**	**<0.05**	**410.7**	**38.6**	**10.6**

[a]The detection limit of VKO is 0.05 ng/ml.
n.d., not determined.

Discussion

Variation of Phenotypes and Underlying Genetic Defects

The present study offers a detailed description of the phenotypes of two unrelated families with a combined hereditary deficiency of the vitamin K-dependent coagulation factors. Molecular analysis of the γ-glutamyl carboxylase gene and increased plasma levels of vitamin K epoxide in the affected probands indicated that a defect in a protein of the VKOR complex is the most likely cause of the disease phenotype. So far only 11 kindreds with a combined deficiency of vitamin K-dependent coagulation factors have been reported in the literature. Some important characteristics of these families are compared to our 2 kindreds in Table 5.

Such rare disorders with suggested autosomal recessive inheritance, occur predominantly in families with consanguineous marriage. However, only in two of the previously published families consanguinity is known [1, 11]. In our family of Lebanese origin consanguinity most likely contributes to the manifestation of the disease. In our second family we found no relation between the parental family branches, but, all grandparents came from a restricted local area. Therefore, a founder mutation may be present.

The degree of deficiency of vitamin K-dependent coagulation proteins varies considerably from very severe forms with activity levels of less than 5% to very mild forms, as in our families, with activity levels ranging from 20% to 60% (Table 5). Interestingly, in some of the families the coagulation factor deficiencies could be completely corrected by oral substitution of vitamin K whereas other families showed only partial or no response.

Table 5. Phenotype characteristics of published families with a combined deficiency of vitamin K-dependent coagulation factors

Reference	Consanguinity	Degree of Deficiency	Correction by Vitamin K	Skeletal Abnormalities	Cause of Phenotype
Fischer and Zweymuller 1966	n.k.	Severe	Partially	n.k.	n.k.
Chung et al. 1979, includes [22]	No	Severe	Partially	No	n.k.
Johnson et al. 1980	No	Mild	No	No	n.k.
Goldsmith et al. 1982	No	Mild	Yes	No	n.k.
Vincente et al. 1984	No	Severe	No	No	n.k.
Ekelund et al. 1986	n.k.	Severe	No	No	n.k.
Pauli et al. 1987, includes [23]	No	Moderate	Partially	Yes	VKOR
Leonard et al. 1988	n.k	n.k.	n.k.	Yes	n.k.
Pechlaner et al. 1992	No	Mild	n.k.	No	n.k.
Boneh and Bar-Ziv 1996	Yes	Moderate	Yes	Yes	n.k.
Brenner et al. 1998, includes [12]	Yes	Moderate	Yes	No	Carboxylase
present study	Yes	Mild	Yes	No	VKOR
present study	(No)	Mild	Yes	No	VKOR

VKOR, Vitamin K epoxidase reductase; n.k., not known or information not given

So far, in three of the families with a moderate to severe deficiency of coagulation factors [2, 9, 11] skeletal abnormalities were associated with the combined decrease of vitamin K-dependent proteins (Table 5). These skeletal abnormalities comprised irregular ossification, nasal hypoplasia, distal digital hypoplasia and mild conductive hearing loss, thus resembling the phenotype of warfarin embryopathy. In contrast, none of the four families with a milder form of the disease showed skeletal abnormalities. Although the phenotype may result from a primary pharmacological effect of coumarine derivates, the report of Pauli et al. (1987) provided evidence that warfarin embryopathy is secondary to the pharmacological effect of warfarin, e.g., inhibition of the VKOR.

In only two of the previously published families were some details of the pathomechanism discussed. Pauli et al. [2] found increased plasma levels of vitamin K epoxide in the affected proband that point to a defect in the VKOR-protein complex. Brenner et al. [1] showed that a missense mutation within the γ-glutamyl carboxylase gene was causative for the disease phenotype. Both families exhibited a moderate decrease of coagulation factor levels that was associated with skeletal abnormalities in case of the family with a putative defect of the VKOR.

Molecular analysis of the γ-glutamyl carboxylase gene and increased vitamin K epoxide levels in the affected probands in both of our families provided evidence that a defect in the VKOR must underlie the mild deficiency of all coagulation proteins. Thus, the families reported herein represent the second and third families with evidence for a defect in the VKOR. Purification and isolation of the VKOR enzyme has been attempted by several groups without success for many years. It now seems that the VKOR represents a multienzyme complex and that purification procedures destroy the protein integrity of this complex and subsequently the VKOR enzyme activity. According to a hypothetical model, the VKOR complex consists at least of the transmembraneous microsomal epoxide-hydrolase and a further protein originating from the glutathione-S-transferase super-family [19, 20]. In the two families reported herein we expect a molecular defect in one of these proteins.

Clinical Aspects

The genetic disorder in both of our families became clinically apparent by severe or even fatal perinatal intracerebral bleedings. Severe bleeding at birth is known to be associated with acquired conditions of combined deficiency of vitamin K-dependent coagulation factors. A hereditary cause is suggested to be extremely rare and may be masked if vitamin K substitution leads to a temporary normalization of coagulation factors. Mild reduction of vitamin K-dependent coagulation factors, at it was present in our families, may also complicate diagnosis.

Another aspect of clinical relevance is the question of vitamin K substitution in the affected individuals. The deficiency of coagulation factors is only mild and silent during every day life. However, there may be two arguments for a regular substitution of vitamin K:
- Bleeding complications, predominantly induced by trauma, might occur at a similar frequency as during oral anticoagulant therapy. Risk of bleeding could be completely prevented by substitution of vitamin K.

– In the previously published family with a defect in the VKOR [2] additional symptoms of skeletal abnormalities could be found.
Recently, Masciotte et al. [21] reported a decreased bone mineralisation in children receiving long-term oral anticoagulation therapy. In our families no skeletal abnormalities were clinically obvious. Nevertheless, it may be safe to substitute vitamin K in order to minimize risk of mineralisation deficits in the growing children.

In conclusion, the present study reports the second and third families with a defect in a protein of the VKOR-multienzyme complex. Future genetic analysis of these and further families with similar phenotypes by means of homozygosity mapping and analysis of candidate genes may be useful towards the identification of the causative gene defects and lead to a better understanding of the vitamin K pathway.

Summary

Hereditary combined deficiency of the vitamin K-dependent coagulation factors is a rare bleeding disorder. To date, only 11 families have been reported in the literature. The phenotype varies considerably with respect to bleeding tendency, response to vitamin K substitution and the presence of skeletal abnormalities, suggesting genetic heterogeneity. In only two of the reported families the cause of the disease has been elucidated as either a defect in the γ-carboxylase enzyme [1] or in a protein of the vitamin K 2,3-epoxide reductase (VKOR) complex [2].
Here we present a detailed phenotypic description of two new families with an autosomal recessive deficiency of all vitamin K-dependent coagulation factors. In both families offspring had experienced severe or even fatal perinatal intracerebral hemorrhage. The affected children exhibit a mild deficiency of the vitamin K-dependent coagulation factors that could be completely corrected by oral substitution of vitamin K. Sequencing and haplotype analysis excluded a defect within the γ-carboxylase gene. The finding of highly increased amounts of vitamin K epoxide in all affected members of both families indicated a defect in a protein of the VKOR-multienzyme complex. Further genetic analysis of such families will provide the basis for a more detailed understanding of the structure-function relation of the enzymes involved in vitamin K metabolism.

Acknowledgements. This study was supported by grants of the Stiftung Hämotherapie-Forschung, the Gesellschaft für Thrombose und Hämostaseforschung and the DFG (OI 100/3–1) to JO and CRM.

References

1. Brenner B, Sanchez-Vega B, Wu SM, Lanir N, Stafford DW, Solera J. A missense mutation in γ-Glutamyl Carboxylase gene causes combined deficiency of all vitamin K-dependent blood coagulation factors. Blood 1998; 92: 4554–4559

2. Pauli RM, Lian JB, Mosher DF, Suttie JW. Association of congenital deficiency of multiple vitamin K-dependent coagulation factors and the phenotype of the warfarin embryopathy: Clues to the mechanism of teratogenicity of coumarin derivates. Am J Hum Genet 1987; 41: 566–583

3. Fischer M, Zweymuller E. Kongenitaler kombinierter Mangel der Faktoren II, VIII und X. Zeitschrift für Kinderheilkunde 1966; 95: 309–323

4. Chung KS, Bezeaud A, Goldsmith JC, McMillan CW, Menache D, Roberts HR. Congenital deficiency of blood clotting factors II, VII, IX and X. Blood 1979; 53: 776–787

5. Johnson CA, Chung KS, McGrath KM, Bean PE, Roberts HR. Characterization of a variant prothrombin in a patient congenitally deficient in factors II, VII, IX and X. Br J Haematol 1980; 44: 461–469

6. Goldsmith GH Jr, Pence RE, Ratnoff OD, Adelstein DJ, Furie B. Studies on a family with combined functional deficiencies of vitamin K-dependent coagulation factors. J Clin Invest 1982; 69: 1253–1260

7. Vincente V, Maia R, Alberca I, Tamagnini GPT, Lopez Borrasca A. Congenital deficiency of vitamin K-dependent coagulation factors and protein C. Thromb Haemost 1984; 51: 343–346

8. Ekelund H, Lindeberg L, Wranne L. Combined deficiency of coagulation factors II, VII, IX and X: A case of probable congenital origin. Ped Hematol Oncol 1986; 3: 187–193

9. Leonard CO. Vitamin K responsive bleeding disorder: A genocopy of the warfarin embryopathy. Proceedings of the Greenwood Genetic Center 1988; 7: 165–166

10. Pechlaner C, Vogel W, Erhart R, Pümpel E, Kunz F. A new case of combined deficiency of vitamin K-dependent coagulation factors. Thromb Haemost 1992; 68: 617

11. Boneh A, Bar-Ziv J. Hereditary deficiency of vitamin K-dependent coagulation factors with skeletal abnormalities. Am J Med Gen 1996; 65: 241–243

12. Brenner B, Tavori S, Zivelin A, Keller CB, Suttie JW, Tatarsky I, Seligsohn U. Hereditary deficiency of all vitamin K-dependent procoagulants and anticoagulants. Br J Haematol 1990; 75: 537–542

13. Hauschka PC, Lian JB, Cole DE, Gundberg CM. Osteocalcin and matrix Gla protein: vitamin K-dependent proteins in bone. Physiol Rev 1989; 69: 990–1047

14. Sperling R, Furie BC, Blumenstein M, Keyt B, Furie B. Metal binding properties of γ-carboxyglutamic acid. J Biol Chem 1978; 253:3898–3906

15. Kuo WL, Stafford DW, Cruces J, Gray J, Solera J. Chromosomal localization of gamma-glutamyl carboxylase gene at 2p12. Genomics 1994; 25: 746

16. WU SM, Cheung WF, Frazier D, Stafford DW. Cloning and expression of the cDNA for human γ-glutamyl carboxylase. Science 1991; 254:1634–1636

17. WU SM, Stafford DW, Frazier D, Fu YY, High KA, Chu K, Sanchez-Vega B, Solera J. Genomic sequence and transcription start site for the human γ-glutamyl carboxylase. Blood 1997; 89: 4058–4062

18. Thijssen HHW, Drittij-Reijnders MJ. Vitamin K metabolism and vitamin K1 status in human liver samples: a search for inter-individual differences in warfarin sensitivity. Brit J Haematol 1993; 84:681–685

19. Cain D, Hutson SM, Wallin R. Assembly of the warfarin-sensitive vitamin K 2,3-epoxide reductase enzyme complex in the endoplasmic reticulum membrane. J Biol Chem 1997; 272: 29068–29075

20. Guenthner TM, Cai D, Wallin R. Co-purification of microsomal epoxide hydrolase with the warfarin-sensitive vitamin K1 oxide reductase of the vitamin K cycle. Biochem Pharmacol 1998; 55: 169–175

21. Masciotte P, Julian J, Webber C, Charpentier K. Osteoporosis: A potential complication of longterm warfarin therapy (abstract). Thromb Haemost 1999 (Suppl): 422

22. McMillan CW, Roberts HR. Congenital combined deficiency of coagulation factors II, VII, IX and X. N Eng J Med 1966; 274: 1313–1315

23. Hall JG, Pauli RM, Wilson KM. Maternal and fetal sequelae of anticoagulation during pregnancy. Am J Med 1980; 68: 122–140

Twenty-Two Novel Mutations
of Factor VII Gene in Factor VII Deficiency

K. Wulff, F.H. Herrmann

Introduction

The human FVII gene comprises 9 exon regions spanning 12 kb (O'Hara et al. 1986) and is located at chromosome 13q34. FVII is a modular protein similar to factors IX and X. FVII is synthesized with a 38 amino acid pre-pro leader sequence containing a hydrophobic translocation signal and a pro-sequence containing highly conserved residues important for gamma-carboxylation. Exon 2 encodes the propeptide and the Gla domain. The Gla domain is followed by a short hydrophobic region, referred to as the aromatic stack helix, that is encoded by exon 3. This exon links to the first and second epidermal growth factor-like (EGF) domains, encoded by exons 4 and 5, respectively. Exons 6 through 8 provide the genetic information for the activation and serine protease catalytic domain (Tuddenham et al. 1994). Hereditary factor VII deficiency is usually transmitted as an autosomal recessive disorder with an incidence of 1 per 500,000 in the general population. The hemorrhagic diathesis in affected patients can be highly variable and does not necessarily correlate with plasma factor VII activity levels (Ragni et al. 1981; Mariani et al. 1981; Triplett et al. 1985; Cooper et al. 1997). Plasma levels of factor VII vary significantly in the general population (Lane et al. 1992) due to genetic polymorphisms that are located in the promoter region and the exons of the FVII gene that encode for the mature protein (Green et al. 1991; Marchetti et al. 1993; Mariani et al. 1994). A number of reports have described the molecular basis of FVII deficiency. So far, 36 different mutations responsible for FVII deficiency have been characterized (Cooper et al. 1997; HGMD FVII data base) . In the »Greifswald study factor VII deficiency« we investigated the molecular basis for inherited factor VII deficiency in 64 unrelated patients from medical centers of Germany.

Materials and Methods

The study group consisted of 64 unrelated subjects with FVII activities from <1% to 41% of the normal range. The identification of patients with FVII deficiency and the analysis of the hemostasiological parameters were carried in the home hospitals (see Acknowledgements).

I. Scharrer/W. Schramm (Ed.)
30th Hemophilia Symposium Hamburg 1999
© Springer-Verlag Berlin Heidelberg 2001

DNA Isolation

Ten milliliters EDTA-blood was collected of patients with FVII deficiency. DNA was extracted of white blood cells by NaCl extraction method (Miller et al. 1988).

Mutation Detection

PCR primers for the FVII gene, derived from the FVII gene sequence of O'Hara et al. (1987), were designed and used for amplification of all coding regions and exon-intron boundaries of patients DNA. The polymerase chain reaction (PCR) was carried out in a 50 µl reaction volume containing 300 ng genomic DNA, 1 µmol/l external primers, 200 µmol/l of each deoxyribonucleotide, 5% dimethyl-sulfoxide (DMSO vol/vol) and 1.25 U Taq DNA polymerase in 1x reaction buffer (GIBCO-BRL). Samples were initially denatured for 3 min at 94°C and than amplified 30 cycles, each consisting of 40 s denaturing at 94°C, 40 s annealing at 58°C, 60°C, or 65°C, and 90 s extension at 72°C. A sample of the amplified DNA was electrophoresed on 2% NuSieve agarose gel.

Sequencing

The double-stranded PCR products were purified and concentrated in Microcon 100 concentrators (Amicon GmbH). The sequence reaction was performed as a cycle sequencing procedure using Taq Dye Deoxy-terminator Cycle sequencing kit (PE/Applied Biosystems). All sequences were determined at least twice.

Results

In »Greifswald study factor VII deficiency« the molecular defects in the factor VII gene in 64 unrelated individuals were detected. Thirty-two different mutations were analyzed in the coding regions or splice sites of the FVII gene (Table 1). Twenty-two of these mutations are novel, previously unreported mutations (Cooper et al. 1997, HGMD FVII data base 1999) that cause FVII deficiency. Twenty-nine (91%) lesions were single nucleotide-substitutions, 22 (69%) were missense mutations, 2 (6%) nonsense mutations, and 5 (16%) mutations occurred in the splice sites of exons 2, 4, and 7. Three (9%) mutations are deletions of one, four or 15 bp in intron 7 or in the catalytic domain of FVII in exon 8 (Table 1). The mutations were localized in different exon regions of the FVII gene (Wulff et al. 2000).
Fifteen of 32 reported mutations have been noted only once (Table 1); 12 (38%) of the mutations are transition within CpG dinucleotides, which are known as mutation hot spots.
   Fourteen of the identified mutations affected the protease domain of FVII, indicating that loss of protease function is the most common cause for the clinical phenotype. The most frequent lesion Ala294Val was detected in 21 unrelated

Table 1. Molecular defects in factor VII gene of inherited factor VII deficiency

Codon	Exon	Nucleotide no. and change	Amino acid change	CpG	Protein domain	No. mutant alleles/ no. un-related patients
−35	1a	10C>T	[a]Gln>stop	No	Pre-pro-leader	1/1
−20	1a	56T>C	[a]Leu>Pro	No	Pre-pro-leader	1/1
−17	1a	64G>A	[a]Val>Ile Splice site?	No	Pre-pro-leader	2/1
4	2	3832T>C	[a]Phe>Leu	No	Gla	2/1
IVS2+1	Intron 2	3935G>C	[a]Donor splice	No		1/1
IVS2+5	Intron 2	3938G>T	[a]Donor splice site	Yes		1/1
IVS3−1	Intron 3	5956G>A	[a]Acceptor splice site	No		1/1
60	4	5998T>C	[a]Ser>Pro	No	EGF 1	1/1
68	4	6023A>G	[a]Tyr>Cys	No	EGF 1	1/1
IVS4+1	Intron 4	6071G>A	Donor Splice site	Yes		2/1
94	5	7815G>A	[a]Glu>Lys	Yes	EFG 2	2/1
135	6	8909T>C	[a]Cys>Arg	No	Activation	3/2
152	6	8960C>T	[a]Arg>stop	Yes	Activation	2/2
152	6	8961G>A	Arg>Gln	Yes	Activation	1/1
156	6	8973G>A	[a]Gly>Asp	No	Activation	1/1
194	7	9683G>A	[a]Cys>Tyr	No	Activation	1/1
206	7	9717G>A	[a]Ala>Thr	Yes	Activation	2/2
9729–9732 del GGGT	Intron 7	Del 4 bp	Donor Splice site	No		1/1
213–217	8	10554–10568 del 15 bp	[a]Inframe	No	Catalytic	2/2
242	8	10641G>C	[a]Asp>His	Yes	Catalytic	1/1
244	8	10648C>T	Ala>Val	Yes	Catalytic	2/1
247	8	10656C>T	[a]Arg>Cys	Yes	Catalytic	1/1
252	8	10671G>A	[a]Val>Met	Yes	Catalytic	3/3
265	8	10710G>A	Gly>Lys	Yes	Catalytic	1/1
281	8	10758G>T	[a]Val>Phe	No	Catalytic	4/4
294	8	10798C>T	Ala>Val	No	Catalytic	21/19
298	8	10811G>A	Met>Ile	No	Catalytic	3/3
303	8	10825C>T	[a]Pro>Arg	No	Catalytic	4/4
310	8	10846G>T	Cys>Phe	No	Catalytic	2/2
343	8	10944G>C	[a]Asp>His	No	Catalytic	1/1
359	8	10993C>T	Thr>Met	Yes	Catalytic	1/1
404;294	8	11128delC; 10798C>T	Frameshift; Ala294 Val	No	Catalytic	6/5

[a]Novel mutation according HGMD data base FVII mutations, 1999.

patients in our study including one patient from Hungary and one patient from Romania. This mutation is also prevalent in Polish and Italian patients (Arbini et al. 1994; Bernardi et al. 1994), indicating that this represents the most frequent mutation in European populations.

A frequent novel mutation in the German population is the G>T transversion with substitution Val281 by Phe in exon 8 of the FVII gene. This mutation was detected in four FVII alleles of four unrelated probands in combination with the FVII mutations Cys135 Arg or Ala294 Val (three patients). In four unrelated patients the novel mutation Pro303 Arg was analyzed. This lesion in the catalytic domain was identified in two heterozygous probands with FVII activities of 29% and 48%.

It is known that clinical features of inherited FVII deficiency are quite variable. The correlation between reported coagulation activity and clinical bleeding tendency is rather poor. The clinical phenotype in patients is generally more severe in homozygous versus compound heterozygous patients whilst heterozygous are most asymptomatic (Herrmann et al. 2000).

Summary

Factor VII is a vitamin K-dependent coagulation protease essential for the initiation phase of normal hemostasis. The human factor VII spans 13 kb and is located on chromosome 13, 2.8 kb upstream of the factor X gene. We investigated in the »Greifswald study factor VII deficiency« the molecular basis for inherited factor VII (FVII) deficiency in 64 unrelated patients with FVII coagulant activities (FVII:C) <1% to 48%. All exons and exon-intron-boundaries of the FVII gene were amplified by PCR and directly sequenced. In 84 unrelated mutant FVII alleles were found 32 different independent FVII mutations; 22 of these lesions represent novel types of factor VII mutations, 29 (91%) lesions were single nucleotide-substitutions, 22 (69%) were missense mutations, 2 (6%) nonsense mutations, and 5 (16%) mutations occurred in the splice sites of the exons 2, 3, 4, and 7. Three (9%) mutations are deletions of one, four, or 15 bp in intron 7 or in the catalytic domain of FVII in exon 8. Whereas 15 mutations were noted only once, the missense mutation Ala294 Val in exon 8 was the most common mutation, causing deficiency in 21 FVII alleles of 19 unrelated patients. This study shows the great spectrum of different mutations as risen for FVII deficiency in Germany.

Acknowledgements. We thank our clinical co-workers for providing blood samples from patients with FVII deficiency and the report of clinical and hemostasiological data: Auberger, K./Munich; Auerswald, G./Bremen; Aumann, V./Magdeburg; Barthels, M./Hanover; Bergmann, F./Hamburg; Bergmann, K./Eisenach; Bratanoff, E./Erfurt; Eifrig, B./Hamburg; Franke, D./Magdeburg; Grundeis, M./Eisenach; Heinrichs/Bergen; Heinrichs, M./Berlin; Konrad, H./Rostock; Kreuz, W./Frankfurt; Lenk, H./Leipzig; Losonczy, H./Pecs, Hungary; Maak, B./Saalfeld; Marx /Hamburg; Mauz-Körholz/Düsseldorf; Pollmann/Münster; Reinhardt, U.-M./Greifswald; Scheel, H./Leipzig; Schenk, J./Homburg; Serban, M./Timisovare, Romania; Schobeß/Halle; Sutor, A./Freiburg; Syrbe, G./Stadtroda; Vogel, G./Erfurt; Vollmann, D./Aschersleben; Weinstock, N./Karlruhe; Wendisch, J./Dresden; Wenzel, E./Homburg; Wittenstein, B./Hamburg; Wolf, K./ Chemnitz.

References

Arbini AA, Bodkin D, Lopaciuk S, Bauer KA. 1994. Molecular analysis of Polish patients with factor VII deficiency. Blood 84: 2214–2220

Bernardi F, Castaman G, Redaelli R, Pinotti M, Lunghi B, Rodeghiero F, Marchetti G. 1994. Topologically equivalent mutations causing dysfunctional coagulation factors VII (294Ala→Val) and X (334Ser→Pro). Hum Mol Genet 3: 1175–1177

Broze GJ, Majerus PW. 1980. Purification and properties of the human coagulation factor VII. J Biol Chem 255: 1242

Cooper DN, Millar DS, Wacey A, Banner DW, Tuddenham EGD. 1997. Inherited factor VII deficiency: Molecular genetics and pathophysiology. Thromb Haemost 8: 151–160

Green F, Kelleher C, Wilkes H, Temple A, Meade T, Humphries S. 1991. A common genetic polymorphism associated with lower coagulation factor VII levels in healthy individuals. Arterioscler Thromb 11: 540–546

HGMDDatabase FVII Mutation 1999. htttp://europium.mrc.rpms.ac.uk/usr/WWW/WebPages/FVII/database.dir/referenc.htm

Herrmann FH, Wulff K, Auberger K, Aumann V, Bergmann F, Bergmann K, Bratanoff E, Franke D, Grundeis M, Kreuz W, Lenk H, Losonczy H, Maak B, Marx G, Mautz-Körholz C, Pollmann H, Schenk J, Serban M, Sutor H, Syrbe G, Vogel G, Weinstock N, Wenzel E, Wolf U. 2000. Molecular biology and clinical manifestation of hereditary factor VII deficiency. Semin Thromb Hemost, in press

Marchetti G, Petracchini P, Papacchini M, Ferrati M, Bernardi F. 1993. A polymorphism in the 5´ region of coagulation factor VII gene (F7) caused by an inserted decanucleotide. Hum Genet. 90: 575–576

Mariani G, Mazzucconi MG, Hermans J, Ciavarella N, Faiella A, Hassan HJ, Mannucci PM, Nenci GG, Orlando M, Romoli D, Mandelli F 1981: Factor VII deficiency: immunological characterization of genetic variants and detection of carriers. Br J Haematol 48: 7

Mariani G, Marchetti G, Arcieri P, Bernardi F.1994. The role of factor VII gene polymorphism in determining FVII activity and antigen plasma level. Blood 84: 86a

Miller M, Dykes DD, Polesky HF. 1988. A simple salting out procedure for extracting DNA from human nucleated cells. Nucleic Acids Res 16: 121

O'Hara PJ, Grant FJ, Haldemann BA, Gray CL, Insley MY, Hagen FS, Murray MJ. 1987. Nucleotide sequence of the gene coding for human factor VII, a vitamin K-dependent protein participating in blood coagulation. Proc Natl Acad Sci USA 84: 5158–5162

Ragni MV, Lewis JH, Spero JA, Hasiba U. 1981. Factor VII deficiency. Am J Hematol 10: 79–88

Triplett DA, Brandt JT, Batard MA, Dixon JS, Fair DS 1985. Hereditary factor VII deficiency: Heterogeneity defined by combined functional and immunochemical analysis. Blood 66: 1284

Tuddenham EGD, Cooper DN 1994. The molecular genetics of haemostasis an its inherited disorders. Oxford University

Wulff K, Herrmann F H. 2000. Twenty two novel mutations in factor VII deficiency. Hum Mutat, 15: 489–496

Prevalence of Common Mutations and Polymorphisms of the Genes of FII, FV, FVII, FXII, FXIII, MTHFR and ACE – Identified As Risk Factors for Venous and Arterial Thrombosis – in Germany and Different Ethnic Groups (Indians, Blacks) of Costa Rica

F.H. Herrmann, L. Salazar-Sanchez, K. Wulff, R. Grimm, G. Schuster, G. Jimmez-Aru, M. Chavez, W. Schröder

Introduction

Several genetic variants are currently identified as risk factors for venous and arterial thrombosis (deep venous thrombosis, myocardial infarction and stroke). Activated protein C resistance due to the factor V Leiden (FVL) and the 20210 G>A mutation in the factor II (FII, Prothrombin) gene are well-established causes of thrombophilia. Concerning the risk of myocardial infarction and stroke the results are different: There are studies reporting positive (Ma et al. 1996; Montaruli et al. 1996; Nabavi et al. 1998; Simioni et al. 1995; Arruda et al. 1997; Doggen et al. 1998; Rosendaal et al. 1997; Watzke et al. 1997; Corral et al. 1997) or neutral influences (Ardissino et al. 1996; Sanchez et al. 1997; Schröder et al. 1999; Corral et al. 1997; Kapur et al. 1997; Eikelboom et al. 1998; Ferraresi et al. 1997; Prohaska et al. 1999). The 677C>T mutation in the methylenetetrahydrofolate reductase gene (677C>T MTHFR), which caused a mild hyperhomocysteinemia is considered as a risk factor for coronary heart disease (Kluijtmans et al. 1996; Morita et al. 1997), venous thrombosis and stroke (Margaglione et al. 1998; Kluijtmans et al. 1999), but the results are controversial.

For some new variants of clotting factors FVII, F XII and FXIII associations with venous and arterial thrombosis were reported. Within FVII gene eight polymorphisms are known (Herrmann et al. 1998), three of them influence the level of FVII activity: the insertions polymorphism of the promoter (Marchetti et al. 1993), a tandem repeat unit polymorphism within intron 7 (O'Hara et al. 1988; Marchetti et al. 1991; de Knijff et al. 1994; Mariani et al. 1994) and the Arg353 Gln polymorphism of exon 8 (Green et al. 1991). Recently Iacoviello et al. (1998) have demonstrated in patients with myocardial infarction and family history of cardiovascular diseases, that the Gln353 allele of the Arg353Gln polymorphism and the H7 allele of the tandem repeat unit polymorphism of the hypervariable region 4 within intron 7 might have a protective effect on the risk of myocardial infarction. These alleles independently showed an effect in reducing the risk and both were associated with the lower levels of FVII (Iacoviello et al. 1998; Green et al. 1991; Mariani et al. 1994).

For the G>T transition in exon 2 of the FXIIIa subunit gene was recently reported a protective effect against myocardial infarction (Kohler et al. 1998a, b) and thrombosis (Franco et al. 1999; Catto et al. 1999), but an increased predisposition to primary intracerebral hemorrhage (Catto et al. 1998; Franco et al. 1999).

I. Scharrer/W. Schramm (Ed.)
30th Hemophilia Symposium Hamburg 1999
© Springer-Verlag Berlin Heidelberg 2001

For severe factor XII deficiency an increased predisposition has been reported for venous thromboembolic diseases and myocardial infarction. Some cohort studies have shown a high prevalence of slightly reduced FXII levels in patients of deep venous thrombosis or coronary heart diseases (Mannhalter et al. 1987; Halbmayer et al. 1992, 1994; Winter et al. 1995), but more association studies in this field are necessary. The recently described C>T mutation at nucleotide 46 in the 5'untranslated region of FXII (FXII 46C>T) (Kanaij et al. 1998) is associated with a diminished plasma FXII level and the role of this polymorphism as a thrombophilic risk factor is under discussion.

Recently new polymorphic markers of FV gene were described by the group of Bernardi (Bernardi et al. 1997b; Lunghi et al. 1996; Castoldi et al. 1997). A specific factor V gene haplotype (HR2) was defined by five restriction polymorphisms in exon 13 and a sequence variation located in exon 16. The exon 13 markers included the *RsaI* polymorphic site, the rare allele of which (R2) has been previously found to be associated with partial FV deficiency in the Italian population (Lunghi et al. 1996). The nucleotide change 4070 G>A underlying the R2 allele gives rise to an amino acid change His to Arg at position 1299. Bernardi et al. (1997) demonstrated that the FV gene marked by the HR2 haplotype, which was invariantly found to underlie the R2 marker, is both able to contribute by itself to determine a mild APC resistance phenotype and to interact synergically with the FV Leiden mutation Arg506Gln to produce a severe APC resistance phenotype. Carriers of the R2 allele are more frequent among patients of carotid endarterectomy (Marchetti et al. 1999) and the carriership of the R2 allele is associated with an increased risk for coronary artery disease (Hoekema et al. 1999) and venous thromboembolism (Faioni et al. 1999).

Many epidemiological studies have been performed to associate the presence (insertion, I) or absence (deletion, D) of a 287 bp Alu repeat element in intron 16 of the ACE gene to the level of the circulating enzyme or cardiovascular pathophysiology. Some reports have found that the D allele confers increased susceptibility to cardiovascular diseases and myocardial infarction, others found no such association or even beneficial effect (for references see Rieder et al. 1999; Ludwig et al. 1994; Lindpaintner et al. 1995). The same is true for cerebrovascular diseases, stroke or stenosis of carotids. Markus et al. (1995) reported that the DD genotype is a risk factor for lacunar stroke but not for carotid atheroma. However, the precise role of the I/D polymorphism is not clear, so more association studies are necessary.

In order to estimate the role of these factors mentioned above as risk factors in a certain population it is necessary to know their prevalences as far as they can vary widely in different populations worldwide (Perry et al. 1997; Sacchi et al. 1997; Kluijtmans et al. 1998; Rosendaal et al. 1998; Herrmann et al. 1999; Schröder et al. 1999; Song et al. 1999). Only few studies are known about its frequencies in different ethnic groups.

In this study we determined the prevalences of the following mutations/polymorphisms in different ethnic groups of Costa Rica (Indians, Blacks and Caucasians) and in healthy Germans: FII 20210G>A, FV Leiden, FV His1299 Arg (R2), FVII 73G>A, FVII Arg353 Gln, FVII repeat polymorphism in intron 7, FXII 46C>T, FXIII Val34 Leu as well as MTHFR 677C>T and the insertion/deletion polymorphism of the ACE gene.

Subjects and Methods

Blood samples were obtained from blood donors from Germany and Costa Rica (San Jose) as well as from different ethnic group from Costa Rica: Blacks from the area of Limon ($n=74$) and Guanacaste ($n=44$) and Indians from five tribes (Malecos, Bribri, Cabecar, Guaymi and Chorotegas).

DNA Extraction

Genomic DNA was extracted from blood samples by standard methods (Miller et al. 1988). For some analyses blood samples soaked onto filter paper cards from the probands were used for PCR as described previously (Schröder et al. 1996; Herrmann et al. 1997).

Determination of Mutations and Polymorphisms

FVL, FII 20210 G>A, MTHFR 677C>T

For the DNA analysis of the variants of FV, FII and MTHFR blood samples soaked onto filter paper cards from the probands were used for PCR. The analysis of the three molecular markers has been performed by standard methods by PCR and restriction analysis as described elsewhere (Bertina et al. 1994; Poort et al. 1996; Frosst et al. 1995).

Factor V HR2

The HR2 haplotype was analyzed by PCR amplification of the exon 13 RsaI polymorphic site and digestion with RsaI as described by Bernardi et al. 1997b. Primers were directed against nt 3579–3600 and nt 4280–4261 of the factor V gene sequence (Lunghi et al. 1996).

Factor XII 46C>T

The polymorphism 46C>T in the promoter (Kanaji et al. 1998) of the FXII gene was analyzed by PCR amplification and digestion with Hsp 92 I or directly by sequencing. Primer were designed from the FXII sequence (Cool and MacGillivray 1987).

FXIII Val 34 Leu

The 163G>T polymorphism caused an amino acid exchange of Val34 to Leu in exon 2 of the FXIII gene (Kohler et al. 1998b). This variation was analyzed by PCR amplification and heteroduplex analysis (Wulff et al. 1997). Two samples of the each genotype (G/G, G/T and T/T) were identified by direct sequencing of the PCR products.

ACE Insertion/Deletion Polymorphism

The analysis of the I/D polymorphism in intron 16 of the ACE gene was performed according to the protocols described by Rigat et al. (1992). To prevent mistyping of the DD genotype a second PCR with insertion specific primers was performed to control DD types as described by Odawara et al. (1997).

FVII Polymorphisms

Single Nucleotide Polymorphism 73G>A

By the 73G>A mutation a restriction site for *MspI* was destroyed. The novel polymorphism 73G>A in intron 1a (Herrmann et al. 1998) was analyzed by PCR amplification and digestion with *MspI* or directly by sequencing. Primers were designed from the FVII sequence (O'Hara et al. 1988).

Repeat Variation Within Intron 7

The hypervariable region 4 of intron 7 of the FVII gene was analyzed by PCR amplification according to a modification of Marchetti et al. (1991). Primer were designed from the FVII sequence (O'Hara et al. 1988). Five alleles were identified: a common allele with 6 monomers of 37 bp length (b), a less frequent allele with 7 monomers (a) and the very rare allele with five monomers (5) (Iacoviello et al. 1998), and the new variations with eight (8) and nine monomers (9).

Single Nucleotide Polymorphism Arg353 Gln

The polymorphism Arg353 Gln (Green et al. 1991) in exon 8 was analyzed by PCR amplification and digestion with *MspI* or by sequencing. PCR primers were designed from the FVII sequence (O'Hara et al. 1988).

Statistic Analysis

Allele frequencies were calculated by counting genes from the observed genotypes. The genotypes among different ethnic groups were determined and allele frequencies were compared by the chi-square test.

Results

The prevalence of various mutations and polymorphisms of cardiovascular risk factors were studied in blood donors from northeastern German and from blood donors from San Jose, Costa Rica, as well as from Indians and Blacks from Costa Rica. The allele frequencies and prevalence of their genotypes are summarized in Tables 1–3.

FV Leiden (Table 1)

Only 4 out of 195 Costa Rican blood donors carried the FV Leiden mutation in heterozygous form, which gives a prevalence of 2% (allele frequency of 0.01). In comparison to the study group of northeastern Germany (heterozygous prevalence

Table 1. Prevalences of mutations/polymorphisms of FV, FII and MTHFR in Germany and Costa Rica

| | Northeastern Germany Caucasians | | Costa Rica | | | | | |
| | | | Blood donors | | Indians | | Blacks | |
	n	%	n	%	n	%	n	%
FV Leiden								
Genotypes	170		195		143		117	
1691 G/G	159	93.5	191	97.9	143	100	117	100
1691 G/A	11	6.5	4	2.1	–	–	–	–
1691 A/A	–		–		–	–	–	–
Allele frequencies								
1691 G		0.967		0.990		1.00		1.00
1691 A		0.033		0.010	–	–	–	–
FV-HR 2 His 1299 Arg								
Genotypes	170		188		135		118	
R1R1	143	84.1	143	76.0	67	49.6	104	88.2
R1R2	27	15.9	43	22.9	63	46.7	13	11.0
R2R2	–	–	2	1.1	5	3.7	–	–
R1R3	–	–	–	–	–	–	1	0.8
Allele frequencies								
R1		0.921		0.875		0.730		0.941
R2		0.079		0.125		0.270		0.055
FII Prothrombin								
Genotypes	170		192		143		116	
20210 G/G	168	98.8	189	98.4	143	100	116	100
20210 G/A	2	1.2	3	1.6	–	–	–	–
20210 A/A	–		–	–	–		–	–
Allele frequencies								
20210 G		0.994		0.992		1.00		1.00
20210 A		0.006		0.008	–	–	–	–
MTHFR								
Genotypes	170		194		137		118	
677 C/C	84	49.4	85	43.8	7	5.1	62	52.5
677 C/T	73	42.9	64	33.0	55	40.1	42	35.6
677 T/T	13	7.7	45	23.2	75	54.8	14	11.9
Allele frequencies								
677 C		0.709		0.603		0.252		0.703
677 T		0.291		0.397		0.748		0.297

6.5%, allele frequency 0.03) the FV Leiden mutation is very rare in Costa Rica. It is significantly lower in Costa Rican blood donors than in German controls (χ^2=13.4, $p \leq$0.0002). None of the 143 Indians and 117 Blacks studied carried this mutation.

FV-His1299 Arg (HR2) (Table 1)

The R2 allele was found in 27 subjects among 170 German Caucasians (15.9%, allele frequency 0.079). Comparable to this is the R2 frequency in Blacks from Costa Rica (13 out of 118, allele frequency 0.055). However, the frequency is very different between Blacks from Limon (5.4% R1R2 heterozygous and Guanacaste 20.45% R1R2 heterozygous). In Blacks from Limon the very rare R3 allele could additionally be detected. It was already described by Lunghi et al. (1998) that this new R3 polymorphism His1254Arg mimics the R2 polymorphism His1299Arg in subjects of African origin.

In Costa Rica blood donors the prevalence of HR2 haplotype is significantly higher than in German controls (R2 allele frequency 0.125 versus 0.079, χ^2=3.9, $p \leq$0.045) but it was found to be extremely high in Costa Rican Indians (R2 allele frequency 0.270) compared to Germany (χ^2=39.9, $p \leq$0.001) and compared to Costa Rican blood donors (χ^2=21.9, $p \leq$0.001).

Heterozygous carriers for the R2 allele are extremely frequent in Indians (46.7%) and in the blood donors from Costa Rica; five homozygous (R2R2) in Indians and two among the blood donors were detected.

Because FV Leiden is absent in Indian and Black populations no compound-heterozygous could be detected. In northeastern Germany double heterozygote carriers comprise 1.76% of all subjects investigated, 11.11% of all R2 carriers or 27.27% of all FVL carriers.

FII 20210 G>A (Table 1)

The prothrombin mutation 20210G>A was found in 2 subjects among 170 Germans (prevalence of heterozygous 1.2%). Among the blood donors from Costa Rica we found 3 heterozygous out of 192 subjects (prevalence 1.6%). This mutation is absent in 143 Indians as well as in 116 Blacks.

MTHFR Mutation

The prevalence of the 677C>T MTHFR mutation in northeastern Germany and various ethnic groups of Costa Rica is given in Table 1. The allele frequency of the mutant allele in the blood donors and in the Blacks from Costa Rica is similar (677 T 0.397 and 0.297, respectively), but very high in Indians (0.748), being the highest prevalence in a population so far investigated. This frequency is significant different from the northeastern German population (χ^2=126.6, $p \leq$0.0001) and from the Costa Rica control group (χ^2=79.7, $p \leq$0.001).

Concerning the homozygous TT the prevalence in northeastern Germany is 7.7%, 23.2% in the group of blood donors from Costa Rica and 11.9% among the Blacks, but extremely high in the Indian population (54.8%).

FXII 46C>T Mutation (Table 2)

The allele frequency of the common genetic polymorphism (46C>T substitution) in the 5'untranslated region of factor XII was originally described to be 0.20 (Kainaji 1998). In the German population we have determined a similar allele frequency (0.19); 6.2% of all German subjects were homozygous for the 46 T allele.

In the Costa Rica the allele frequency of the 46 T allele is higher: 0.30 in the blood donor group (χ^2=5.2, p=0.022) and 0.25 in the Indian population. The highest allele frequency of 0.46 was determined in Blacks, which was significantly different

Table 2. Prevalences of mutations/polymorphisms of FXII, FXIII, ACE in Germany and Costa Rica

| | Northeastern Germany Caucasians | | Costa Rica | | | | | |
| | | | Blood donors | | Indians | | Blacks | |
	n	%	n	%	n	%	n	%
FXII								
Genotypes	97		55		84		114	
46 C/C	67	69.1	24	43.6	43	51.2	33	28.9
46 C/T	24	24.7	29	52.7	40	47.6	56	49.2
46 T/T	6	6.2	2	3.7	1	1.2	25	21.9
Allele frequencies								
46 C		0.814		0.700		0.750		0.535
46 T		0.186		0.300		0.250		0.465
FXIII								
Genotypes	276		57		57		117	
Val 34/Val34	144	52.1	22	38.6	29	50.1	67	57.3
Val 34/Leu34	112	40.6	33	57.9	18	31.6	47	40.2
Leu34/Leu34	20	7.3	2	3.5	10	17.5	3	2.5
Allele frequencies								
Val 34		0.725		0.67		0.67		0.773
Leu 34		0.275		0.33		0.38		0.226
ACE								
Genotypes	170		192		138		117	
II	31	18.2	38	19.8	96	69.6	14	11.9
ID	89	52.4	103	53.6	40	29.0	69	59.0
DD	50	29.4	51	26.6	2	1.4	34	29.1
Allele frequencies								
I		0.444		0.466		0.841		0.415
D		0.556		0.534		0.159		0.585

from the northeastern German and from the blood donors from Costa Rica (χc^2=36, 6, p>0.0001 and Cc^2=8, 31, p=0.0039). Among the Blacks 21.9% of all subjects were homozygous for the 46 T allele, whereas in the blood donors and in the Indians from Costa Rica only 3.7% and 1.2% were homozygous for the less frequent 46 T allele, respectively.

FXIII Val34 Leu Substitution (Table 2)

The allele frequency of the less frequent Leu34 allele of the Val34Leu FXIII polymorphism is almost similar in the various populations studied and ranges between 0.24 and 0.33. Differences were observed in the genotype frequencies. Homozygosity for the less frequent Leu34 allele was determined in 7.3% of the Germans, 3.5% of the blood donors and 2.5% of the Blacks of Costa Rica. But 17.5% of all Indians are homozygous for the Leu34 allele.

ACE I/D Polymorphism (Table 2)

Among the Germans the I and D alleles had frequencies of 0.44 and 0.56, respectively. These frequencies as well as the frequencies of the genotypes II, ID and DD (18.2%, 52.4%, and 29.4%, respectively) are virtually comparable to those previously published for European Caucasians or US whites (for references see Rigat et al. 1992; Lindpaintner et al. 1995; Ludwig et al. 1995).

In blood donors from Costa Rica allele frequencies (I:0.47 and D:0.53) and genotype frequencies (II:19.79%, ID:53.65% and DD:26.65%) are not significantly different from those found in the German control group. In Blacks no statistic significant differences were found compared to German or Costa Rica control group (I:0.41, D:0.59, II 12%, ID 59%, DD 34%).

In contrast, the frequency of the D allele is very low in Indians (I:0.84, D:0.16). Homozygous DD carriers are very rare in the population (II 69.6%, ID 29%, DD 1.4%). The differences in allele frequencies are statistically significant compared to German controls (χ^2=101.6, p≤0.001) or Costa Rica controls (χ^2=95, 7, p≤0.001).

Polymorphisms of F VII Gene (Table 3)

We have studied the prevalence of two well known frequent polymorphisms influencing the FVII activity as well as the recently described novel polymorphism within the promoter of the FVII gene:

FVII IVS1a Polymorphism 73G>A

The influence of the G>A transition at nucleotide 73 in the intron 1a (Herrmann et al. 1998) of the FVII level is nowadays unknown. In a control group of 95 unrelated Caucasians blood donors the frequency of the rare mutant allele (73 A) is

Table 3. Prevalence of FVII Polymorphisms in Germany and in ethnic groups of Costa Rica

	Northeastern Germany Caucasians		Costa Rica Blood donors		Indians		Blacks	
	n	%	n	%	n	%	n	%
FVII+73 G>A								
Genotypes	72		5		65		112	
73 G/G	53	73.6	34	66.7	65	100	70	62.5
73 G/A	19	26.4	16	31.4			36	32.1
73 A/A			1	1.9			6	5.4
Allele frequencies								
73G		0.87		0.824		1.00		0.79
73A		0.13		0.176				0.21
FVII Arg353Gln								
Genotypes	96		56		92		93	
Arg353Arg M1, M1	71	74.0	41	73.2	89	96.7	72	77.4
Arg353Gln M1, M2	22	22.9	14	25.0	3	3.3	19	20.4
Gln353Gln M2, M2	3	3.1	1	1.8	–	–	2	2.2
Allele frequencies								
Arg353 M1		0.854		0.857		0.984		0.88
Gln353 M2		0.146		0.143		0.016		0.12
FVII Intron 7 37 bp repeats								
Genotypes	76		49		94		115	
6/6 b/b	33	43.4	19	38.8	41	43.6	37	32.2
7/6 a/b	32	42.1	24	49.0	31	33.0	54	47.0
7/7 a/a	8	10.5	6	12.2	22	23.4	18	16.7
6/5 b/5	3	3.9	–	–	–	–		
8/6 8/b	–	–	–	–	–	–	4	3.5
8/7 8/a	–	–	–	–	–	–	1	0.9
9/6 9/b	–	–	–	–	–	–	1	0.9
Allele frequencies								
5		0.02	–	–	–	–	–	–
b		0.66		0.633		0.601		0.578
a		0.316		0.367		0.399		0.396
8	–	–			–	–		0.022
9	–	–			–	–		0.002

0.13. Heterozygous were found in 24.2% of all subjects, but only one individual was homozygous for the mutant alleles. In the Costa Rican blood donors and Costa Rican Blacks the 73 A allele frequencies are similar (0.18 and 0.21, respectively). In the group of Costa Rican Indians the 73 A is absent.

FVII Repeat Polymorphism in Intron 7

The repeat polymorphism of the hypervariable region 4 in intron 7 varied in our study between the investigated ethnic groups. The Costa Rican Indians had a higher prevalence (23.4%) of the A (6 repeat) allele in comparison to the Caucasians (10.5%), the Costa Rican blood donors (12.2%) and Blacks (16.7%). The five monomers with a high risk for myocardial infarction (Iacoviello et al. 1999) were only found in the German blood donors. The novel repeat polymorphisms of 8 and 9 monomers were found in the Blacks in a prevalence of 2.2% and 0.4%.

FVII Polymorphism Arg353 Gln

The Arg353Gln substitution is caused by a G>A mutation in exon 8 of the FVII gene. In the German control group the frequency of the mutant Gln353 allele (M2) is 15%.

The allele frequency of the mutant allele M2 is 14% in the Costa Rican control group and 12% in Blacks. The Gln353 allele is less frequent (2.0%) in Indians. None homozygous mutant genotype M2 was found among the Indians.

Because from each Indian tribe blood samples of only a relatively small number of individuals were screened further studies are necessary to determined the prevalence of the polymorphism in the various tribes of Indians and in the different populations of Blacks from Costa Rica. It seems that for some polymorphisms (MTHFR, ACE) intertribal heterogeneity exists, which might be caused by the isolation of small groups and a high degree of consanguinity. These studies are under way.

Discussion

The prevalence of various mutations and polymorphisms of vascular risk factors was studied in blood donors, Indians and Blacks from Costa Rica and compared with the results from northeastern Germans. Concerning the prevalence of DNA polymorphisms of these risk factors there are clear differences in Indians and Blacks of Costa Rica compared with Caucasian populations.

The FV Leiden mutation and the 20210 A mutation of prothrombin are known in Caucasians as risk factors for venous thrombosis (thrombophilia) and discussed as risk factor for arterial thrombosis. Both polymorphisms are absent in Indians and Blacks. In contrast to the absence of these polymorphisms the recently described His1299Arg polymorphism of the FV gene haplotype HR2 is more frequent in blood donors of Costa Rica and extremely high in Indians. Carriership of the R2 allele (1299 Arg) is associated with lower APC resistance (Bernardi et al. 1997b; Hoekema et al. 1999) and interacts with the FV Leiden mutation to produce a severe APC resistance phenotype (Hoekema et al. 1999; Faioni et al. 1999; de Visser et al.1999; Schroeder et al. 1999).The R2 allele seems to be associated with carotid artery disease (Marchetti et al. 1999), coronary artery disease (Hoekema et al. 1999) and venous thrombosis (Faioni et al. 1999; Mingozzi et al. 1999). In Indians and blood donors of Costa Rica seven homozygous for the R2 allele were also determined. Hoekema et al. (1999) have shown in an APC resistance test, quantifying the ability of FV to act as cofactor in APC-catalyzed FVIII(a) inactivation, that the APC sensitivity ratios for homozygous carriers are significantly lower than in controls.

These data indicate that R2-FV has reduced ability to act as a cofactor in the APC catalyzed FVIII(a) inactivation. This may provide a mechanistic explanation for the increased risk for coronary artery disease. Whether the observed homozygosity of the R2 allele in Indians and controls of Costa Rica is associated with a higher risk has to be estimated in further clinical studies which a larger number of homozygous individuals.

In 1 out of 119 Blacks the very rare R3 allele was determined. This polymorphism was firstly described in subjects of Somali (6 out of 40 persons) and in 1 out of 146 Greek Cypriots. This new R3 polymorphism mimics the R2 polymorphism in subjects of African origin (Lunghi et al. 1998).

The extremely high prevalence of homozygous for the mutant allele of the 677C>T polymorphism of the MTHFR gene in Costa Rica (Indians and blood donors) is remarkable, particularly under the point of view that homozygosity is discussed as a risk factor for cardiovascular diseases caused by mild homocysteinemia. Clinical studies are necessary to clear up the influence of this genotype on the prevalence of CVD in various ethnic groups and in relation to their different life style.

Several case reports of severe FXII deficient subjects with thrombotic events or myocardial infarctions, cohort studies and case control studies (Goodnough et al. 1983; Mannhalter et al. 1987; Halbmayer et al. 1992; Winter et al. 1995; Pandita et al. 1997) have reported an increased predisposition to vascular thrombosis. Other authors did not find a decrease of FXII as determinant of thrombosis (Koster et al. 1984; Lämmle et al. 1991; von Känel et al. 1992) and coronary artery disease (Kelleher et al. 1992; Merlo et al. 1994; Kohler et al. 1999).

The recently described FXII 46 C>T mutation diminished the plasma FXII level in homozygous and heterozygous carriers in comparison with normal individuals, homozygous tend to have lower levels than heterozygous. The decreased translation efficiency of the mutant messenger RNA causes these low plasma FXII levels (Kanaii et al. 1998). The FXII 46C>T mutation exhibits an ethnic variability that might contribute to the racial differences observed in FXII plasma levels. In Orientals the FXII level is lower than in Caucasians; the allele frequency of 46 C/T was estimated to be 0.27/0.73 in Orientals, and 0.8/0.2 in Caucasians. Franco et al. (1999) observed an allele T frequency of 0.25 in Whites and 0.32 in Blacks ($n=19$) and Mulattos ($n=15$).

In our study the observed allele frequency in northeastern Germany (0.186) is in the range of other Caucasians (Kohler et al. 1999, 0.28; Kanaij et al. 1998, 0.20). In Costa Rica we determined a significant higher frequency for the FXII46 T allele in blood donors in comparison to the German population (0.300 versus 0.186). The frequency in Indians is in the normal range 0.250. However, the highest frequency of 0.465 for the 46 T Allele was observed in the studied Black populations. About half of the control population of Costa Rica as well as of the Indians and Blacks are heterozygous, and homozygosity of the mutant allele is extremely high in the Blacks, more than 20% are homozygous. That is the highest rate reported until now.

The role of this mutation as a risk factor in these populations is unclear and further studies are necessary. The possibility of interactive effects of FXII mutation with other genetic effects associated with vascular thrombosis/coronary artery disease has to be studied. Franco et al. (1999) discussed that this mutation alone is probably not a major risk factor for venous thrombotic disease. Recently, Zeerleder et al. (1999) have shown that hereditary partial and probably severe FXII deficiency does not constitute a thrombophilic condition.

The factor XIII Val34Leu polymorphism was originally described in a Finnish population with a 34 Leu allele frequency of 0.23 in 600 normal controls. Similar frequency is reported from other Caucasian populations (Mikkola et al. 1994; Suzuki et al. 1996; Kohler et al. 1998a, b; Balogh et al. 1999). In healthy South Asians the frequency of the protective 34 Leu allele was less frequent (0.13) than in Whites (0.289) (Kain et al. 1999). Recently, Franco et al. (1999) have detected the allele frequencies in different ethnic groups of Brazil. The allele frequency among Whites (0.267%) was similar to the reported frequencies in other Caucasians. On the basis of a relatively small number of Blacks (n=19) and Mulattos (n=15) the allele frequency of 0.205 was calculated. In our studies we are able to study the frequency in large groups of Caucasians (Germany) and Indians and Blacks from Costa Rica. Our data showed a significantly increased frequency among the Indians. The homozygous state of FXIII 34 Leu was found to have an extremely higher prevalence among Indians (17,5) compared to other studied groups from Costa Rica (2.5% in Blacks, 3.5% in blood donors).

From several studies it is known, that homozygosity of the 34 Leu allele bears a strong protection against myocardial infarction (Kohler et al. 1998a), intracerebral hemorrhage (Catto et al. 1998), as well as venous thrombosis (Catto et al. 1999; Franco et al. 1999; Rosendaal et al. 1999). These findings support the hypothesis that the factor XIII34Leu is involved in the production of weaker fibrin structures, which might thereby protect against clot formation and predispose to hemorrhage (Kohler at al. 1998; Catto et al. 1999). The mechanism underlying this protective effect is still unclear. The FXIII 34 Leu variant gives rise to increased FXIII specific activity (Aware et al. 1999). Rosendaal et al. (1999) described activities for FXIIIGG (Val Val) of 96%, FXIII GT (Val Leu):131% and FXIII TT (Leu Leu): 152%.

McCormack et al. (1998) determined in healthy Caucasian control subjects 41% heterozygous and 7% homozygous and a mutant allele frequency of 0.28. In Pima Indians from the Gila River Indian Community in Arizona a higher prevalence of the protective mutation was found (48% heterozygous, 16% homozygous, mutant allele frequency 0.40). In Asian Indians a lower prevalence of the mutation was determined (17.5% heterozygote, 3.75 homozygote, allele frequency 0.13) (Nelson et al. 1990; Dhawan et al. 1994). In both Pima and Asian Indians populations there is a high incidence of type II diabetes (Nelson et al. 1990; Dhawan et al. 1994). Non insulin-dependent diabetes is associated with a high risk of myocardial infarction (MI) in Caucasians. In Asian Indians the incidence of MI is correspondingly high (Marmot et al. 1985). However the Pima Indians have a low incidence of fatal coronary heart disease (CHD) despite the world's highest reported prevalence of type II diabetes, suggesting vascular disease is not an inevitable consequence of diabetes, and genetic and environmental factors must cause the differences in disease prevalence. According to McCormack et al. (1998) the observed differences in factor XIII genotype frequencies suggest that the mutation might contribute to the contrasting cardiovascular risk in these populations.

In the Indians the frequency of the D-allele of the ACE polymorphism was very low in comparison to the Blacks, blood donors and the German control group. This deletion allele is known as risk factor for CHD. Because of the low prevalence, this factor seems not to be important as a risk factor in Indians.

Epidemiological studies have shown that high blood levels of FVII were associated with an increased risk of ischemic heart disease. Many environmental and biochemical factors influence the plasma level of FVII. Age, gender, body mass index, insulin resistance, use of oral contraceptives have been associated with FVII levels (Balleisen et al. 1985). Dietary fats and blood lipids are important determinants of FVII levels (Miller et al. 1991; Hoffman et al. 1992; Mennen et al. 1996). Recent studies have demonstrated that three polymorphisms of the FVII gene can directly influence the FVII levels and also modulate its response to environmental stimuli. Iacoviello et al. (1998) have recently demonstrated in patients with myocardial infarction and family history of CVD, that the alleles 353Gln and H7 of the Arg353Gln and the hypervariable region 4 (HRV4) polymorphism, respectively, had a protective effect on the risk of MI. The alleles showed an independent effect in reducing the risk and were both associated with low levels of FVII.

The Gln allele frequencies of the Arg353Gln polymorphism in Northeastern Germany, blood donors and Blacks of Costa Rica were similar to those described by other studies (Bernardi et al. 1996; Bernardi et al. 1997a; Di Castelnuovo et al. 1998). However the frequency of this allele was very rare in Indians (0.020). Such low frequency is known from North European populations at high risk of myocardial infarction (de Maat et al. 1997; Lane et al. 1992; de Knijff et al. 1994.) Individuals with the Gln Gln genotype have a decreased risk for myocardial infarction, they have the lowest level of FVII activity and FVII antigens in comparison to the Arg Gln and homozygous Arg genotype (Iacoviello et al. 1998). Recently, Iacoviello et al. (1999) has shown, that smoking, which was confirmed as an important risk factor for myocardial infarction, was much less so in subjects carrying the 353Gln allele. Among 92 Indians no homozygote Gln Gln genotype was found. Concerning the HVR4 polymorphisms it is known, that the combined H7H5 and H6H5 genotypes were associated with the highest risk, followed in descending order by the H6H6, H6H7 and H7H7 genotypes (Iacoviello et al. 1998). The prevalence of the H7 allele is in a similar range (0.32/0.37) in the studied populations of Germany and blood donors of Costa Rica and slightly higher in Indians and Blacks (0.40/0.396), but the H7H7 genotype is very high in Indians (23.4%) and Blacks (16.7%) in comparison to Germans (10.5%) and blood donors of Costa Rica (12.2%). In Indians the potential higher risk, caused by the absence of the protective homozygous Gln genotype seems to be compensated by the high frequency of the H7H7 genotype.

The 353Gln variant of the FVII gene has consistently been associated with lower levels of FVII in white Europeans (Humphries et al. 1994), Gujarati Indians (Lane et al. 1992), Afrocaribbeans in Britain (Lane et al. 1992; Temple et al. 1997) and Japanese (Kario et al. 1995).

Conclusions

Cardiovascular diseases and venous thrombosis are multifactorial diseases. Risk factors resulting from genetics, environment and behavior. The concept of the multicausal disease has received much attention in the last years. One of the reasons is that some of the genetic risk factors concern single point mutations that are quite common in the general populations. The search for molecular risk factors remains intensive. There are known molecular factors that increase the relative risk for the disease, and others that have protective effects. The genetic background is given by the combination of all these molecular markers and their interaction. The general risk is then the result of the interaction of this genetic background with the common environmental risk factors (e.g. surgery, use of contraceptives, pregnancy, etc. for thrombosis and dietary habit, mild hyperhomocysteinemia, age, sex, smoking, etc. for CVD). We need more information about the relationship between the genetic background, common risk factors, and clinical phenotype.

Our studies have shown, that there are clear differences in the genetic background of different populations/subpopulations in Costa Rica. In Indians the prevalence of some established risk factors is lower than in Caucasians (D allele of ACE) or absent (FV Leiden, FII polymorphism), and on the other side protective mutations have a higher prevalence (FXIII 34 Leu, FVII H7H7). However, concerning the FVII polymorphism the protective genotype H7H7 was extremely frequent in Indians, but the protective homozygous 353Gln genotype was absent.

These results indicate, that we have to detect not only one molecular risk factor for determination of the risk/predisposition for a given disease, but we have to study a panel of these molecular risk factors as genetic background for trying to answer the questions for genetic predisposition of a subject. Additional clinical studies are necessary to study the influence of the different genetic background in relation to the environmental factors for the prevalence of cardio- and cerebrovascular diseases in the given population. It is known that the dietary habits modify the relationship between homocysteine level and MTHFR mutation as well as triglyceride levels and FVII polymorphism for example. Under these circumstances the study of the life style of the subpopulations and ethnic groups should be very useful for understanding the differences in the epidemiology of diseases between these populations.

Summary

Several genetic variants are currently identified as risk factors for venous and arterial thrombosis (deep venous thrombosis, myocardial infarction and stroke). The factor V Leiden (FVL) and the 20210 G>A mutation in the factor II (FII, Prothrombin) gene are well established causes of thrombophilia, concerning the risk of myocardial infarction and stroke but the results are different. The 677C>T mutation in the methylenetetrahydrofolate reductase gene (677C-T MTHFR) is considered as a risk factor for coronary heart disease, venous thrombosis and stroke, but the results are controversial. For some new variants of clotting factors FV, FVII,

FXII and FXIII associations with venous and arterial thrombosis were reported. Many epidemiological studies have been performed to associate the presence (insertion, I) or absence (deletion, D) of a 287 bp Alu repeat element in intron 16 of the ACE gene to cardiovascular pathophysiology. Some reports have found that the D allele confers increased susceptibility to cardiovascular diseases and myocardial infarction, others found no such association or even beneficial effect.

In order to estimate the role of these factors mentioned above as risk factors in a certain population it is necessary to know their prevalences as far as they can vary widely in different populations worldwide. Only few studies are known about its frequencies in different ethnic groups.

In this study we determined the prevalences of ten different mutations/polymorphisms in healthy Germans and in different ethnic groups of Costa Rica: (Indians, Blacks and Caucasians): FII 20210G>A, FV Leiden, F V His1299 Arg (R2), FVII 73G>A, FVII Arg353 Gln, FVII repeat polymorphism in intron 7, FXII 46C>T, FXIII Val34 Leu as well as MTHFR 677C>T and the insertion/deletion polymorphism of the ACE gene.

There are well-known molecular factors which increase the relative risk for the disease and others who have protective effects. The genetic background is given by the combination of all these molecular markers and their interaction. The general risk is the result of the interaction of this genetic background with the common environmental risk factors (e.g., surgery, use of contraceptives, pregnancy, etc. for thrombosis and dietary habit, mild hyperhomocysteinemia, age, sex, smoking, etc. for CVD). Our studies have shown, that there are clear differences in the genetic background of the populations from Germany and Costa Rica. In comparison to the German population the prevalence of established risk factors in Indians are lower (D-Allele of ACE) or absent (FV Leiden, FII polymorphism), and on the other side protective mutations have a higher prevalence (FXIII34Leu, FVII H7H7). However, concerning the FVII polymorphisms the protective genotype H7H7 was extremely frequent in Indians, but the protective homozygous 353Gln genotype was absent.

The reported differences of the prevalences of risk and protective factors in the populations indicate, that we have to analyse a panel of molecular markers as genetic background for the determination of the genetic predisposition.

References

Anwar R, Gallivan L, Edmonds SD, Markham AF. Genotype/phenotype correlations for coagulations factor XIII: specific normal polymorphisms are associated with high or low factor XIII specific activity. Blood 1999; 93: 897–905

Ardissino D, Peyvandi F, Merlini PA, Colombi E, Mannucci PM. Factor V (Arg506→Glu) mutation in young survivors of myocardial infarction. Thromb Haemost 1996; 75: 701–701

Arruda VR, Annichino-Bizzacchi JM, Goncalves MS, Costa FF. Prevalence of the prothrombin gene variant (nt20210 A) in venous thrombosis and arterial disease. Thromb Haemost 1997; 78: 430–3

Balleisen L, Bailey J, Epping P-H, Schulte H, van de Loo J. Epidemiological study on factor VII, factor VIII and fibrinogen in an industrial population: I. baseline data on the relation to age, gender, body-weight, smoking, alcohol, pill-using, and menopause. Thromb Haemost 1985; 54: 475–9

Balogh I, Póka R, Pfiegler G, Dékány M, Bereczky Z, Muszbek L. Prevalence of genetically determined major thrombosis risk factors in Eastern-Hungary. Thromb Haemost 1999; 82 (Suppl) 667

Bernardi F, Aricieri P, Chiarotti F, Corral J, Pinotti M, Prydz H, Samama M, Sandset PM, Strom R, Vincente Garcia V, Mariani G. Contribution of factor VII genotype to activated FVII levels. Differences in genotype frequencies between northern and southern european populations. Arterioscler Thromb Vasc Biol 1997a; 17: 2548–53

Bernardi F, Faioni EM, Castoldi E, Lunghi B, Castaman G, Sacchi E, Mannucci PM. A factor V gene component differing from factor V R506Q contributes to the activated protein C resistance phenotype. Blood 1997b; 90: 1552–1557

Bernardi F, Marchetti G, Pinotti M, Aricieri P, Baroncini C, Papacchini M, Zepponi E, Ursicino N, Chiarotti F, Mariani G. Factor VII gene polymorphisms contribute about one third of the factor VII level variation in plasma. Arterioscler Thromb Vasc Biol 1996; 16: 72–7

Bertina RM, Koeleman BC, Koster T, Rosendaal RF, Dirven RJ, Ronde de H, Velden van der PA, Reitsma PH. Mutation in blood coagulation factor V associated with resistance to activated protein C. Nature 1994; 369: 64–7

Carew A, Pollak ES, High KA, Bauer KA. Severe factor VII deficiency to a mutation disrupting an Sp1 binding site in the factor VII promoter. Blood 1998: 92: 1639–1645

Castoldi E, Lunghi B, Mingozzi F, Ioannou I, Marchetti G, Bernardi F. New coagulation factor V gene polymorphisms define a single and infrequent haplotype underlying the factor V Leiden mutation in Mediterranean populations and Indians. Thromb Haemostas 1997; 78:1037–1041

Castoldi E, Rosing J, Lunghi B, Hoekema L, Girelli D, Mingozzi F, Ferraresi P, Friso S, Corrocher R, Tans G, Bernardi F. Factor V gene mutations (R2 gene) are associated with coronary artery disease in elderly people. Thromb Haemost 1999; 82 (suppl.): 509

Catto AJ, Kohler HP, Bannan S, Stickland M, Carter A, Grant PJ. Factor XIII Val34Leu. A novel association with primary intracerebral hemorrhage. Stroke 1998; 29: 813–6

Catto AJ, Kohler HP, Coore J, Mansfield MW, Stickland MH, Grant PJ. Association of a common polymorphism in the factor XIII gene with venous thrombosis. Blood 1999; 93: 906–8

Cool DE, MacGillivray RTA. Characterization of the human blood coagulation factor XII gene. Intron/exon gene organization and analysis of the 5'-flanking region. J Biol Chem 1987; 262: 13.662–13.673

Corral J, Gonzalez-Conejero R, Lozano ML, Rivera J, Heras I, Vicente V. The venous thrombosis risk factor 20210 A allele of the prothrombin gene is not a major risk factor for arterial thrombotic risk. Br J Haematol 1997;99: 304–7

de Knijff P, Green F, Johansen LG, Grootendorst D, Temple A, Cruickshank JK, Humphries JE, Jespersen J, Kluft C. New alleles in F7 VNTR. Hum Molec Genet 1994; 3:384

de Maat MPM, Green F, de Knijff P, Jespersen G, Kluft C. Factor VII polymorphisms in populations with different risk of cardiovascular disease. Arterioscler Thromb Vasc Biol 1997; 17: 1918–23

de Visser MCH, Guasch JF, Kamphuisen PW, Vos HL, Rosendaal FR, Bertina RM. The HR2 haplotype of factor V: effects on factor V levels, normalized APR sensitivity ratios and the risk of venous thrombosis. Thromb Haemost 1999; 82 (suppl.): 203–4

Dhawan J, Bray CL, Warburton R, Ghambhir DS, Morris J. Insulin resistance, high prevalence of diabetes, and cardiovascular risk in immigrant Asians. Genetic or environmental effect? Br Heart J 1994; 72: 413–21

Di Castelnuovo A, D'Orazio A, Amore C, Falanga A, Kluft C, Donati MB, Iacoviello L. Genetic modulation of coagulation factor VII plasma levels: contribution of different polymorphisms and gender-related effects. Thromb Haemost 1998; 80: 592–7

Doggen CJ, Cats VM, Bertina RM, Rosendaal FR. Interaction of coagulation defects and cardiovascular risk factors: increased risk of myocardial infarction associated with factor V Leiden or prothrombin 20210 A. Circulation 1998; 97: 1037–41

Eikelboom JW, Baker RI, Parsons R, Taylor RR, van Bockxmeer FM. No association between the 20210G/A prothrombin gene mutation and premature coronary artery disease. Thromb Haemost 1998; 80: 878–80

Faioni EM, Franchi F, Bucciarelli P, Margaglione M, de Stefano V, Castaman G, Finazzi G, Casorelli I, Mannucci PM. The HR2 haplotype in the factor V gene confers an increased risk of venous thromboembolism to carriers of factor V R506Q. Thromb Haemost 1999; 82: 418

Ferraresi P, Marchetti G, Legnani C, Cavallari E, Castoldi E, Mascoli F, Ardissino D, Palareti G, Bernardi F. The heterozygous 20210G/A prothrombin genotype is associated with early venous thrombosis in inherited thrombophilias and is not increased in frequency in artery disease. Arterioscler Thromb Vasc Biol 1997; 17: 2418–22

Fisher M, Fernandez JA, Ameriso SF, Xie D, Gruber A, Paganini HA, Griffin JH. Activated protein C resistance in ischemic stroke not due to factor V arginine 506 → glutamine mutation. Stroke 1996; 27: 1163–1166

Franco RF, Reitsma PH, Lourenco D, Maffei FH, Morelli V, Tavella MH, Araújo AG, Piccinato CE, Zago MA. Factor XIII Val34Leu is a genetic factor involved in the etiology of venous thrombosis. Thromb Haemost 1999; 81: 676–9

Frosst P, Blom HJ, Milos R, Goyette P, Sheppard CA, Matthews RG, Boers GJ, den Heijer M, Kluijmans LAJ, van den Heuvel LP, Rozen R. A candidate genetic risk factor for vascular diseases: a common mutation in methylenetetrahydrofolate reductase. Nat Genet 1995; 10: 111–3

Goodnough LT, Saito H, Ratnoff OD. Thrombosis or myocardial infarction in congenital clotting factor abnormalities and chronic thrombocytopenias: a report of 21 patients and a review of 50 previously reported cases. Medicine 1983; 62: 248–55

Green F, Kelleher C, Wilkes H, Temple A, Meade T, Humphries S. A common genetic polymorphism associated with lower coagulation factor VII level in healthy individuals. Arterioscler Thromb 1991; 11:540–546

Halbmayer WA, Haushofer A, Radek J, Schön R, Deutsch M, Fischer M. Prevalence of factor XII (Hageman factor) deficiency among 426 patients with coronary heart disease awaiting cardiac surgery. Coron Artery Dis 1994; 5:451–4

Halbmayer WA, Mannhalter C, Feichtinger C, Rubi K, Fischer M. The prevalence of factor XII deficiency in 103 orally anticoagulated outpatients suffering from recurrent venous and/or arterial thrombosis. Thromb Haemost 1992; 68: 285–90

Henry M, Morange PE, Canavy I, Alessi MC, Juhan-Vague I. Rapid detection of factor XIII Val34Leu by allele specific PCR. Thromb Haemost 1999; 81: 463

Herrmann FH, Schröder W, Altman R, Jimenez Bonilla R, Perez-Requejo JL, Singh JR. Zur Prävalenz des G20210A-Prothrombin-Polymorphismus, der C677T-Mutation-Gens und der Faktor V-Leiden Mutation in Nordostdeutschland, Argentinien, Venezuela, Costa Rica und Indien. In: I. Scharrer/W. Schramm (Hrsg.) 28. Hämophilie-Symposium Hamburg 1997. Springer-Verlag Berlin Heidelberg 1999: 305–9

Herrmann FH, Koesling M, Schröder W, Altman R. Jimenez Bonilla R, Lopaciuk S, Perez-Requejo JL, Singh JR. Prevalence of factor V Leiden mutation in various populations. Genet Epidemiol 1997; 14: 403–411

Herrmann FH, Wulff K. Molekulare Genanalyse und Gendiagnostik bei Hämophilie B und Faktor VII Mangel. Hämostaseologie 1998;18:129–139

Hoekema L, Castoldi E, Tans G, Manzato F, Bernardi F, Rosing J. Characterization of blood coagulation factor V (a) encoded by the R2-gene. Thromb Haemost 1999; 82 (suppl.): 684

Hoffman CJ, Miller RH, Hultin MB. Correlation of factor VII activity and antigen with cholesterol and triglycerides in healthy young adults. Arterioscler Thromb 1992; 12: 267–70

Humphries SE, Lane A, Green FR, Cooper J, Miller GJ. Factor VII coagulant activity and antigen levels in healthy men are determined by interaction between factor VII genotype and plasma triglyceride concentration. Arterioscler Thromb 1994; 14: 193–8

Iacoviello L, Di Castelnuovo A, De Knijff P, D'Orazio A, Amore C, Arboretti R, Kluft C, Donati MB. Polymorphisms in the coagulation factor VII gene and the risk of myocardial infarction. N Engl J Med 1998; 338: 79–85

Iacoviello L, Di Castelnuovo A, D'Orazio A, Donati MB. Cigarette smoking doubles the risk of myocardial infarction in carriers of a protective polymorphism in the blood coagulation factor VII gene. Thromb Haemost 1999; 81: 658

Kain K, Catto A, Kohler HP, Grant PJ. Haemostatic risk factors in healthy white and South Asian populations in U.K. Thromb Haemost 1999; 82 (Suppl.) 185

Kanaji T, Okamura T, Osaki K, Kuroiwa M, Shimoda K, Hamasaki N, Niho Y. A common genetic polymorphism (46 C to substitution) in the 5'-untranslated region of the coagulation factor XII gene is associated with low translation efficiency and decrease in plasma factor XII level. Blood 1998; 91: 2010–4

Kapur RK, Mills LA, Spitzer SG, Hultin MB. A prothrombin gene mutation is significantly with venous thrombosis. Arterioscler Thromb Vasc Biol 1997; 17: 2875–9

Kario K, Narita N, Matsuo T, Kayaba K, Tsutsumi A, Matuso M, Miyata T, Shimada K. Genetic determinants of plasma FVII activity in the Japanese. Thromb Haemost 1995; 73: 617–22

Kelleher CC, Mitropoulos KA, Imeson J, Meade TW, Martin JC, Reeves BEA, Hughes LO. Hageman factor and risk of myocardial infarction in middle-aged men. Atherosclerosis 1992; 97: 67–73

Kluijtmans LAJ, den Heijer M, Reitsma PH, Heil SG, Blom HJ, Rosendaal FR. Thermolabile methylenetetrahydrofolate reductase and factor V Leiden in the risk of deep-vein thrombosis. Thromb Haemost 1998; 79: 254–8

Kluijtmans LAJ, Kastelein JJP, Lindemans J, Boers GHJ, Heil SG, Bruschke AVG, Jukema JW, VandenHeuvel LPWJ, Trijbels JMF, Boerma GJM, Verheugt FWA, Willems F, Blom HJ. Thermolabile methylenetetrahydrofolate in coronary artery disease. Circulation 1999 (accepted)

Kluijtmans LAJ, van den Heuvel LPWJ, Boers GHJ, Frosst P, Stevens EMB, van Oost BA, den Heijer M, Trijbels FJM, Rozen R, Blom HJ Molecular genetic analysis in mild hyperhomocysteinemia: A common mutation in the methylenetetrahydrofolate reductase gene is a genetic risk factor for cardiovascular disease. Am J Hum Genet 1996; 58: 35–41

Kohler HP, Futers TS, Grant PJ. FXII (46 C→T) polymorphism and in vivo generation of FXII activity. Thromb Haemost 1999; 81: 745–7

Kohler HP, Grant PJ. Clustering of haemostatic risk factors with FXIIIVal34Leu in patients with myocardial infarction. Thromb Haemost 1998a; 80: 862

Kohler HP, Stickland MH, Ossei-Gerning N, Carter A, Mikkola H, Grant PJ. Association of a common polymorphism in the factor XIII gene with myocardial infarction. Thromb Haemost 1998b; 79: 8–13

Koster T, Rosendaal FR, Briet E, Vandenbroucke JP. John Hageman's factor and deep vein thrombosis: Leiden Thrombophilia Study. Br J Haematol 1994; 87: 422–4

Lämmle B, Wuillemin WA, Huber I, Krauskopf M, Zürcher C, Pflugshaupt R, Furlan M. Thromboembolism and bleeding tendency in congenital factor XII deficiency – A study on 74 subjects from 14 Swiss families. Thromb Haemost 1991; 65: 117–21

Lane A, Cruickshank JK, Mitchell J, Henderson A, Humphries S, Green F. Genetic and environmental determinants of factor VII coagulant activity in ethnic group at differing risk of coronary heart disease. Atherosclerosis 1992; 94: 43–50

Lindpaintner K, Pfeffer MA, Kreutz R, Stamper MJ, Grodstein F, LaMotte F, Buring J, Hennekens CH. A prospective evaluation of an angiotensin-converting enzyme gene polymorphism and the risk of ischemic heart disease. New Engl J Med 1995; 32: 706–711

Ludwig E, Corneli PS, Anderson JL, Marshall HW, Lalouel JM, Ward RH. Angiotensin-converting enzyme gene polymorphism is associated with myocardial infarction but not with development of coronary stenosis. Circulation 1995; 91: 2120–2124

Lunghi B, Castoldi E, Mingozzi F, Bernardi F. A new factor V gene polymorphism (His1254Arg) present in subjects of African origin mimics the R2 polymorphism (His1299Arg). Blood 1998; 91: 364–5

Lunghi B, Iacoviello L, Gemmati D, DiIasio MG, Castoldi E, Pinotti M, Castaman G, Redaelli R, Mariani G, Marchetti G, Bernardi F. Detection of new polymorphic markers in the factor V gene: Association with factor V levels in plasma. Thromb Haemost 1996; 75 :45–48

Ma J, Stamfer MJ, Hennekens CH, Frosst P, Selhub J, Horsford J, Malinow MR, Willet WC, Rozen R. Methylenetetrahydrofolate reductase polymorphism, plasma folate, homocysteine and risk of myocardial infarction in US physicians. Circulation 1996; 94: 2410–2416

Mannhalter C, Fischer M, Hopmeier P, Deutsch E. Factor XII activity and antigen concentrations in patients suffering from recurrent thrombosis. Fibrinolysis 1987; 1: 259–63

Marchetti G, Ferraresi P, Quaglio S, Taddia C, Chiozzi A, Cataldi A, Bernardi F, Mascoli F. Study of FV genetic markers in carotid artery disease. Thromb Haemost 1999; 82 (suppl.): 450

Marchetti G, Gemmati D, Patracchini P, Pinotti M, Bernardi F. PCR detection of a repeat polymorphism within the F7 gene. Nucleic Acids Res 1991; 19:4570

Marchetti G, Petracchini P, Papacchini M, Ferrati M, Bernardi F. A polymorphism in the 5'region of coagulation factor VII gene (F7) caused by an inserted decanucleotide. Hum Genet 1993; 90:575–576

Margaglione M, D'Andrea G, d'Addedda M, Giuliani N, Cappucci G, Iannaccone L, Vecchione G, Grandone E, Brancaccio V, Minno G. The methylenetetrahydrofolate reductase TT677 genotype is associated with venous thrombosis independently of the coexistence of the FV Leiden and the prothrombin A^{20210} mutation. Thromb Haemost 1998; 79: 907–911

Mariani G., Marchetti G., Arcieri P., Bernardi F. The role of factor VII gene polymorphism in determining FVII activity and antigen plasma level. Blood 1994; 84, Suppl. 1: 86a

Markus HS, Barley J, Lunt R, Bland JM, Jeffery S, Carter ND, Brown, MM. Angiotensin-converting enzyme gene deletion polymorphism – A new risk factor for lacunar stroke but not carotid atheroma. Stroke 1995; 26:1329–1333

Marmot M, Adelstein A. Immigrant mortality in England and Wales 1970–1978. Population Trends 1985; 33: 14–7

McCormack LJ, Kain K, Catto AJ, Kohler HP, Stickland MH, Grant PJ. Prevalence of FXIII V34L in populations with different cardiovascular risk. Thromb Haemost 1998; 80: 523–4

Mennen LJ, Schouten EG, Grobbee DE, Kluft C. Coagulation factor VII dietary fat and blood lipids: a review. Thromb Haemost 1996; 76: 492–9

Merlo C, Furlan M, Sulzer I, Kremer Hovinga J, Binder BR, Lämmle B. Contact activation factors in 200 survivors of myocardial infarction. Thromb Haemost 1994 (abstr.); 73: 1410a

Mikkola H, Syrjälä M, Rasi V, Vahtera E, Hämäläinen E, Peltonen l, Paotie A. Deficiency in the A-subunit of coagulation faxtor XIII: two novel point mutations demonstrate different effects on transcript levels. Blood 1994; 84:517–25

Miller GJ, Martin JC, Mitropoulos KA et al. Plasma factor VII is activated by postbrandial triglyceridemia, irrespective of dietary fat composition. Atherosclerosis 1991; 86: 163–71

Miller M, Dykes DD, Polesky HF. A simple salting out procedure for extracting DNA from human nucleated cells. Nucleic Acids Res 1988; 16:121

Mingozzi F, Lunghi B, Ferraresi P, Gastoldi E, Legnani C, Gemmati D, Pancani C, Palareti G, Marchetti G, Bernardi F. Factor V markers for the detection of genetic components of APC-resistance in venous thrombosis. Thromb Haemost 1999; 82 (suppl.): 404

Montaruli B, Voorberg J, Tamponi G, Borchiellini A, Muleo G, Pannocchia A, van Mourik JA, Schinco P (1996) Arterial and venous thrombosis in two Italian families with the factor V Arg506 ->Gln mutation. Eur J Haematol 57: 96–100

Morita H, Taguchi H, Kurihara H, Kitaoka M, Kaneda H, Kurihara Y, Maemura K, Shindo T, Minamino T, Ohno M, Yamaoki K, Ogasawara K, Aizawa T, Suzuki S, Yazaki Y. Genetic polymorphism of 5, 10-methylenetetrahydrofolate reductase (MTHFR) as a risk factor for coronary artery disease. Circulation 1997; 95: 2032–6

Nabavi DG, Junker R, Wolff E, Lüdemann P, Doherty C, Evers S, Droste D, Kessler C, Assmann G, Ringelstein BE. Prevalence of factor V Leiden mutation in young adults with cerebral ischemia: a case control study on 225 patients. J Neurol 1998; 245: 653–658

Nelson RG, Sievers ML, Knowler WC, Swinburn BA, Pettitt DJ, Saad MF, Liebow IM, Howard BV, Bennett PH. Low incidence of fatal coronary heart disease in Pina Indians despite high prevalence of non-insulin-dependent diabetes. Circulation 1990; 81: 987–95

O`Hara PJ, Grant FJ. The human factor VII gene is polymorphic due to variation in repeat copy number in a minisatellite. Gene 1988; 66:147–158

Odawara M, Matsunuma A, Yamashita K. Mistyping frequency of the angiotensin-converting enzyme gene polymorphism and an improved method for its avoidance. Hum Genet 1997; 100: 163–166

Pandita D, Steen P, Potti A. Risk factors for deep venous thrombosis of the upper extremities. Ann Int Med 1997; 127: 1129

Perry DJ, Riddell AF, Pasi KJ, et al. TL-MTHFR and venous thromboembolic disease. Thromb Haemost 1997; 78 Suppl:568

Poort SR, Rosendaal FR, Reitsma PH, Bertina RM. A common genetic variation in the 3'-untranslated region of the prothrombin gene is associated with elevated plasma prothrombin levels and an increase in venous thrombosis. Blood 1996; 88: 3698–3703

Prohaska W, Schmidt M, Mannebach H, Gleichmann U, Kleesiek K. The prevalence of the prothrombin 20210G→A mutation is not increased in angiographically confirmed coronary artery disease. Thromb Haemost 1999; 81: 161–2

Ridker PM, Hennekens CH, Lindpaintner K, Stampfer MJ, Eisenberg PR, Miletich JP. Mutation in the gene coding for coagulation factor V and the risk of myocardial infarction, stroke, and venous thrombosis in apparently healthy men. N Engl J Med 1995; 332: 912–917

Rieder M, Scott LT, Clark AG, Nickerson DA. Sequence variation in the human angiotensin converting enzyme. Nature Genetics 1999; 22: 59–62

Rigat B, Hubert C, Corvol P, Soubrier F. PCR detection of the insertion/deletion polymorphism of the human angiotensin converting enzyme gene (DCP 1) (dipeptidyl carboxypepetidase 1). Nucl Acids Res 1992; 20: 1433

Rosendaal FR, Doggen CJ, Zivelin A, Arruda VR, Aiach M, Sisovick DS, Hillarp A, Watzke HH, Bernardi F, Cumming AM, Preston FE, Reitsma PH. Geographic distribution os the 20210 G to A prothrombin variant. Thromb Haemost 1998; 79: 706–708

Rosendaal FR, Grant PJ, Ariens RAS, Poort SR, Bertina RM. Factor XIII Val34Leu, Factor XIII antigen and activity levels and risk of venous thrombosis. Thromb Haemost 1999; 82 (Suppl) 508

Rosendaal FR, Siscovick DS, Schwartz SM, Psaty BM, Raghunathan TE, Vos, HL. A common prothrombin variant (20210 G to A) increased the risk of myocardial infarction in young women. Blood 1997; 90: 1747–50

Sacchi E, Tagliabue L, Duca F, Manucci PM. High freqency of the C677 mutation in the methylenetetrahydrofolate reductase (MTHFR) gene in Northern Italy. Thromb Haemost 1997; 78:963–964

Sanchez J, Roman J, de la Torre MJ, Velasco F, Torres A. Low prevalence of the factor V Leiden among patients with ischemic stroke. Haemostasis 1997; 27: 9–15

Schröder W, Koesling M, Konrad H, Spitzer C, Kessler Ch, Herrmann FH. Molekulare Marker bei Thrombophilie und Schlaganfall. In: F.H. Herrmann (ed.) Molekulare (DNA) Diagnostik Hereditärer Hämostasedefekte. Verlag Pabst Science Publishers Lengerich, Berlin, Düsseldorf, Leipzig, Riga, Scottsdale (USA), Wien, Zagreb (1999) 201–216

Schröder W, Koesling M, Wulff K, Wehnert M, Herrmann FH. Large-scale screening for factor V Leiden mutation in a North-Eastern German population. Haemostasis 1996; 26: 233–236

Simioni P, de Rone H, Prandoni P, Saladini M, Bertina RM, Girolami A. Ischemic stroke in young patients with activated protein C resistance. Stroke 1995; 26: 885–890

Song KS, Park YS, Kim HK, Choi IR. Absence of the prothrombin gene variant in Koreans. Thromb Haemost 1999; 81: 990

Suzuki K, Henke J, Iwata M, Henke L, Tsuji H, Fukumaga GI, Szekelyi M, Ito S. Novel polymorphisms and haplotypes in the human coagulation factor XIII A-subunit gene. Hum Genet 1996; 98: 393–5

Temple A, Luong LA, Cruickshank K, Humphries SE. The 10-base-pair insertion in the promoter of the factor VII gene is not associated with lower levels of factor VIIc in Afro-Carribeans. Thromb Haemost 1997; 77: 212–24

von Känel R, Wuillemin WA, Furlan M, Lämmle B. Factor XII clotting activity and antigen levels in patients with thromboembolic disease. Blood Coagul Fibrinolysis 1992; 3: 555–61

Watzke HH, Schuttrümpf J, Graf S, Huber K, Panzer S. Increased prevalence of a polymorphism in the gene for human prothrombin in patients with coronary heart disease. Thromb Res 1997; 87: 521–6

Winter M, Gallimore M, Jones DW. Should factor XII assays be included in thrombophilia screening. Lancet 1995; 346–52

Wulff K, Ebener U, Wehnert CH-S, Ward PA, Reuner U, Hiebsch W, Herrmann FH, Wehnert M. Direct molecular genetic diagnosis and heterozygous identification in X-linked Emery-Dreifuss muscular dystrophy by heteroduplex analysis. Disease Markers 1997; 13: 77–86

Zeerleder S, Schloesser M, Redondo M, Wuillemin WA, Engel W, Furlan M, B Lämmle. Revaluation of the incidence of thromboembolic complications in congenital factor XII deficiency. Thromb Haemost 1999; 82: 1240–6

Factor V Variants – FV Leiden, FV R2 Polymorphism (ex 13), FV *Dde*I Polymorphism (int 16) – Risk Factors for Venous Thrombosis? Results of a Pilot Study

W. Schröder, H. Konrad, R. Grimm, G. Schuster, F.H. Herrmann

Introduction

Inherited resistance to activated protein C (APCR) was identified as a major risk factor for venous thromboembolism. It is caused by a point mutation at nt 1691 G→A in the factor V gene resulting in the replacement of Arg 506 by Gln (FV Leiden mutation; Bertina et al. 1995). The prevalence in our Northeastern German population is about 7%. Among patients with DVT in 30% a FV Leiden mutation was evident. However, in approximately 5–10% of thrombosis patients with an APC resistance no Factor V Leiden mutation can be observed. Other factors like an elevated FVIII activity, antiphospholipid antibodies or pregnancy may contribute to a modulated APCR in some of those cases but are not evident in all.

In 1997 a new haplotype of the factor V gene – HR2 – was described by Bernardi et al. This haplotype is characterized by five polymorphic markers in exon 13 of the factor V gene and one polymorphism in exon 16. It was shown, that all these polymorphisms are in a strong linkage disequilibrium not only in Caucasians but also in populations of Southern India and Somalia (Bernardi et al. 1997).

Thus, the determination of only one of the markers – 4070 A(R1)/G(R2) – is sufficient to characterize this haplotype. The rare allele of this polymorphism (R2) has been found to be associated with partial FV deficiency as well as with lower APC ratios in patients with venous thrombosis and in a healthy control group. Additionally, it was found to be more frequent in patients with APC ratios below the 15th percentile than in those with higher APC ratios or in normal controls (Lunghi et al. 1996).

It has been discussed in the literature that this FV haplotype is both able to contribute by itself to determine a mild APC resistance phenotype in patients without FVL and to interact synergically with the FVL mutation to produce a severe APCR phenotype.

The FV *Dde*I-polymorphism (alleles D1/D2) in intron 16 is a worldwide common haplotype. The D2 allele is discussed to be a very old ancestral allele, probably older than the FVL allele as it was shown by Castoldi et al. (1997) in populations from Italy, Cyprus, Somalia and Southern Indians. The FV Leiden mutation is strongly associated with the D2 allele in different populations supporting the hypothesis of a single origin of the FVL mutation. Data for German populations have not previously been recruited.

With the characterization of the FV polymorphisms mentioned above in a patients group as well as in a control from Northeastern Germany we contribute to a large population study.

I. Scharrer/W. Schramm (Ed.)
30th Hemophilia Symposium Hamburg 1999
© Springer-Verlag Berlin Heidelberg 2001

Material and Methods

Patients

The factor V polymorphisms G 1691 A (exon 10; FVL), A 4070 G (exon 13; R2) and the G→A polymorphism (*DdeI*) nt 12 in intron 16 have been characterized in 170 healthy control persons. Also included in the study were 183 patients with deep venous thrombosis (courtesy of Prof. Konrad in Rostock). The FVL and the HR2 haplotype could be characterized in all 183 patients with deep venous thrombosis, the *DdeI* polymorphism in intron 16 was determined in 145 patients.

DNA-Preparation and Genotyping

DNA was isolated by the »salting out« method according to Miller et al. (1988). If no isolated DNA was available, PCR was done immediately from dried filter paper blood spots as described earlier (Schröder et al. 1996).

All FV polymorphisms were detected by PCR, digestion with the appropriate restrictase (*MnlI* for FVL, *RsaI* for HR2, *DdeI* for the polymorphism in int 16) and fragment detection on NuSieve agarose (3%). [FVL: Bertina et al. (1994) Nature (Lond) 369:64–66; HR2: Lunghi et al. (1996) Thromb Haemost 75:45–48; *DdeI*: Castoldi et al. (1997) Thromb Haemost 78:1037–41.]

Results

FV Leiden G 1691 A

The prevalence of the factor V Leiden mutation in the regional control group was with 6.5% in the expected range. In patients with deep venous thrombosis we found a prevalence of 25.4% heterozygous and 1.7% homozygous (Tables 1, 2), which corresponds with our previous data (Schröder et al. 1996; Herrmann et al. 1998)

HR2 Haplotype (ex 13)

For the R2 allele representative for the HR2 haplotype a frequency of 8% in the control group and 7.2% in the DVT patients (Tables 1, 2) was evident. This is in the same range as reported for other populations (Italy 8%; Somalia 8%, India 10%). Heterozygote carriers were observed with a prevalence of 13.9% among the patients group and 15.6% in the control group. No homozygous R2/R2 have been observed neither in the patients group nor in the controls.

In our study there was only one patient with an APCR without an FVL genotype. No R2 allele was evident in this patient. A lupus antibody was not detected; FVIII:C had not been determined in this patient at the time of the study.

Table 1. FV Leiden and the HR2 genotype in patients with venous thrombosis

	R1/R1	R1/R2	R2/R2	Total
	n	*n*	*n*	*n*
FVL wt	174 (61.5%)	32 (11.3%)	0	206 (72.7%)
FVL hz	63 (22.3%)	9 (3.2%)	0	72 (25.4%)
FVL ho	5 (1.7%)	0	0	5 (1.7%)
	242 (86%)	41 (13.9%)	0	283

Table 2. FVL and HR2 genotypes in a control group

	R1/R1	R1/R2	R2/R2	Total
	n	*n*	*n*	*n*
FVL wt	135 (79.5%)	24 (14.1%)	0	159 (93.6%)
FVL hz	8 (4.7%)	3 (1.8%)	0	11 (6.5%)
FVL ho	0	0	0	0
	143 (84.4%)	27 (15.6%)	0	170

Double Heterozygous

Combined heterozygosity of FVL and R2 is more common in the patients group. In the control group 1.8% (3/170) of probands were double heterozygote for FVL and R2. In the patients group 3% (9/283) were double heterozygote (Tables 1, 2). However, this difference was not statistically significant.

All but one of the nine patients with double heterozygosity had developed more than one deep vein thrombosis. The patient with only one thrombotic event was 25 years old. In five patients a positive family anamnesis was evident.

*Dde*I Polymorphism (int 16)

The allele frequency for the more rare allele D2 is 7% in the controls and 21% in the patient group. All probands without exception with an FVL allele also have the *Dde*I-2 allele (Tables 3, 4).

Table 3. FVL and *Dde*I (int 16) genotypes in patients with venous thrombosis

	D1/D1	D1/D2	D2/D2	Total
	n	*n*	*n*	*n*
FVL wt	91 (62.7%)	12 (8.3%)	1 (0.7%)	104 (71.7%)
FVL hz	0	35 (24.1%)	4 (2.7%)	39 (26.8%)
FVL ho	0	0	2 (1.4%)	2 (1.4%)
	91 (62.7%)	47 (32.4%)	7 (4.8%)	145

Table 4. FVL and *Dde*I (int 16) genotypes in a control group

	D1/D1 n	D1/D2 n	D2/D2 n	Total n
FVL wt	146 (85.9%)	13 (7.6%)	0	159 (93.5%)
FVL hz	0	11 (6.5%)	0	11 (6.5%)
FVL ho	0	0	0	0
	146 (85.9%)	24 (14.1%)	0	170

Conclusions

In our study we could not confirm the role of the HR2 haplotype as an independent risk factor for thrombosis. A low APCR was only found in combination with a FVL but not with an independent HR2. Similar results were also presented by Luddington et al. (2000) who did not find any association between the R2 allele and FV levels or APC sensitivity ratios in a large case control study.

Thus, we conclude that the R2 allele alone is not associated with an increased risk of venous thrombosis. However, in combination with FVL it seems to be responsible for a more severe APCR phenotype. In the literature a three- to fourfold increase in the relative risk for venous thrombosis is discussed for double heterozygote carriers (Faioni et al. 1999).

The D2 allele is more common in the patient group due to the strong linkage to the FV Leiden mutation. The *Dde*I-polymorphism itself does not contribute to the APCR phenotype. Our findings support the hypothesis, that FVL is younger than the D2 allele of the *Dde*I polymorphism and that a founder effect has occurred spreading the mutation in Caucasians.

References

Bernardi F, Faioni EM, Castoldi E, Lunghi B, Castaman G, Sacchi E, Mannucci PM (1997) A factor V genetic component differing from factor V R506 Q contributes to the activated protein C resistant phenotype. Blood 90: 1552–1557
Bertina RM, Reitsma PH, Rosendaal FR, Vandenbroucke JP (1995) Resistance to activated protein C and factor V Leiden as risk factors for venous thrombosis. Thromb Haemost 74: 449–453
Castoldi E, Lunghi B, Mingozzi F, Ioannu P, Marchetti G, Bernardi F (1997) New coagulation Factor V gene polymorphism define a single and infrequent haplotype underlying the factor V Leiden mutation in Mediterranean populations and Indians. Thromb Haemost 78:1037–41
Faioni EM, Franchi F, Bucciarelli P, Margaglione M, de Stefano V, Castaman G, Finazzi G, Mannucci PM (1999) Coinheritance of the HR2 haplotype in the factor V gene confers an increased risk of venous thromboembolism to carriers of factor V R506Q (factor V Leiden). Blood 94: 3062–3066
Herrmann FH, Schröder W, Altmann R, Jimenez-Bonilla R, Perez-Requejo JL, Singh JR (1998) Zur Prävalenz des G20210 A Prothrombin Polymorphismus, der C677T-Mutation des MTHFR-Gens und der Faktor V Leiden Mutation in Nordostdeutschland, Argentinien, Venezuela, Costa Rica und Indien. In 28. Hämophilie Symposion Hamburg 1997,

Verhandlungsberichte. Scharrer I., Schramm (Hrsg.). Springer, Berlin, Heidelberg, New York, Tokio

Lunghi B, Iacoviello L, Gemmati D, Dilasio MG, Castoldi E, Pinotti M, Castaman G, Redaelli R, Mariani G, Marchetti G, Bernardi F (1996) Detection of new polymorphic markers in the factor V gene: Association with factor V levels in plasma. Thromb Haemost 75: 45 –48

Luddington R, Jackson A, Pannerselvam S, Brown K, Baglin T (2000) The factor V R2 allele: risk of venous thromboembolism, factor V levels and resistance to activated protein C. Thromb Haemost. 83: 204–208

Miller SA, Dykes DD, Polesky HF (1988) A simple salting out procedure for extracting DNA from nucleated cells. Nucleic Acids Res 16: 1215–20

Schröder W, Koessling M, Wulff K, Wehnert M, Herrmann FH (1996) Large scale screening for factor V Leiden mutation in a North-Eastern German population. Haemostasis 26: 233–236

Relation Between Prothrombin Mutation 20210 G→A, Prothrombin Time, Factor V Leiden, and Prothrombin Level

A. Siegemund, S. Köhler, T. Siegemund

Introduction

It has been known since the first description of the prothrombin mutation 20210 G→A by Poort et al. (1996) that this mutation is accompanied by elevated levels of prothrombin. These elevated prothrombin levels (>115%) are associated with a higher risk of thrombosis; however, the mechanism causing the elevated prothrombin levels remains unknown. To identify the carriers of the mutation it is necessary to detect the 20210 A-allele by PCR; the measurement of prothrombin levels alone is insufficient to discriminate between carriers and non-carriers. The aim of our study is to develop a highly sensitive screening test for the prothrombin mutation in order to reduce the amount of DNA testing required.

Patients

More than 900 patients with venous and arterial occlusions, respectively, have been tested over the last 2 years. Of these, 125 patients were heterozygous carriers of the prothrombin mutation 20210 GA, and 1 patient was a homozygous carrier (20210 AA). Eighteen patients were carriers of both the prothrombin mutation and the factor V (FV) Leiden. In some cases, patients were tested repeatedly (with/without heparin, with/without oral anticoagulation).

The control group included patients (tested for thrombogenic risk factors in our laboratory) without the prothrombin mutation, and 114 blood donors, respectively.

Methods

Prothrombin levels were determined using a clotting assay (Thromborel R, FII-deficient plasma, Dade Behring), APC resistance with ProC Global FV (Dade Behring, FV-deficient plasma Haemachrom Diagnostica), prothrombin time (PT) with Immunoplastin HIS (Progen), prothrombin mutation 20210 G→A by PCR (Medipro), and FV Leiden by PCR (Medipro; only in cases of positive screening test with INR<0.7). The interpretation of the results was based on the ratio between FII and PT. The endogenous thrombin potential (ETP) was measured according to Wielders et al. (1997). Pefabloc FG (Loxo) was used as a clot inhibitor.

I. Scharrer/W. Schramm (Ed.)
30th Hemophilia Symposium Hamburg 1999
© Springer-Verlag Berlin Heidelberg 2001

Table 1. Ratio FII-PT in the Relationship between factor V Leiden and the prothrombin mutation

Factor V	Prothrombin 20210	Mean (all patients)	n	Mean PT>30%	n	Mean PT>70%	n
GG	GA	1.22	421	1.24	328	1.24	162
GA	GA	1.08	118	1.14	80	1.15	43
GG	GG	0.95	315	0.97	276	0.99	189
GA	GG	0.89	78	0.91	66	1.0	43

Results

We found significant differences between carriers of the prothrombin mutation 20210 G→A and non-carriers (Fig. 1). In patients with FV Leiden the prothrombin levels were decreased, and therefore the ratios are also lowered (Table 1). The differences between patients with prothrombin mutation and patients with FV Leiden (group 1/2 to group 3/4) are statistically significant ($p<0.0001$); the differences between the groups 1/3 ($p=0.001$) and 1/4 ($p=0.017$) are also significant. This means that in the case of the prothrombin mutation an imbalance exists between FII and the other factors influencing the PT. FV Leiden influences the PT in the opposite direction. Assuming the prothrombin level remains unchanged in patients with both mutations, other mechanisms must be involved for increasing PT. This method is also applicable for patients undergoing oral anticoagulation therapy, the differences between the different groups also being significant (group 1/3, $p=0.001$; group 1/2 to group 3/4, $p=0.002$). The distribution of the ratio FII/PT with and without FV Leiden as second mutation are shown in Figures 2 and 3.

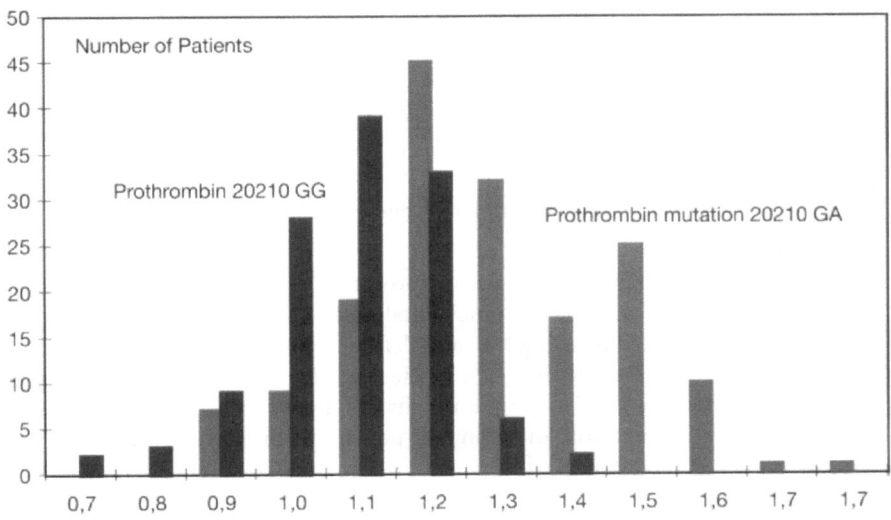

Fig. 1. Distribution of the ratio F II-PT in patients with 20210 GG/20210 GA

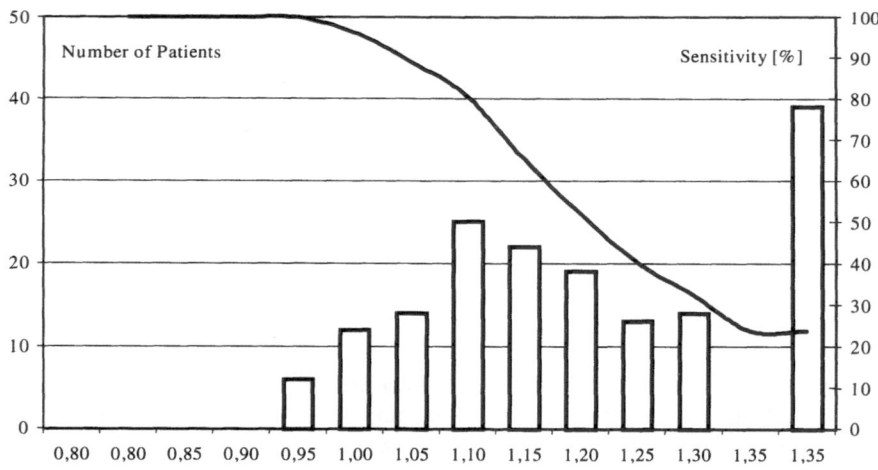

Fig. 2. Ratio FII-PT in patients with 20210 GA, FV-Leiden wildtype, PT>70%

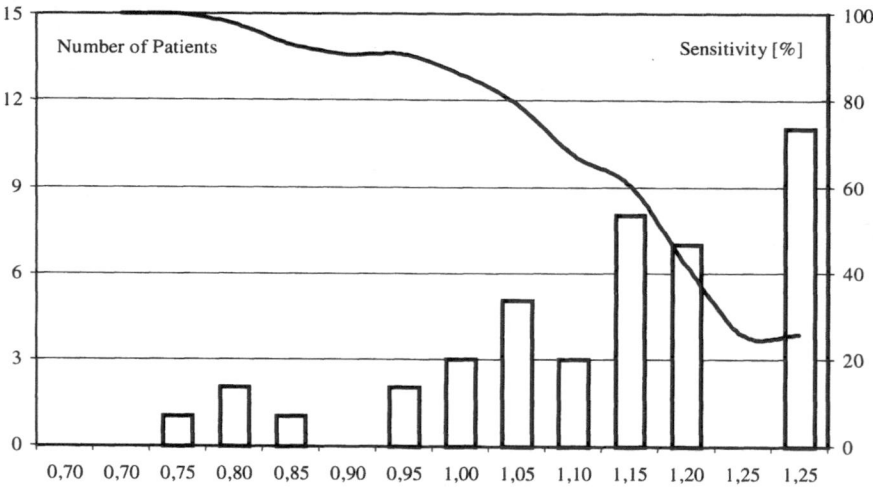

Fig. 3. Ratio FII-PT in patients with prothrombin mutation and FV-Leiden, PT>70

This screening method for detection of the prothrombin mutation carriers is influenced negatively if FV Leiden is a coincidental mutation, but the sensitivity of this method can be enhanced by using the ratio defined above. Using a cut-off of 1.0 for the ratio we found a sensitivity of 94.5% (patients with PT>70%). The non-detected patients ($n=6$) had a ratio of 0.95, meaning that a ratio <0.95 excludes the presence of the prothrombin mutation. Including all patients with PT>30% the sensitivity was 83.9%. This will be improved by excluding all patients with unstable oral anticoagulation and disorders of liver functions.

The relation between sensitivity and specificity using this ratio in comparison to using only FII measurements is shown in Figure 4.

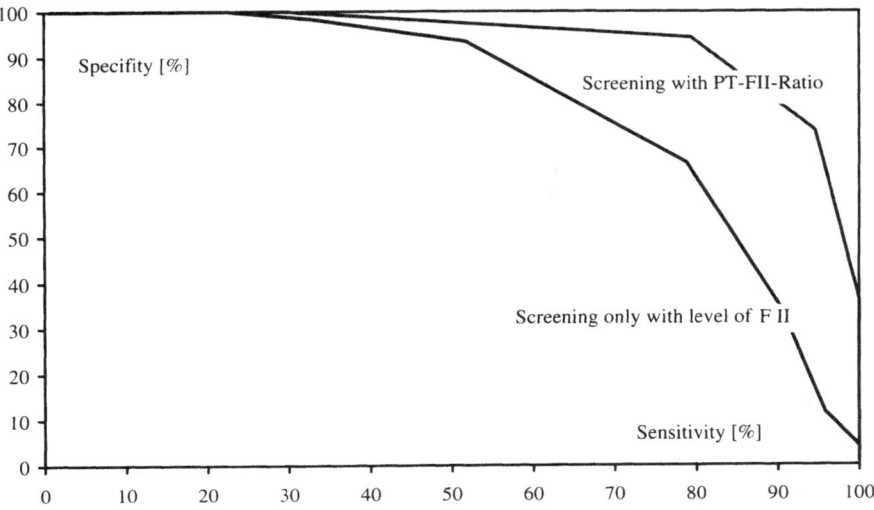

Fig. 4. Sensitivity and specificity – comparison between FII and ratio FII/PT

Our investigations show significant differences (p=0.003) in ETP between patients and controls with and without the prothrombin mutation, respectively. In cases where the ratio FII/PT>1, with elevated ETP, and excluding other inhibitor defects (e.g. AT III deficiency), the probability of the prothrombin mutation 20210 G→A is very high.

Conclusions

Using a ratio from the single factor test (FII) and the global test (PT) the sensitivity for detecting the prothrombin mutation 20210 G→A may be substantially increased. There exists an imbalance between the single clotting factors with a predominance of FII resulting in increased thrombin potential. However, the simultaneous existence of FV Leiden reduces this imbalance between FII and the other clotting factors influencing the PT. The ratio method is also suitable for the investigation of other hypercoagulable conditions, for example in the case of high levels of FIX (patent 1998/B007–1175).

References

Poort SR, Rosendaal FR, Reitsma PH, Bertina. A common genetic variation in the 3'-untranslated region of the prothrombin gene is associated with elevated plasma prothrombin levels and an increase in venous thrombosis. Blood 1996; 88: 3698–703.

Wielders S, Mukherjee M, Michiels J, Rijkers DTS, Cambus JP, Knebel RWC, Kakkar V, Hemker HC. The routine determination of the endogenous thrombin potential: first results in different forms of hyper- and hypocoagulability. Thromb. Haemost. 1997; 77: 629–36.

Localization and Characterization of Mutations Within the Factor VIII Gene in a Cohort of 212 Patients with Hemophilia A

J. Schröder, V. Ivaskevicius, S. Rost, A. Müller, H.-H. Brackmann,
W. Effenberger, W. Kreuz, C. Escuriola Ettingshausen,
I. Scharrer, H. Lenk, C. Mauz-Körholz, C.R. Müller, R. Schwaab,
J. Oldenburg

Introduction

The clinical manifestation of hemophilia A is heterogeneous and characterized by a great variety of mutations within the factor VIII gene. The knowledge of the different mutations is of particular interest in understanding the pathophysiology of hemophilia A. It is important for prognosis of the course of the disease (inhibitor formation) [1,2] and also for genetic counseling. The goal of this study was to establish a fast and effective method for the large-scale mutation screening of hemophilia A patients.

Methods

Mutation analysis was performed by different methods. At first a Southern blot technique was used to investigate the most prevalent intron-22 inversion [3]. Patients that showed no abnormality were screened for mutations by using denaturing gradient gel electrophoresis (DGGE) in exons 1–13, 15–26 and three hotspots inside exon 14. If no mutation could be found by DGGE patients were screened for the whole exon 14 by chemical mismatch cleavage (CMC) [4]. Mutations localized by the screening methods were finally characterized by direct sequence analysis.

Results and Discussion

Overall, 212 patients affected with various degrees of severity of hemophilia A were included in the study. In 188 (88.7%) patients we identified the causative mutation for hemophilia A. The results are shown in Figure 1 with respect to the method used and in Figure 2 as a mutation profile. 63 (29.7%) of the mutations were found by Southern blot analysis. A total of 117 (54.6%) mutations could be identified in exons 1–13, 15–26 and three hotspots within exon 14. Only 8 (3.8%) mutations were found in the other regions of exon 14. Apart from the prevalent intron-22 inversions (about 30%) nearly every family shows its own specific mutation. A third of the mutations were unknown in the hemophilia database.

I. Scharrer/W. Schramm (Ed.)
30th Hemophilia Symposium Hamburg 1999
© Springer-Verlag Berlin Heidelberg 2001

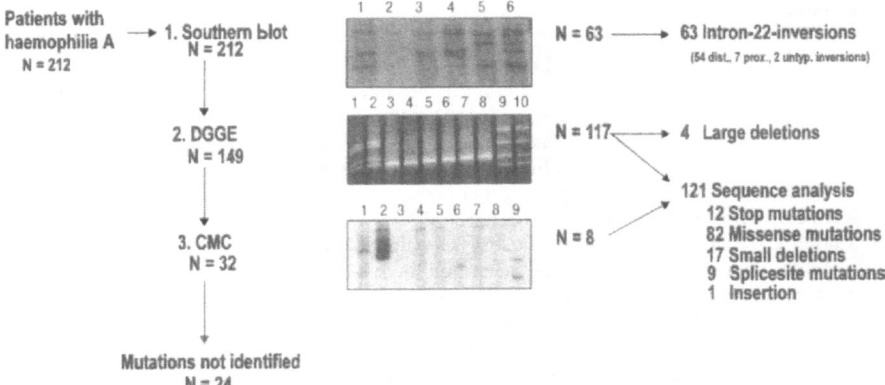

Fig. 1. Analysis of the factor VIII gene. *1.* Southern blot: *Lanes 1 and 2:* normal pattern; *lane 3:* distal inversion; *lane 4:* distal inversion heterozygous; *lane 5:* proximal inversion; *lane 6:* proximal inversion heterozygous. *2.* DGGE. *Lanes 1 and 2:* mutations; *lanes 3–8:* wildtype; *lanes 9 and 10:* positive controls. *3.* CMC. *Lane 1:* length standard; *lane 2:* negative control; *lanes 6 and 9:* mutations; *lanes 4, 5, 7 and 8:* wildtype

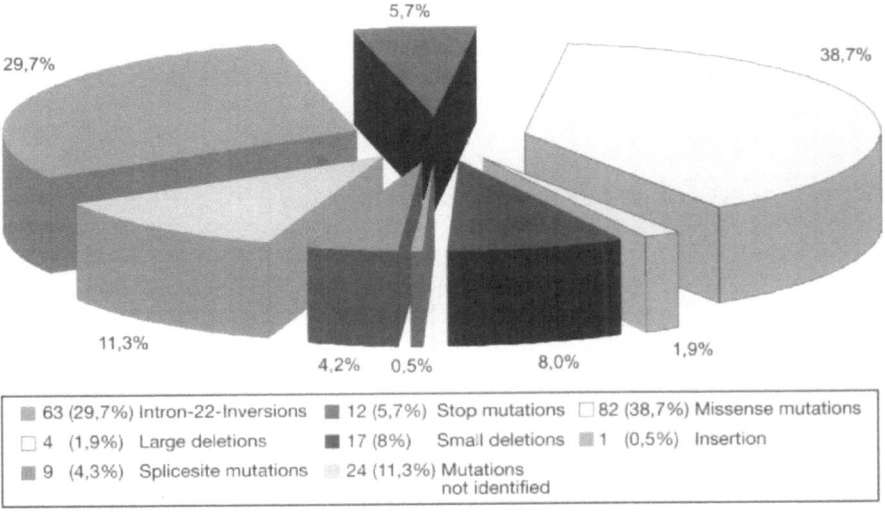

Fig. 2. Mutation profile in 212 patients with hemophilia A

Conclusions

The strategy shown in this study enables a fast and effective large-scale detection of causative mutations in hemophilia A patients. The sensitivity of 90% of the methods so far used may be increased by applying new techniques such as DHPLC (denaturing high-performance liquid chromatography) and complete sequencing of the factor VIII gene.

References

1. Schwaab R, Brackmann H-H, Meyer C, Seehafer J, Kirchgesser M, Haack A, Olek K, Tuddenham EGD, Oldenburg J: Haemophilia A: Mutation Type determines risk of inhibitor formation. Thromb Haemost (1995) 74: 1402–1406
2. Kreuz W, Becker S, Lenz E, Martinez-Saguer I, Escuriola Ettingshausen C, Funk M, Ehrenforth S, Auerswald G, Kornhuber B Factor VIII Inhibitors in Patients with Hemophilia A: Epidemiology of Inhibitor Development and Induction of Immune Tolerance for Factor VIII. Sem Thromb Haemost (1995) 21: 382–389
3. Lakich D, Kazazian HH, Antonarakis SE, Gitchier J: Inversions disrupting the factor VIII gene are a common cause of severe haemophilia A: Nature genetics, vol. 5 (1993): 236–41
4. Becker J, Schwaab R, Moller-Taube A, Schwaab U, Schmidt W, Brackmann H-H, Grimm T, Olek K, Oldenburg J: Characterization of the factor VIII defect in 147 patients with sporadic hemophilia A: family studies indicate a mutation type-dependent sex ratio of mutation frequencies: Am J Hum Genet 1996 Apr; 58(4): 657–670

Genomic Diagnosis of Hemophilia A in Hungarian Patients

Á. Nagy, M. Kescskés, B. Meng, E. Denicke, W. Schröder,
F.H. Herrmann, H. Losonczy

Introduction

Hemophilia A (factor VIII deficiency) is an X-linked inherited bleeding disorder of blood coagulation. In most of the European countries hemophilia occurs in 13–18 out of 100,000 males. Hemophilia A accounts for about 85% of the cases. According to current statistics 711 patients with hemophilia A have been registered in Hungary. The factor VIII gene is 186 kb at Xq28, and is characterized by very high mutational heterogeneity. The size and complexity of the gene makes the causal mutation detection extremely difficult, apart from the identification of large deletions, and nucleotide substitutions affecting restriction enzyme sites. From detailed studies it is now clear that almost 50% of hemophilia A result from inversions [2,4]. Behind the most important rearrangement a common recurrent mechanism is an illegitimate cross-over between a copy of gene F8 A sequence in intron 22 and one of two extragenous but highly homologous copies of gene F8 A in opposite orientation, resulting in an aberrant Southern pattern. This defect result in gene disruption separating exon 1 from exon 22, which leads to the lack of intact factor VIII. Cross-over between the most distal extragenic sequence A and its IVS22 homologue results in a type 1 inversion, while cross-over between the proximal sequence and its intronic homologue gives a type 2 inversion. The rare types of inversions (3 A, 3B) are characterized by different Southern blot diagnostic patterns [2].

Ten useful polymorphisms also have been identified within or flanking the factor VIII gene. Ethnic variation in heterozygosity is less marked than seen for factor IX. The two most useful ones are the CA repeat VNTRs found within introns 13 and 22 [5].

According to an epidemiological study 82.5% of the affected Hungarian families require prenatal diagnosis for hemophilia A [3].

We report the first Hungarian data having applied the genomic diagnostics in Hungary. In the present study 60 patients with severe hemophilia A (<2% factor VIII activity) and some female relatives also have been screened for the inversion of the factor VIII gene in order to investigate the frequency of this defect. Eleven out of them required further screening for family members using three different Southern blot based indirect methods (BglII, KpnXba/intron22, KpnXba/DXS 115) for polymorphism analysis.

I. Scharrer/W. Schramm (Ed.)
30th Hemophilia Symposium Hamburg 1999
© Springer-Verlag Berlin Heidelberg 2001

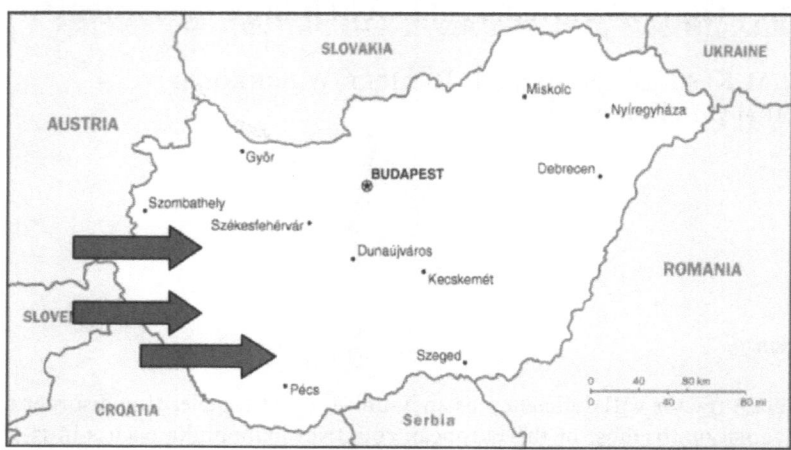

Fig. 1. Hemophilia centers and regions involved in the Hungarian hemophilia study (participant areas are shown by *black arrows*)

Materials and Methods

Blood Sampling

Samples were collected with the help of different regional hemophilia centers of the country (Fig. 1). After providing detailed instructions, around 30% of the families with hemophilia A agreed to participate in our study.

Method

DNA was isolated from 5 ml K_3-EDTA anticoagulated blood using a standard salting-out method.

For inversion mutation detection the standard protocols were used, as previously described by Lakich [4].

Polymorphism analysis for hemophilia A patients and families was carried out using the basic procedures: BglII according to Antonarakis et al.[1], Xba/intron 22 and Xba/DXS 115 described by Wion et al. [7] and Vivian et al. [6].

Results

Among the 60 patients investigated inversion was found in 27 cases (45%). By far the greatest number were carrying type I, while the rare types of inversion (3 A, 3B) were not detectable (Table 1).

Circulating inhibitors were present in only three subjects out of total (Table 2). In contrast to previous publications, the low prevalence of inhibitor formation is not

Table 1. Frequency of inversion among hemophilic patients

	Number of patients
Inversion type I	20 (33.3%)
Inversion type II	7 (11.5%)
Patient without inversion	33 (55%)

Table 2. The presence of circulating inhibitor among patients with severe hemophilia A

Number of patients	Inhibitor+	Inhibitor-
Inversion type I and type II (n=27)	1 (3.7%)	26
Patient without inversion (n=33)	2 (6%)	31

correlated to the existence of inversion among the subjects studied . Mothers of six patients with inversion were also studied (data not shown). Five of them proved to be heterozygous for the same defect, but one was not a carrier. Eleven siblings were also studied. Four out of them carried the inversion of intron 22.

For the polymorphism analysis 89 subjects were involved in order to overestimate the heterozygosity rates.

Table 3 records the gene frequencies and the heterozygosity rate of the examined polymorphisms of factor VIII gene. The expected heterozygosities were calculated from the gene frequencies and compared with those observed in reference to the Caucasians.

Table 3. Gene frequencies and heterozygosity of factor VIII polymorphisms (data within the parentheses refer to the Caucasians)

No. of subjects: 89 (23 women)	No. of chromosomes, p(+):q(−)	Heterozygosity expected 2pq/observed frequency
BglII (DX13)	112 0.54:0.46	0.49/0.39 (0.50)
Xba/intron22	112 0.52:0.48	0.50/0.35 (0.42–0.58)
Xba/DXS 115	108 0.18:0.82	0.30/0.35 (0.41–0.59)

In the 11 siblings examined the complete pedigrees and parental blood samples were available. On the basis of their results, 4 siblings proved to be carriers and in 5 cases the carrier state could be excluded. The inversion mutation analysis provided informative for only 1 subject, and none of the methods used yielded information for the remaining 1 subject.

Prenatal Screening

In two cases the family also required prenatal screening. One mother decided to keep the child before the termination of the diagnostic procedure for religious reasons. Later, she gave birth to a healthy boy. In the second case the prenatal genetic screening resulted in the diagnosis of a healthy fetus and the boy was born without any complication.

Discussion

We have introduced the application of some widely used methods for genomic diagnosis as the first attempt to introduce routine carrier screening in Hungary. Samples were collected mainly from the western part of the country. 8% of the total registered (711) patients and their families affected by hemophilia A participated in the study.

According to our data the incidence of intron 22 inversions is 45% among the Hungarian patients with hemophilia A, which correlates well to the European data (37-53%) with reference to Antonarakis et al [2]. The most frequent abnormality was the distal type (type I) inversion in 20 out of 60 cases (33.3%), which is apparently the most common inversional event according to large-scale investigations.

The presence of a genetic abnormality increases the risk for inhibitor formation, which is a major problem for the replacement therapy of patients. Usually the occurrence of clotting factor VIII inhibitor is 10-30% among severe hemophiliacs. The simultaneous appearance of inhibitor formation and intron 22 inversion was found in 20% of the examined subjects by Antonarakis et al. [2]. Interestingly, we detected low frequency of circulating inhibitor (5% among severe hemophiliacs). The cause of this finding has not been determined so far.

The combined use of the three different polymorphism analyses gave results with over 90% certainty. These analyses provide useful, indispensable data for those families, who are negative by inversion detection.

References

1. Antonarakis S.E., Copeland K.L., Carpenter R.J. et al. (1985) Prenatal diagnosis of Haemophilia A Lancet 1: 1-9.
2. Antonarakis S.A., Rossiter J.P., Young M. (1995) Factor VIII gene inversions in severe haemophilia A Results of an international consortium study Blood 86 (6): 2206-2212)
3. Istvan I., Czeizel A., Kerényi M., et al. (1990) Genetic-Epidemiologic Study of Haemophilia A and B in Hungary (Human hered., 20: 29-33
4. Lakich D., Kazazian H.H., Antonarakis S.E., Gitschier J.(1993) Inversions disrupting the factor VIII gene are a common cause of severe haemophilia A Nat. Gen. 5: 236-241
5. Peake I: (1995) Molecular Genetics and Counselling in Haemophilia Thromb. Haemost., 74 1: 40-44
6. Vivian C., Tong T.M.F., Chan T.P.T., Tang M., Wan C.W., Chan F.Y., Chu Y.C.(1989) Multiple XbaI polymorphisms for carrier detection and prenatal diagnosis of haemophilia Brit. J. Haemat. 73: 497-500
7. Wion K.L., Tuddenham E.G.D., Lawn R.M. (1986) A new polymorphism in the factor VIII gene for prenatal diagnosis of haemophilia A Nucl.Ac.Res. 14 .11: 4535-4542

Indirect Genomic Diagnosis
of Hungarian Hemophilia B Patients

M. Kecskés, Á. Nagy, T. Vidra, H. Losonczy

Introduction

Hemophilia B (factor IX deficiency) is an X-linked inherited bleeding disorder of blood coagulation. Hungary belongs to the Caucasians with its 10 million citizens. According to current statistics 179 patients with hemophilia B have been registered. The families involved often require genetic counseling: carrier screening and subsequent prenatal diagnosis. Nowadays, precise human genetic diagnostics based on genomic examination (direct or indirect) and pedigree analysis also assume an important role in modern diagnostics in our country.

The cloning and detailed analysis of the factor IX gene has resulted in the detection of both polymorphisms and mutations within the gene. Since the 35-kb factor IX gene at Xq27.1 has been completely sequenced, rapid PCR-based methods have been established for all known polymorphisms. Ten particularly useful ones have been described with marked ethnic variations in frequency (Peake 1992, 1995). Since no diallelic polymorphism can be informative more than 50%, a combined use of them must be available. We report the first Hungarian data after having applied indirect genomic diagnostics in Hungary. 22 patients and family members of 14 of them were analyzed using PCR-based methods. Four polymorphisms have been examined in the same population (*Xmn*I, *Taq*I, *Dde*, *Hha*I). The combined use of them in carrier detection, the heterozygosity rate, the haplotype frequencies were recorded and compared with the international data referring to Caucasians.

Materials and Methods

Blood Sampling

Samples were collected with the help of different regional hemophilia centers of the country (Fig. 1). More than one third of the Hungarian patients attend them. After providing detailed instructions around 30% of the families agreed to participate in our study.

Methods

DNA was prepared from 400 µl K_3-EDTA anticoagulated blood using the standard phenol method. Basic PCR procedures were used (Winship et al. 1989; Reiss et al. 1990; Bowen et al. 1991) with some minor modifications.

I. Scharrer/W. Schramm (Ed.)
30th Hemophilia Symposium Hamburg 1999
© Springer-Verlag Berlin Heidelberg 2001

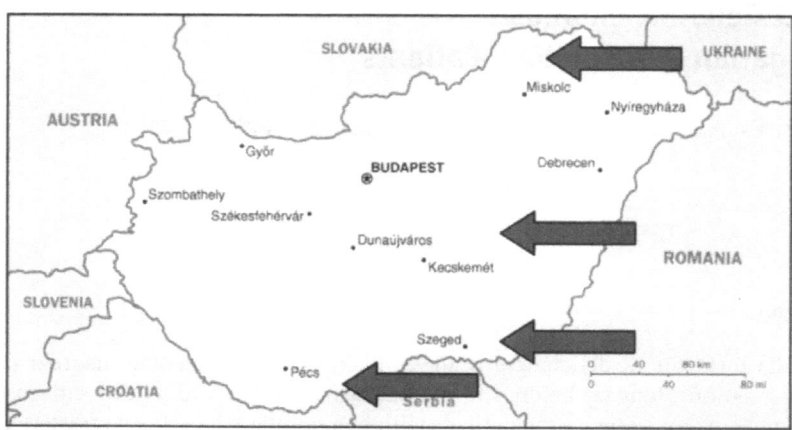

Fig. 1. Hemophilia centers and regions involved in the Hungarian hemophilia study (participant areas are shown by *black arrows*)

Results

Table 1 shows the gene frequencies and the heterozygosity rate of the examined polymorphisms of factor IX gene. The expected heterozygosities were calculated from the gene frequencies and compared with those observed in reference to the Caucasians. It is worth noticing that there was a large proportion of *Taq*I homozygous (+,+) women in the sample (39%), which could skew the genotype frequency.

The observed frequency of the *Hha*I and *Xmn*I heterozygosity was less than expected according to the literature (Graham et al. 1991).

20 siblings within families affected with hemophilia B were interested in the determination of their carrier state. 75% of them were given definite diagnoses using the indirect genetic methods detailed above. The carrier state was established in 7 cases and excluded in 8 subjects. For the remaining participants studied the absence of the parental DNA sample caused uncertainty, while in 2 cases none of the

Table 1. Gene frequencies and heterozygosity of factor IX polymorphisms

No. of subjects: 54 (31 women)	Hemophilia B	
RFLP	No. of chromosomes, p(+):q(−) of polymorphism	Heterozygosity expected (2pq)/observed frequency[a]
*Taq*I (intron 4)	84 0.47:0.53	0.49/0.31 (0.45)
(intron 1)	84 0.78:0.22	0.34/0.32 (0.36)
*Hha*I (3' flanking)	84 0.33:0.67	0.44/0.26 (0.48)
*Xmn*I (intron 3)	84 0.20:0.80	0.32/0.28 (0.41)

[a]Data in parentheses refer to Caucasians

analyzed RFLPs was informative. DNA of 1 patient could not be amplified where the direct diagnosis of gene deletion was highly suspected.

Discussion

We have introduced the application of some widely used methods for genomic diagnosis as the first attempt to introduce routine carrier screening in Hungary. Samples were collected from the eastern part of the country. 12% of the total registered patients and their families affected by hemophilia B participated in the study. It was a common limiting factor for the blood sampling that only 30% of the hemophilia families showed any interest. The patients who participated in the study were interested in the clinically more serious factor of deficiency.

The indirect genetic methods have proved to be sufficient and well suited for routine carrier screening. The examined factor IX gene polymorphisms were informative with a high degree of certainty, and insufficient informativity was responsible only for those 10% of failed diagnosis. One possible explanation behind the lower heterozygosity rate of $XmnI$ and $HhaI$ polymorphisms is that the investigated female family members and their affected relatives did not carry the positive alleles in most cases (63%). In contradiction, the positive Hha site was more frequent among those remaining patients investigated (50%) where no family member required any screening. However, the overall heterozygosity rate would be increased by testing other common polymorphisms such as $MnlI$ or $MseI$ (Winship et al. 1993).

References

1. Graham G.B., Kunkel G.R., Egilmez N.K., Wallmark A., Fowlkes D.M., Lord T.S.: The Varying Frequencies of Five DNA Polymorphisms of X-linked Coagulant Factor IX in Eight Ethnic Groups (Am.J.Hum.Genet. 1991: 49: 537–544)
2. Peake I: Molecular Genetics and Counselling in Haemophilia (Thromb. Haemost. 1995, 74 (1):40–44)
3. Peake I.: Registry of DNA Polymorphisms Within or Close to the Human Factor VIII and IX Genes (Thromb. Haemost. 1992, 67 (2):277–280)
4. Reiss J., Neufeldt U., Wieland K., Zoll B.: Diagnosis of Haemophilia B using the Polymerase Chain Reaction (Blut, 1990, 60:31–36)
5. Winship P.R., Rees D.J.G., Alkan M.: Detection of Polymorphisms at Cytosine Phosphoguanidine Dinucleotides and Diagnosis of Haemophilia B Carriers (The Lancet 1989, March 25. 631–634)
6. Winship P.R., Nichols C.E., Chuansumrit A, Peake I.: An MseI RFLP in the 5 flanking region of the factor IX gene: its use for haemophilia B carrier detection in Caucasian and Thai population (Br.J.Haemat. 1993, 84: 101–105)
7. Bowen D.J., Thomas P., Webb C.E., Bignell P., Peake J., and Bloom A.L.: Facile and rapid analysis of three DNA polymorphisms within the human factor IX gene using the polymerase chain reaction (Br.J.Haemat. 1991, 77:559–560)

IX.d Poster: Pediatrics

Relation of Cardiovascular Fitness, Hemostatic and Metabolic Risk Factors for Coronary Heart Disease in Obese Children and Adolescents

S. Gallistl, K. Sudi, M. Borkenstein, M. Tröbinger, G. Weinhandl, W. Muntean

Introduction

Several studies dealing with risk factors for coronary heart disease (CHD) in children and adolescents provide evidence that prevention of CHD should begin during childhood [1,2]. Beside metabolic disturbances, which have been shown to be correlated with atherosclerotic lesions in even young children [3], epidemiological evidence indicates that several markers of hemostatic and thrombotic function are potent predictors of risk for both myocardial infarction and stroke [4,5,6]. Impaired fibrinolysis (tissue-type plasminogen activator, plasminogen activator inhibitor, D-dimer) was found to predict future rates of cardiovascular morbidity and mortality [7–10]. In the Northwick Park Heart Study, both the levels of factor VII coagulant activity and plasma fibrinogen were associated with an increased risk of non-fatal myocardial infarction and ischemic heart disease death among middle-aged men [11]. Additional hemostatic markers for arterial thrombosis comprise increased plasma levels of factor VIII and von Willebrand factor [12], prothrombin fragment 1+2 and thrombin-antithrombin complexes [13].

It has been demonstrated that physical activity and cardiovascular fitness significantly reduce the risk of CHD by improvement of the metabolic state, lipoprotein profile, and hemostatic markers in adults [14,15]. The relationships between fitness and metabolic cardiovascular risk factors in children are very similar to those in adults [16,17]. There is no data on the relation of cardiovascular fitness and hemostatic risk factors in children and adolescents. We therefore investigated a possible association between hemostatic risk factors for CHD and cardiovascular fitness in otherwise healthy obese children and adolescents.

Methods

Participants

The study comprised 35 obese (body mass index above the 85th percentile for age and sex [18]) children and adolescents (18 male, 17 female) aged 4.4–17.5 years (median 12.2 years). At admission, a medical history was taken and physical examination performed to ensure that the participants were healthy. All children and adolescents had normal liver and renal function as assessed by standard clinical chemistry analysis. No participants were taking medications known to affect lipid

I. Scharrer/W. Schramm (Ed.)
30th Hemophilia Symposium Hamburg 1999
© Springer-Verlag Berlin Heidelberg 2001

284 S. Gallistl et al.

metabolism or the coagulation system. Informed consent was obtained from each child and a legal guardian. The study protocol was approved by the investigation review board of the University of Graz, Austria.

Analytical Methods

Venous blood samples were taken after an overnight fast between 7:30 a.m. and 9:30 a.m. in order to further minimize any effect on hemostatic and fibrinolytic variables through the diurnal rhythm. Lipid analyses were performed on the first 3–4 ml blood. Total cholesterol, triglycerides, and glucose levels were determined using automated enzymatic methods (Hitachi 937, Roche Diagnostics, Austria). HDL cholesterol and VLDL were determined after precipitation of the lipoproteins by dextran sulfate. LDL cholesterol was calculated using the Friedewald formula. Insulin and C-peptide were assessed by means of RIA (Linco Research, Mo., USA).

Blood samples for the measurements of hemostatic parameters were drawn into plastic tubes containing 0.1 mol l⁻¹ sodium citrate. The plasma was separated by centrifugation at 3000 g at 4°C for 10 min and stored at –70°C. Factor VII coagulant activity (VII:C) and factor VIII coagulant activity (VIII:C) were determined using one-stage clotting assays and deficient plasmas for factor VII and factor VIII, respectively (Behring, Germany). The plasma level of fibrinogen was assayed by a thrombin time method according to Clauss [19]. Von Willebrand factor antigen (Boehringer, Germany), prothrombin fragment 1+2 (Behring, Germany), and tissue-type plasminogen activator antigen (t-PA-Ag, Kabi, Austria) were determined using commercially available enzyme-linked immuno-assay kits.

Measurement of Body Composition

Measurement of body composition was performed by means of bioelectrical impedance (BIA Akern-RJL 101/S) with an applied current of 50 kHz. Measurements were performed in the fasting state after children had been resting in supine position for 10 min. Fat-free mass (FFM) was calculated [20] and fat mass (FM) was estimated as the difference between body weight and calculated FFM.

Determination of Cardiovascular Fitness

Twenty-five patients were eligible for assessment of cardiovascular fitness. The nature and the risk of the experimental procedures were explained in detail, and written informed consent was obtained. Within 1 week after the blood sampling and assessment of routine laboratory parameters participants underwent an incremental cycle ergometer exercise [21] (ECB PRO Ergometer 850, Tunturi, Austria) starting at 35 W and increments of 10–15 W every minute until voluntary exhaustion. Power output was calculated as watts per kilogram body weight, and in order to disentangle power output from body FM, in watts per kilogram FFM.

Statistical Analysis

Data not normally distributed were log_{10}-transformed (BMI, VLDL, triglycerides, glucose, insulin, C-peptide, and fibrinogen). Unpaired t-test and analysis of variance were used to compare parameters between groups where appropriate. Correlations between variables of interest were calculated using Pearson's correlation coefficient and partial correlation was performed to adjust for the influence of confounding variables. The independence of variables was tested by multiple regression analysis. The magnitude of significant contribution to the variance of the dependent variable was tested in a stepwise, multiple-regression model. The significance level of p values was set at 5%. Calculations were performed using SPSS for Windows (SPSS, Chicago) and WinStat 3.1. (Kalmia).

Results

Results in the Whole Study Population

The whole study consisted of 35 subjects (18 male, 17 female). Body mass index was above the 85th percentile for age and sex in all individuals and above the 95th percentile in 31 individuals. The main clinical characteristics and biological parameters are given in Table 1.

Table 1. Characteristics of the study population

	Median	Range
Age (years)	12.2	4.4–17.5
BMI (kg m^{-2})	29.1	20.2–45.8
Fat-free mass (kg)	37	19–58
Fat mass (kg)	30.5	11.8–66.8
Percentage fat mass	47.1	29.6–59.4
Triglycerides (mmol l^{-1})	1.06	0.38–3.58
Cholesterol (mmol l^{-1})	4.66	3.43–7.17
HDL cholesterol (mmol l^{-1})	1.18	0.52–1.92
LDL cholesterol (mmol l^{-1})	2.53	1.21–4.56
VLDL (mg dl^{-1})	89	16.1–380
Glucose (mmol l^{-1})	5.5	4.5–7.7
Insulin (mU l^{-1})	15.5	4.6–82
C-peptide (mU l^{-1})	2.25	0.6–9.4
Factor VII:C (%)	88	60–120
Factor VIII:C (%)	140	68–193
vWF-Ag (%)	127	54–173
Fibrinogen (g l^{-1})	3.37	2.11–5.89
t-PA-Ag (μg l^{-1})	3.6	1.6–6.3
F1+2 (nmol l^{-1})	0.61	0.26–1.46
W kg^{-1} bw	2.77	1.8–3.6
W kg^{-1} FFM	5.1	3.9–5.9

Table 2. Relation between fat mass and risk factors for CHD

	Fat mass	
VII:C	$r=0.34$	$p=0.027$
Log triglycerides	$r=0.44$	$p=0.004$
Log VLDL	$r=0.41$	$p=0.007$
Log insulin	$r=0.68$	$p<0.0001$
Log C-peptide	$r=0.73$	$p<0.0001$

Body FM correlated significantly with factor VII coagulant activity (VII:C), log triglycerides, log VLDL, log insulin, and log C-peptide (Table 2). No correlation was found between FM and total cholesterol, LDL cholesterol, and HDL cholesterol, tissue type plasminogen activator antigen (t-PA-Ag), log fibrinogen, factor VIII coagulant activity (VIII:C), von Willebrand factor antigen (vWF-Ag), and prothrombin fragments 1+2 (F1+2).

Relation Between Cardiovascular Fitness, Hemostatic and Metabolic Risk Factors

Of the 35 individuals, 25 were eligible for determination of cardiovascular fitness assessed by incremental cycle ergometer exercise. Children with power output (expressed as watt/kg body weight) below the median (≤ 2.77 W kg^{-1}) were compared to children with power output above the median (>2.77 W kg^{-1}). Results are shown in Table 3. Individuals with lower power output had significantly higher levels of body fat mass, factor VII:C, log fibrinogen, t-PA-Ag, log triglycerides, log VLDL, log insulin, and log C-peptide. Pearson's correlation revealed a significant inverse correlation between power output (watt/kg bw) and t-PA-Ag ($r=-0.62$, $p=0.001$), log insulin ($r=-0.69$, $p<0.0005$), and log C-peptide ($r=-0.64$, $p<0.001$). Factor VII:C ($r=-0.31$, $p=0.08$), log fibrinogen ($r=-0.32$, $p=0.08$), and log VLDL ($r=-0.35$, $p=0.056$) tended to be correlated inversely with power output. When cardiovascular fitness was disentangled from body fat mass by expressing the power output in watt/kg FFM, and patients were divided in two groups by the median

Table 3. Relation between power output and risk factors for CHD

	A	B	
VII:C	100	79	$p=0.005$
Log fibrinogen	0.56	0.47	$p=0.017$
t-PA-Ag	4.1	3.1	$p=0.048$
Log triglycerides	0.15	-0.04	$p=0.009$
Log VLDL	2.2	1.9	$p=0.007$
Log insulin	1.5	1.1	$p=0.0015$
Log C-peptide	0.57	0.2	$p=0.0015$

A$\leq$2.77 W kg^{-1} B>2.77 W kg^{-1}
Mean values are shown; units as presented in Table 1

again (5.14 W kg^{-1} FFM), no differences were found between the groups with respect to the above mentioned parameters. However, power output was significantly correlated with HDL cholesterol ($r=0.4$, $p<0.05$) after adjustment for FM.

Relation Between Hemostatic and Metabolic Risk Factors

Factor VII:C was significantly correlated with, log insulin, log C-peptide, log VLDL, factor VIII:C, and log fibrinogen (Table 4). We found a weak, but not significant correlation between factor VII:C and log triglycerides. After stepwise multiple regression analysis log C-peptide, log insulin and log fibrinogen contributed independently and significantly to the variance of factor VII:C ($R^2=0.66$, $p<0.001$). T-PA-Ag correlated significantly with log triglycerides ($r=0.32$, $p=0.02$) and log fibrinogen ($r=0.31$, $p=0.04$), and tended to be correlated with log VLDL ($r=0.25$, $p=0.07$) and factor VII:C ($r=0.27$, $p=0.06$). In multiple linear regression analysis, only log triglycerides explained independent significant proportions of the variance of t-PA-Ag ($R^2=0.15$, $p=0.012$). Log fibrinogen correlated significantly with factor VII:C and showed a weak, but not significant relation to log triglycerides ($r=0.27$, $p=0.055$). Factor VII:C contributed to 25% of the variance of log fibrinogen ($p=0.002$). VWF-Ag was significantly related to glucose ($r=0.39$, $p=0.012$) and log insulin ($r=0.3$, $p=0.036$). After adjustment for fat mass this correlation remained significant. Factor VIII:C and F1+2 were not correlated with metabolic risk factors.

Table 4. Relation between factor VII:C, other hemostatic and metabolic risk factors

	Factor VII:C	
Log insulin	$r=0.4$	$p=0.008$
Log C-peptide	$r=0.63$	$p<0.001$
VLDL	$r=0.33$	$p=0.024$
Log triglycerides	$r=0.27$	$p=0.056$
Factor VIII:C	$r=0.33$	$p=0.026$
Log fibrinogen	$r=0.5$	$p=0.001$

Discussion

In the present study we demonstrate for the first time an unfavorable interrelation between cardiovascular fitness, hemostatic and metabolic risk factors for coronary heart disease (CHD) in obese children and adolescents. FM correlated significantly with higher levels of triglycerides, VLDL, insulin, C-peptide. FM was also correlated to factor VII:C, but did not contribute to the variance of hemostatic risk factors for CHD in our study population. The variance of t-PA-Ag was significantly explained by triglycerides, the variance of factor VII:C mainly by markers of hyperinsulinism, suggesting that unfavorable metabolic changes might precede hemostatic disturbances. In addition, von Willebrand factor antigen (vWF-Ag) correlated significantly with glucose and insulin. In agreement with our results, in adults suffering from non-insulin-dependent diabetes mellitus a correlation between the insulin-resistance syndrome and vWF-Ag and factor VII has been described [22]. Since vWF reflects endothelial cell dysfunction [23-25] our results support the notion that obesity in childhood lays the metabolic groundwork for adult CHD.

Children with low power output showed significantly higher levels of hemostatic and metabolic risk factors, when power output was expressed in a body-weight-dependent manner. This correlation disappeared when power output was disentangled from FM. Several studies demonstrated improvement of hemostatic risk factors and decreased risk of cardiovascular morbidity and mortality associated with physical activity in adults [26-28]. However, when FM was included in multiple regression analyses, cardiovascular fitness failed to explain the variation in the levels of some hemostatic risk factors [29]. It has been shown that physical activity was correlated with favorable levels of t-PA in adults [30]. When triglycerides were taken into account, the correlation was no longer significant. In agreement with our results Gutin et al. have shown that only fatness explained significant independent proportions of the variance in the atherogenic index and insulin levels in non-obese healthy children [31].

Physical training not only alters the serum profile of risk factors for CHD. In obese children, physical training has been shown to alter cardiac autonomic function favorably by reducing the ratio of sympathetic to parasympathetic activity [32]. However, it was not possible to determine the degree to which it was the increase in fitness or the reduction in fatness elicited by the physical training that caused the favorable changes in autonomic balance. It is not known whether fitness exerts an independent effect on the risk factors, beyond its effect in reducing fatness. In children and adolescents the favorable CHD risk profile associated with improved cardiovascular fitness seems to be mainly determined by reduction of fatness caused by physical activity [17]. In our study, after adjustment for FM, only HDL cholesterol was significantly correlated with cardiovascular fitness. This observation is in accordance with the finding that regular physical activity improves HDL cholesterol levels in adults [14].

In summary, our study demonstrates a close relationship between cardiovascular fitness and hemostatic risk factors in pediatric patients with adiposity. Hemostatic risk factors were closely related to metabolic disturbances, known to precede cardiovascular morbidity and mortality. Cardiovascular fitness, in favor of fatness, failed to significantly explain independent proportions of the variance in t-PA-Ag, factor VII:C, fibrinogen and metabolic risk factors for CHD. However, since physical activity provokes improvement in body composition this study might contribute to force public health interventions for primary prevention of risk factors for CHD in childhood.

Summary

Beside metabolic disturbances hemostatic risk factors have been demonstrated to be predictive for coronary heart disease (CHD) in adults. It has been shown that physical activity might have a favorable influence on these parameters. Nothing is known about a possible relation between cardiovascular fitness and hemostatic risk factors in obese children. From 35 obese children and adolescents (18 male, 17 female, age 11.4±3 years, BMI: 29.2±5.2 kg m^{-2}), who were screened for metabolic and hemostatic risk factors for CHD, 25 (11 male, age 13.2±2.5 years, BMI: 29.2±4 kg m^{-2}; 14 female, age 12.3±1.6 years, BMI: 30.3±4.6 kg m^{-2}) were eligible for assessment of cardiovascular fitness by means of incremental cycle ergometer exercise. When patients were divided in two groups by the median of power output (watts/kg body weight), children with lower power output ($\leq$2.77 W kg^{-1}) showed significantly higher values for BMI, FM, factor VII:C, fibrinogen, and tissue type plasminogen activator antigen (t-PA-Ag), triglycerides, VLDL, insulin, and C-peptide. After adjustment for FM only HDL cholesterol correlated significantly with power output. In multiple linear regression analysis, only triglycerides explained significant independent proportions of the variance of t-PA-Ag. Factor VII:C was explained by C-peptide, insulin, and fibrinogen. Our data suggest that in obese children and adolescents the unfavorable CHD risk profile associated with low cardiovascular fitness seems to be mainly determined by changes in the metabolic state, probably caused by higher levels of fatness due to an increasingly sedentary lifestyle.

Acknowledgements. The study was supported by a grant from the Gesellschaft zur Foerderung der Gesundheit des Kindes.

References

1. Gidding SS, Leibel RL, Daniels S, Rosenbaum M, Van Horn L, Marx GR (1996) Understanding obesity in youth. A statement for healthcare professionals from the Committee on Atherosclerosis and Hypertension in the Young of the Council on Cardiovascular Disease in the Young and the Nutrition Committee, American Heart Association. Writing Group. Circulation 94: 3383–3387
2. Gidding SS, Bao W, Srinivasan SR, Berenson GS (1995) Effects of secular trends in obesity on coronary risk factors in children: the Bogalusa Heart Study. J Pediatr 127: 868–874
3. Berenson GS, Srinivasan SR, Bao W, Newman WP 3rd, Tracy RE, Wattigney WA (1998) Association between multiple cardiovascular risk factors and atherosclerosis in children and young adults. The Bogalusa Heart Study. N Engl J Med 338: 1650–1656
4. Smith FB, Lee AJ, Fowkes FG, Price JF, Rumley A, Lowe GD (1997) Hemostatic factors as predictors of ischemic heart disease and stroke in the Edinburgh Artery Study. Arterioscler Thromb Vasc Biol 17: 3321–3325
5. Ridker PM, Hennekens CH (1991) Hemostatic risk factors for coronary heart disease. Circulation 83: 1098–1100
6. Hennekens CH (1998) Increasing burden of cardiovascular disease – current knowledge and future directions for research on risk factors. Circulation 97: 1095–1102
7. Salomaa V, Stinson V, Kark JD, Folsom AR, Davis CE, Wu KK (1995) Association of fibrinolytic parameters with early atherosclerosis. The ARIC Study. Atherosclerosis Risk in Communities Study. Circulation 91: 284–290
8. Van der Bom JG, de Knijff P, Haverkate F et al. (1997) Tissue plasminogen activator and risk of myocardial infarction. The Rotterdam Study. Circulation 95: 2623–2627
9. Ridker PM, Hennekens CH, Cerskus A, Stampfer MJ (1994) Plasma concentration of cross-linked fibrin degradation product (D-Dimer) and the risk of future myocardial infarction among apparently healthy men. Circulation 90: 2236–2240

10. Juhan Vague I, Alessi MC (1997) PAI-1, obesity, insulin resistance and risk of cardiovascular events. Thromb Haemost 78: 656–660
11. Meade TW, Ruddock V, Stirling Y, Chakrabarti R, Miller GJ (1993) Fibrinolytic activity, clotting factors, and long-term incidence of ischaemic heart disease in the Northwick Park Heart Study. Lancet 342: 1076–1079
12. Folsom AR, Wu KK, Rosamond WD, Sharrett AR, Chambless LE (1997) Prospective study of hemostatic factors and incidence of coronary heart disease: the Atherosclerosis Risk in Communities (ARIC) Study. Circulation 96: 1102–1108
13. Bauer KA, Rosenberg RD (1987) The pathophysiology of the prethrombotic state in humans: insights gained from studies using markers of hemostatic system activation. Blood 70: 343–350
14. Hsieh SD, Yoshinaga H, Muto T, Sakurai Y (1998) Regular physical activity and coronary risk factors in Japanese men. Circulation 97: 661–665
15. Wannamethee SG, Shaper AG, Walker M (1998) Changes in physical activity, mortality, and incidence of coronary heart disease in older men. Lancet 351: 1603–1608
16. Craig SB, Bandini LG, Lichtenstein AH, Schaefer EJ, Dietz WH (1996) The impact of physical activity on lipids, lipoproteins, and blood pressure in preadolescent girls. Pediatrics 98: 389–395
17. DuRant RH, Baranowski T, Rhodes T et al (1993) Association among serum lipid and lipoprotein concentrations and physical activity, physical fitness, and body composition in young children. J Pediatr 123: 185–192
18. Must A, Dallal GE, Dietz WH (1991) Reference data for obesity: 85th and 95th percentiles of body mass index (wt/ht2) and triceps skinfold thickness [published erratum appears in Am J ClinNutr 1991 Nov, 54(5): 773]. Am J Clin Nutr 53: 839–846
19. Clauss A (1957) Gerinnungsphysiologische Schnellmethode zur Bestimmung des Fibrinogens. Acta Haemat 17: 237–246
20. Schaefer F, Georgi M, Zieger A, Scharer K (1994) Usefulness of bioelectric impedance and skinfold measurements in predicting fat-free mass derived from total body potassium in children. Pediatr Res 35: 617–24
21. Hofmann P, Pokan R, von Duvillard SP, Seibert FJ, Zweiker R, Schmid P (1997) Heart rate performance curve during incremental cycle ergometer exercise in healthy young male subjects. Med Sci Sports Exerc 29: 762–768
22. Juhan Vague I, Alessi MC, Vague P (1996) Thrombogenic and fibrinolytic factors and cardiovascular risk in non-insulin-dependent diabetes mellitus. Ann Med 28: 371–380
23. Stehouwer CD, Fischer HR, van Kuijk AW, Polak BC, Donker AJ (1995) Endothelial dysfunction precedes development of microalbuminuria in IDDM. Diabetes 44: 561–564
24. Borkenstein MH, Muntean WE (1982) Elevated factor VIII activity and factor VIII-related antigen in diabetic children without vascular disease. Diabetes 31: 1006–1009
25. Muntean WE, Borkenstein MH, Haas J (1985) Elevation of Factor VIII coagulant activity over Factor VIII coagulant antigen in diabetic children without vascular disease. A sign of activation of the Factor VIII coagulant moiety during poor diabetes control. Diabetes 34: 140–144
26. DeSouza CA, Jones PP, Seals DR (1998) Physical activity status and adverse age-related differences in coagulation and fibrinolytic factors in women. Arterioscler Thromb Vasc Biol 18: 362–368
27. Koenig W, Sund M, Doring A, Ernst E (1997) Leisure-time physical activity but not work-related physical activity is associated with decreased plasma viscosity: Results from a large population sample. Circulation 95: 335–341
28. Stratton JR, Chandler WL, Schwartz RS, et al (1991) Effects of physical conditioning on fibrinolytic variables and fibrinogen in young and old healthy adults. Circulation 83: 1692–1697
29. Tanaka H, Clevenger CM, Jones PP, Seals DR, DeSouza CA (1998) Influence of body fatness on the coronary risk profile of physically active postmenopausal women. Metabolism 47: 1112–1120

30. Eliasson M, Asplund K, Evrin PE (1996) Regular leisure time physical activity predicts high activity of tissue plasminogen activator: The Northern Sweden MONICA Study. Int J Epidemiol 25: 1182–1188
31. Gutin B, Owens S, Treiber F, Islam S, Karp W, Slavens G (1997) Weight-independent cardiovascular fitness and coronary risk factors. Arch Pediatr Adolesc Med 151: 462–465
32. Gutin B, Owens S, Slavens G, Riggs S, Treiber F (1997) Effect of physical training on heart-period variability in obese children. J Pediatr 130: 938–943

Inverse Correlation Between Thyroid Function and Hemostatic Risk Factors for Coronary Heart Disease in Obese Children and Adolescents

S. Gallistl, K. Sudi, M. Borkenstein, B. Leschnik, W. Muntean

Introduction

Obesity in youth is associated with unfavorable levels of metabolic and hemostatic risk factors for coronary heart disease (CHD) in later life [1–8]. It has been demonstrated that up to 25% of obese children show hypothyroidism [9]. Hypothyroidism is also associated with increased risk of CHD through high levels of serum lipids and hemostatic abnormalities [10,11]. Factor VII coagulant activity and fibrinogen have been shown to be related to an increased risk of non-fatal myocardial infarction and ischemic heart disease death among middle-aged men in the Northwick Park Heart Study [12]. The Physicians Health Study and the European Concerted Action on Thrombosis (ECAT) study demonstrated tissue-type plasminogen activator antigen (t-PA-Ag) and plasminogen activator inhibitor type 1 antigen (PAI 1-Ag) to be independent predictors of future coronary thrombosis [13,14]. Furthermore, the PLAT study revealed a close association between factor VIII coagulant activity, von Willebrand factor antigen (vWF-Ag) and atherothrombotic events [15]. There is conflicting data on the correlation between thyroid function and levels of hemostatic risk factors for CHD. Hypothyroidism may be associated with a bleeding tendency due to low levels of vWF reversible after thyroxin treatment [16,17]. On the other hand, an inverse relationship between fT4 and plasma D-dimer levels has been described in hyperlipidemic adults, which is consistent with the well-known relation between hypothyroidism and thrombotic events [18]. Since obese children may present both thyroid dysfunction and unfavorable levels of CHD risk factors, we investigated obese children and adolescents for a possible correlation between thyroid function and hemostatic markers for CHD.

Methods

Participants

The study comprised 39 obese (body mass index, BMI [19,20] above the 85th percentile for age and sex) children and adolescents (20 male, 19 female) aged

---

Abbreviations. *BMI* body mass index; *CHD*: coronary heart disease; *FM*: fat mass; *PAI 1-Ag*: plasminogen activator inhibitor type 1 antigen; *t-PA-Ag*: tissue-type plasminogen activator antigen; *vWF-Ag*: von Willebrand factor antigen

---

I. Scharrer/W. Schramm (Ed.)
30th Hemophilia Symposium Hamburg 1999
© Springer-Verlag Berlin Heidelberg 2001

4.4–17.5 years (median 12.5 years). At admission, a medical history and physical examination were performed to ensure that the participants were healthy. All children and adolescents had normal liver and renal function as assessed by standard clinical chemistry analyses. No participants were taking medications. Informed consent was obtained from each child and a legal guardian.

Analytical Methods

Venous blood samples were taken after an overnight fast between 8:00 a.m. and 10:00 am in order to further minimize any effect on hemostatic and fibrinolytic variables through the diurnal rhythm. Serum levels of fT4 (normal range: 9–23 pmol l^{-1}), fT3 (normal range: 2–8 pmol l^{-1}), and TSH (normal range: 0.4–4 mU l^{-1}) were determined by means of radio immunoassay (Behring, Germany). Blood samples for the measurements of hemostatic parameters were drawn into plastic tubes containing 0.1 mol l^{-1} sodium citrate. The plasma was separated immediately by centrifugation at 3000 g for 10 min at 4°C and stored at –70°C. Factor VII coagulant activity and factor VIII coagulant activity were determined using one-stage clotting assays and deficient plasmas for factor VII and factor VIII, respectively (Behring, Germany). The plasma level of fibrinogen was assayed by a thrombin time method according to Clauss. VWF-Ag (Boehringer, Germany), t-PA-Ag, and PAI 1-Ag (both Kabi, Austria) were determined using commercially available enzyme linked immuno-assay (ELISA) kits.

Measurement of Body Composition

Measurement of body composition was performed by means of bioelectrical impedance (BIA Akern-RJL 101/S) with an applied current of 50 kHz. Measurements were performed in the fasting state after children had been resting in supine position for 10 min. Fat-free mass was calculated and fat mass (FM) was estimated as the difference between body weight and calculated fat-free mass.

Statistical Analysis

Data not normally distributed were log$_{10}$-transformed (TSH and fibrinogen). Unpaired t-test and analysis of variance were used to compare parameters between groups where appropriate. Correlations between variables of interest were calculated using Pearson's correlation coefficient and partial correlation was performed to adjust for the influence of confounding variables. The significance level of p values was set at 5%. Calculations were performed using SPSS for Windows (SPSS, Chicago) and WinStat 3.1. (Kalmia).

Results

Results in the Whole Study Population

The whole study consisted of 39 subjects (20 male, 19 female). BMI was above the 85th percentile for age and sex in all individuals and above the 95th percentile in 35

Table 1. Clincal characteristics and biological parameters of study population

	Median	Range
Age (years)	12.5	4.4–17.5
BMI (kg m^{-2})	29.5	20.2–45.8
Fat mass (kg)	31	11.8–66.8
TSH (mU l^{-1})	2.7	1.1–16.1
fT3 (pmol l^{-1}))	6.25	4.8–7.2
fT4 (pmol l^{-1}))	14	4.6–21.4
Factor VII (%)	89	60–120
Factor VIII (%)	136	68–193
vWF (%)	127	54–173
Fibrinogen (mg dl^{-1})	337	211–589
t-PA (μg l^{-1})	3.6	1.6–6.3
PAI 1 (ng ml^{-1})	37.2	6.9–88.7

individuals. The main clinical characteristics and biological parameters are given in Table 1. One boy showed primary hypothyroidism due to fT4 concentration below, and TSH concentration above the normal range, respectively. Twelve children showed TSH levels above the normal range, but had euthyroid levels of fT3 and fT4. Log TSH was negatively related to fT4 ($r=-0.5$, $p<0.001$), but was not related to fT3. FT3 correlated inversely with FM ($r=-0.3$, $p=0.04$).

Relation Between Fat Mass and Hemostatic Risk Factors for CHD

FM was related significantly with factor VII ($r=0.43$, $p=0.04$) and PAI 1-Ag ($r=0.53$, $p<0.001$). Factor VII correlated with factor VIII ($r=0.33$, $p=0.026$), log fibrinogen ($r=0.5$, $p=0.001$), and PAI 1-Ag ($r=0.34$, $p=0.017$), and tended to be associated with t-PA-Ag ($r=0.27$, $p=0.06$). After adjustment for FM the relations between factor VII, factor VIII and log fibrinogen remained significant. PAI 1-Ag correlated significantly with t-PA-Ag ($r=0.41$, $p=0.006$), which remained significant after adjustment for FM, although the magnitude of significance decreased ($p=0.01$).

Relation Between Thyroid Function and Hemostatic Risk Factors for CHD

We divided the study population by the median of fT4 (14 pmol l^{-1}) in two groups. Patients with fT4 concentrations ≤14 pmol l^{-1} showed significantly higher levels of factor VII and log fibrinogen than patients with fT4 concentrations above 14 pmol l^{-1} (Table 2). We found no difference regarding factor VIII, vWF-Ag, t-PA-Ag, and PAI 1-Ag between the two groups.

In the whole study population, Pearson's correlation revealed a significant negative correlation between fT4 and factor VII and log fibrinogen (Figs. 1, 2). Factor VIII ($r=-0.26$, $p=0.066$) and vWF-Ag ($r=-0.28$, $p=0.053$) tended to be correlated inversely with fT4. After adjustment for body FM the inverse correlation be-

Table 2. Hemostatic risk factors for CHD in patients with fT4 values ≤14 pmol l⁻¹ (A) compared to patients with fT4 values >14 pmol l⁻¹ (B)

	A	B	p
VII	94.8	84.4	0.03
log fibrinogen	2.59	2.49	0.01
VIII	144	130	n.s.
vWF triglycerides	125	121	n.s.
t-PA VLDL	3.4	3.7	n.s
PAI-insulin	44.4	37.8	n.s.

Data presented as mean
Units: see Table 1
n.s., not significant

tween fT4 and factor VII ($r=-0.34$, $p=0.024$) and log fibrinogen ($r=-0.35$, $p=0.02$) remained significant. FT3 was inversely correlated with factor VII ($r=-0.30$, $p=0.039$) and tended to be correlated inversely with log fibrinogen ($r=-0.27$,

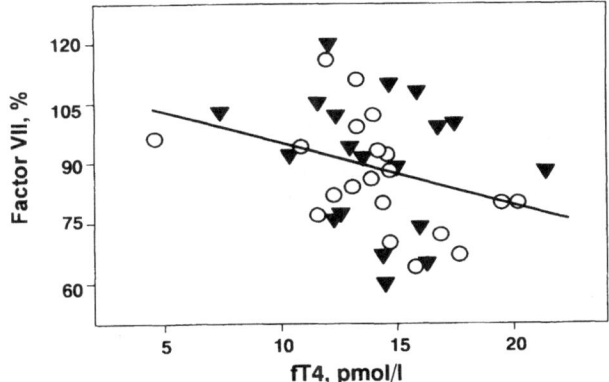

Fig. 1. Correlation between fT4 and factor VII ($r=-0.33$, $p=0.03$); ▼ females, ○ males

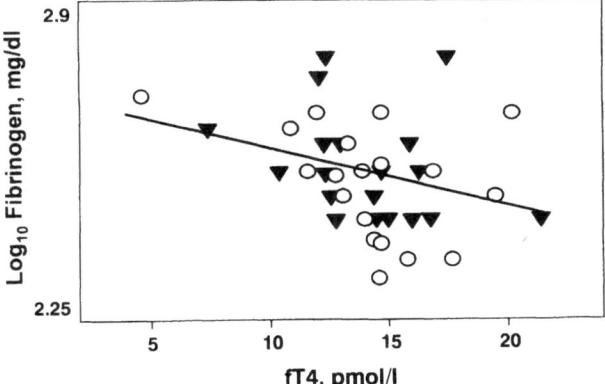

Fig. 2. Correlation between fT4 and log fibrinogen. ($r=-0.35$, $p=0.02$); ▼ females, ○ males

$p = 0.058$). The correlation between fT3 and factor VII was no longer significant after adjustment for FM. We found no relation between TSH and the determined hemostatic risk factors for CHD.

Discussion

Our study demonstrates a close relationship between thyroid function and hemostatic risk factors for CHD in obese children and adolescents, who are known to bear a higher risk of developing CHD in later life [1–3]. In addition, we show a close interrelation of hemostatic risk factors, partially dependent on FM. Low fT4 levels were significantly correlated with higher levels of factor VII and fibrinogen and showed a less impressive correlation with factor VIII and vWF-Ag. The relation was independent of body FM. We found no correlation between thyroid function, t-PA-Ag and PAI 1-Ag. Our results are in agreement with the study of Chadarevian et al., who demonstrated a close inverse relationship between thyroid hormones and hemostatic risk factors in adult hyperlipidemic patients [18]. They suggested that, since thyroid hormones increase synthesis and catabolism of proteins, the unfavorable profile of hemostatic risk factors in euthyroid individuals with lower fT4 indicates a predominate effect on catabolism.

Hemostatic abnormalities have been reported in hypothyroidism including impaired and increased fibrinolytic activity [21], platelet function abnormalities [22], and low levels of several plasma coagulation factors [24]. These observations are partially in contradiction to the well-known fact that atherosclerosis is a major complication of hypothyroidism in adulthood [11] and that atherosclerosis usually is accompanied by increased levels of hemostatic risk factors [25]. Deviations of thyroid hormones in euthyroid individuals might therefore result in different protein metabolism compared to individuals with chronic hypothyroidism, who show impaired protein synthesis [26]. This assumption is supported by the fact that thyroid hormones may provoke acute changes of hemostasis in euthyroid subjects which are not seen in patients suffering from chronic hypothyroidism [24,27].

Although all but one of our patients showed fT3 and fT4 levels within the normal range, 30% had TSH values higher than 4 mU l^{-1}. This observation might be due to a relative unresponsiveness to TSH in our patients, since it has been demonstrated that obese individuals without overt hypothyroidism or myxedema show impaired response to exogenous TSH [28].

With regard to the elevated levels of hemostatic risk factors for CHD in obese children with low fT4, the question arises whether these patients might profit by initiation of treatment with thyroid hormones. Since fT3 was negatively related to body FM in our study population, further studies are needed to clarify whether weight reduction alone might result in improvement of thyroid function and hemostatic risk profile.

In conclusion, our study demonstrates for the first time that lower levels of thyroid hormones are associated with higher levels of hemostatic risk factors for CHD in euthyroid obese children and adolescents, who are at a higher risk of developing CHD.

Summary

Thyroid dysfunction has been shown to be associated with childhood obesity. Both obesity and hypothyroidism are related to increased risk of coronary heart disease (CHD) through high levels of serum lipids and/or hemostatic abnormalities.

Thirty-nine (38 euthyroid, 1 hypothyroid) obese children and adolescents were investigated for thyroid function and risk factors for CHD after overnight fast. Thyroid hormones were measured by means of radioimmunoassay. Factor VII and factor VIII were determined using one-stage clotting assays, fibrinogen was measured according to the method of Clauss, vWF-Ag, t-PA-Ag, and PAI 1-Ag were determined by means of ELISA.

We found a significant inverse correlation between fT4 and factor VII ($r = -0.33$, $p = 0.03$) and fibrinogen ($r = -0.35$, $p = 0.02$), which remained significant after adjustment for body FM. Factor VIII ($r = -0.26$, $p = 0.066$) and vWF-Ag ($r = -0.28$, $p = 0.053$) tended to be correlated negatively to fT4. FT4 did not correlate with t-PA-Ag and PAI 1-Ag. FT3 was inversely related to factor VII ($r = -0.3$, $p = 0.039$), which was not independent of body FM, and showed a less impressive negative correlation with fibrinogen ($r = -0.27$, $p = 0.058$). FT3 did not correlate with vWF-Ag, t-PA-Ag, and PAI 1-Ag. There was no relation between TSH and the determined hemostatic risk factors.

Our study demonstrates a close relationship between thyroid function and hemostatic risk factors for CHD in obese children and adolescents and suggests that thyroid dysfunction is associated with an unfavorable hemostatic state in even pediatric patients.

Acknowledgements. Supported by a grant from the Gesellschaft zur Foerderung der Gesundheit des Kindes.

References

1. Gidding SS, Leibel RL, Daniels S, Rosenbaum M, Van Horn L, Marx GR (1996) Understanding obesity in youth. A statement for healthcare professionals from the Committee on Atherosclerosis and Hypertension in the Young of the Council on Cardiovascular Disease in the Young and the Nutrition Committee, American Heart Association. Writing Group. Circulation 94: 3383–3387
2. Gidding SS, Bao W, Srinivasan SR, Berenson GS (1995) Effects of secular trends in obesity on coronary risk factors in children: the Bogalusa Heart Study. J Pediatr 127: 868–874
3. Berenson GS, Srinivasan SR, Bao W, Newman WP 3rd, Tracy RE, Wattigney WA (1998) Association between multiple cardiovascular risk factors and atherosclerosis in children and young adults. The Bogalusa Heart Study. N Engl J Med 338: 1650–1656
4. Wilmore JH, McNamara JJ (1974) Prevalence of coronary heart disease risk factors in boys, 8 to 12 years of age. J Pediatr 84: 527–533
5. Lauer RM, Connor WE, Leaverton PE, Reiter MA, Clarke WR (1975) Coronary heart disease risk factors in school children: the Muscatine study. J Pediatr 86: 697–706
6. Tershakovec AM, Jawad AF, Stallings VA, Cortner JA, Zemel BS, Shannon BM (1998) Age-related changes in cardiovascular disease risk factors of hypercholesterolemic children. J Pediatr 132: 414–420
7. Ferguson MA, Gutin B, Owens S, Litaker M, Tracy RP, Allison J (1998) Fat distribution and hemostatic measures in obese children. Am J Clin Nutr 67: 1136–1140

8. Cacciari E, Balsamo A, Palareti G, Cassio A, Argento R, Poggi M, Tassoni P, Cicognani A, Tacconi M, Pascucci MG, et al. (1988) Haemorheologic and fibrinolytic evaluation in obese children and adolescents. Eur J Pediatr 147: 381–384

9. Ciovirnache M, Popa M, Florea I, Ionescu V, Popescu H (1980) Somatotyping in the obese children and adolescents. Endocrinologie 18: 193–200

10. Diekman T, Lansberg PJ, Kastelein JJ, Wiersinga WM (1995) Prevalence and correction of hypothyroidism in a large cohort of patients referred for dyslipidemia. Arch Intern Med 155: 1490–1495

11. Ladenson PW (1990) Recognition and management of cardiovascular disease related to thyroid dysfunction. Am J Med 88: 638–641

12. Meade TW, Mellows S, Brozovic M, Miller GJ, Chakrabarti RR, North WR, et al. (1986) Haemostatic function and ischaemic heart disease: principal results of the Northwick Park Heart Study. Lancet 2 (8506): 533–537

13. Ridker PM, Vaughan DE, Stampfer MJ, Manson JE, Hennekens CH (1993) Endogenous tissue-type plasminogen activator and risk of myocardial infarction. Lancet 341 (8854): 1165–1168

14. Juhan Vague I, Pyke SD, Alessi MC, Jespersen J, Haverkate F, Thompson SG (1996) Fibrinolytic factors and the risk of myocardial infarction or sudden death in patients with angina pectoris. ECAT Study Group. European Concerted Action on Thrombosis and Disabilities. Circulation 94: 2057–2063

15. Cortellaro M, Boschetti C, Cofrancesco E, Zanussi C, Catalano M, de Gaetano G, et al. (1992) The PLAT Study: hemostatic function in relation to atherothrombotic ischemic events in vascular disease patients. Principal results. PLAT Study Group. Progetto Lombardo Atero-Trombosi (PLAT) Study Group. Arterioscler Thromb 12: 1063–1070

16. Dalton RG, Dewar MS, Savidge GF, Kernoff PB, Matthews KB, Greaves M, et al. (1987) Hypothyroidism as a cause of acquired von Willebrand's disease. Lancet 1 (8540): 1007–1009

17. Myrup B, Bregengard C, Faber J (1995) Primary haemostasis in thyroid disease. J Intern Med 238: 59–63

18. Chadarevian R, Bruckert E, Ankri A, Beucler I, Giral P, Turpin G (1998) Relationship between thyroid hormones and plasma D-dimer levels. Thromb Haemost 79: 99–103

19. Rosner B, Prineas R, Loggie J, Daniels SR (1998) Percentiles for body mass index in U.S. children 5 to 17 years of age. J Pediatr 132: 211–22

20. Pietrobelli A, Faith MS, Allison DB, Gallagher D, Chiumello G, Heymsfield SB (1998) Body mass index as a measure of adiposity among children and adolescents: a validation study. J Pediatr 132: 204–210

21. Farid NR, Griffiths BL, Collins JR, Marshall WH, Ingram DW (1976) Blood coagulation and fibrinolysis in thyroid disease. Thromb Haemost 35: 415–422

22. Palareti G, Biagi G, Legnani C, Bianchi D, Serra D, Savini R, et al. (1989) Association of reduced factor VIII with impaired platelet reactivity to adrenalin and collagen after total thyroidectomy. Thromb Haemost 62: 1053–1056

23. Edson JR, Fecher DR, Doe RP (1975) Low platelet adhesiveness and other hemostatic abnormalities in hypothyroidism. Ann Intern Med 82: 342–346

24. Van Oosterom AT, Kerkhoven P, Veltkamp JJ (1979) Metabolism of the coagulation factors of the prothrombin complex in hypothyroidism in man. Thromb Haemost 41: 273–285

25. Hennekens CH (1998) Increasing burden of cardiovascular disease: current knowledge and future directions for research on risk factors [published erratum appears in Circulation 1998 May 19; 97 (19): 1995] Circulation 97: 1095–1102

26. Graninger W, Pirich KR, Speiser W, Deutsch E, Waldhausl WK (1986) Effect of thyroid hormones on plasma protein concentration in man. J Clin Endocrinol Metab 63: 407–411

27. Rogers JS, Shane SR (1983) Factor VIII in normal volunteers receiving oral thyroid hormone. J Clin Lab Med 102: 444–449

28. Schmitt T, Luqman W, McCool C, Lenz F, Ahmad U, Nolan S, et al. (1977) Unresponsiveness to exogenous TSH in obesity. Int J Obes 2: 185–190

Heparin-Induced Thrombocytopenia Type II in Three Children and Anticoagulant Therapy with Org 10172 (Orgaran)

B. Zöhrer, W. Zenz, A. Rettenbacher, H. Zotter, P. Covi, H. Kroll, H.M. Grubbauer, W. Muntean

Introduction

In adults, untreated heparin-induced thrombocytopenia type II (HIT type II) with complicating thrombosis has been associated with the death of the patient in up to 28% of cases [4]. For this reason in adults, prompt cessation of heparin and continuance of anticoagulation with Org 10172 (danaparoid sodium, Orgaran) or recombinant hirudin (Refludan) is recommended if thrombocytopenia or a new thrombo embolic event or progression of existing thrombosis has been developed and HIT type II must be suspected [2].

In children with HIT type II, Orgaran has been used only in a few single cases. We report on three children with deep venous thrombosis (DVT) and HIT type II in whom anticoagulant therapy was provided with Orgaran.

Patient 1

A 12-year-old boy with inherited protein S deficiency type I was admitted to our hospital because of DVT of his left lower extremity extending from iliac to calf veins.

Laboratory examination on admission revealed a platelet count of 560×10^9 l^{-1}, cardiolipin IgG antibodies of 27.4 GPL U^{-1} ml^{-1} (normal <23 GPL U^{-1} ml^{-1}), and cardiolipin IgM antibodies of 1.7 MPL U^{-1} ml^{-1} (normal <11 MPL U^{-1} ml^{-1}).

Under intravenous therapy with unfractionated heparin (UFH) (15–20 U kg^{-1} h^{-1}) and thrombolytic therapy with recombinant tissue plasminogen activator (rt-PA) (0.025–0.05 mg kg^{-1} h^{-1}, for 8 days) a new thrombosis occurred at the puncture site of an inferior vena cava filter (right femoral vein) on day 4 of rt-PA therapy (day 6 of heparin therapy). In addition, the need for heparin increased up to 40 U kg^{-1} h^{-1} and platelet count slowly fell down between day 11 and day 14 of heparin therapy. On day 14 of heparin therapy, extension of thrombosis to inferior vena cava (inf.v.c.) up to the renal veins, and thrombocytopenia with a platelet nadir of 80×10^9 l^{-1} was observed.

Evidence of heparin-associated anti-platelet antibodies (Haab) was provided by the heparin-induced platelet aggregation assay (HIPAA).

The patient was administered Orgaran in a dose of 1250 U as bolus intravenously, followed by 400 U h^{-1} and 300 U h^{-1}, respectively, for 4 h each. To maintain therapeutic plasma anti-factor Xa-activity (anti-Xa) levels between 0.5 U ml^{-1} and 0.8 U ml^{-1} doses of 160–250 U h^{-1} were necessary during a treatment period of 16 days.

I. Scharrer/W. Schramm (Ed.)
30th Hemophilia Symposium Hamburg 1999
© Springer-Verlag Berlin Heidelberg 2001

Under this treatment, platelets returned to normal and overlapping oral anti-coagulation was initiated. Computer tomography before discharge displayed no further extension of thrombosis in inf.v.c. and no changing of DVT of iliac and lower limb veins. Since this event the patient continued to have oral anticoagulation over a follow-up period of 4 years.

Patient 2

A 13-year-old girl with highly elevated antiphospholipid antibodies (APA) was admitted to pediatric intensive care unit because of acute pulmonary embolism and a thrombus of 2 cm x 1 cm in diameter localized in the right ventricle.

Laboratory examination on admission revealed a platelet count of 219×10^9 l^{-1}, cardiolipin IgM antibodies of 50.8 MPL U^{-1} ml^{-1} (normal <11 MPL U^{-1} ml^{-1}), and cardiolipin IgG antibodies of 5.8 GPL U^{-1} ml^{-1} (normal <23 GPL U^{-1} ml^{-1}).

Thrombolytic therapy with rt-PA (0.05–0.5 mg kg^{-1} h^{-1}, for 22 h) was performed, and simultaneous intravenous therapy with UFH (15–23 U kg^{-1} h^{-1}) was initiated. Resolution of the intra-cardiac thrombus was observed within 2 days. Administration of heparin was continued for a further 9 days and overlapping oral anti-coagulation was started.

After a short course of heparin because of insufficient oral anticoagulation, a second pulmonary embolism occurred, and again a thrombus in the right ventricle was diagnosed on day 17 of hospital stay. Under intravenous UFH (20–33 U kg^{-1} h^{-1}) temporary clinical improvement was observed. On day 19 of hospital stay, a new thrombus of 1.6 cm x 2 cm in diameter in the right atrium, and left DVT extending from the common iliac to common femoral vein were found. Despite the absence of thrombocytopenia or obvious decrease of platelet count, heparin was substituted for Orgaran because of suspected HIT type II before evidence of Haab in the heparin/platelet factor 4-ELISA was provided.

Under infusion therapy with Orgaran (54–153 U h^{-1}, plasma anti-Xa levels between 0.5 U ml^{-1} and 0.8 U ml^{-1}) partial resolution of both intra-cardiac thrombi, and improvement of peripheral perfusion were observed within a few hours. However, after 24 days of therapy with Orgaran and 10 days of simultaneous oral anticoagulation, thrombosis of left calf veins occurred. Cross-reactivity of Orgaran with Haab was suspected and recombinant hirudin was given for 2 days. Repeat measurement of Haab at this time did not show increased Haab in comparison with previous findings. No extension of thrombosis in the left common iliac and common femoral vein were observed, and echocardiography was normal.

Oral anticoagulation was stopped 1 year post discharge after normalization of APA.

Patient 3

A 9 9/12-year-old girl with APA was admitted to our hospital because of DVT of the left superficial and common femoral veins.

Laboratory examination on admission revealed a platelet count of 241×10^9 l^{-1}, cardiolipin IgG antibodies of 74.0 GPL U^{-1} ml^{-1} (normal <23 GPL U^{-1} ml^{-1}), and cardiolipin IgM antibodies of 3.3 MPL U^{-1} ml^{-1} (normal <11 MPL U^{-1} ml^{-1}).

Under thrombolytic therapy with rt-PA (0.05 mg kg^{-1} h^{-1}, for 19 h) and simultaneous intravenous administration of UFH (22 U kg^{-1} h^{-1}) signs of recanalization were observed. Subsequently, UFH (15–20 U kg^{-1} h^{-1}) was given for a further 3 days.

Starting on day 6 of heparin therapy, a massive drop in platelet count from 184×10^9 l^{-1} to 82×10^9 l^{-1} was observed within 36 h. Suspicion of HIT type II was confirmed by a positive HIPAA as well as by the presence of Haab in the heparin/platelet factor 4-ELISA.

The patient was administered Orgaran in a dose of 1000 U as bolus intravenously, followed by 250 U h^{-1} and 150 U h^{-1}, respectively, for 4 h each. To maintain therapeutic plasma anti-factor Xa-activity (anti-Xa) levels between 0.5 U ml^{-1} and 0.8 U ml^{-1} doses of 100–175 U h^{-1} were necessary during a treatment period of 9 days.

Under this treatment, platelets returned to normal, and overlapping oral anticoagulation was initiated. Ultrasound examination before discharge displayed no new generation of thrombus.

The patient was discharged with subtotal recanalization of left femoral veins. After this event she was on oral anticoagulation for 9 months. APA were persistently elevated during this period.

Discussion

Heparin-induced thrombocytopenia type II (HIT type II) defines a potentially life-threatening immune-mediated adverse event of heparin therapy and occurs in 1–5% of adults treated with heparin for more than 5 days [1].

HIT type II is characterized by a decrease of platelet count (1) which leads to acute thrombocytopenia (below 100×10^9 l^{-1}) or a drop below 50% of the platelet value before the onset of heparin treatment. (2) Thrombocytopenia can not be explained solely by DIC, TTP, lupus anticoagulant syndrome, systemic lupus, sepsis or any other drug, and (3) reverts to a normal count on withdrawal of heparin [4]. The diagnosis is made by the detection of heparin-associated anti-platelet antibodies (Haab).

Approximately 20% of patients with HIT type II may experience new occurrence or extension of a thrombo embolic event [5]. However, some cases of heparin-induced »thrombocytopenia« type II were described showing new thrombosis or a progression of thrombosis together with positive testing for Haab but no decrease of platelets [3].

The symptoms of HIT type II generally occur 5–14 days after the initiation of heparin therapy in a patient not sensitized to heparin, but can occur within a few hours if the patient has previously received heparin [2].

In our three children described HIT type II occurred under a therapy with UFH because of thrombo embolic diseases. Patient 1 developed a new thrombotic event on day 6 of heparin therapy with progression of thrombosis during the following days. Additionally, he showed increasing need of heparin to achieve therapeutic values of PTT, and thrombocytopenia on day 14 of heparin therapy. In patient 2 a progression of thrombosis (i.e., an additional thrombus in the right atrium and DVT) occurred under repeated heparin treatment on day 3 of a new heparin course. The early onset of HIT type II in this case is consistent with a sensitization to heparin she was administered previously. Patient 3 developed thrombocytopenia on day 6 of treatment with UFH. Haab were confirmed in all three patients.

In association with the clinical symptoms the evidence of Haab in a functional or antigen assay is confirmatory for HIT type II, and in adults immediate withdrawal of heparin is recommended. As in most cases the continuation of anticoagulant treatment is necessary a low-molecular-weight heparinoid (Org 10172, danaparoid sodium, Orgaran) or recombinant hirudin (Lepirudin, Refludan) should be administered [2].

Orgaran is a natural low-molecular-weight glycosaminoglycan preparation primarily inactivating activated factor X. For adult patients with acute thromboembolism a »step down« i.v. infusion rate is advised after an initial i.v. bolus injection, e.g., 400 U h^{-1} for 4 h, followed by 300 U h^{-1} for 4 h and then a maintenance infusion rate of 150–200 U h^{-1} to maintain plasma anti-Xa levels between 0.5 U ml^{-1} and 0.8 U ml^{-1} [2].

In our patients we have adjusted the dosage of Orgaran to the body weight. Cessation of heparin and initiation of Orgaran has led to the following findings underlining the diagnosis of HIT type II. In patient 1 we were able to observe a stop of progression of thrombosis as well as the return of platelet counts to normal. In patient 2 – simultaneously with clinical improvement – a visible regression of both intra-cardiac thrombi occurred within a few hours. Thrombosis of the calf veins in this patient might have been caused by the development of a cross-reaction of Orgaran with Haab, but a decreasing Haab titer compared to previous tests at the time of this event made this explanation unlikely. In patient 3, in which Orgaran could be administered before any thrombo embolic complications occurred, normalization of platelet counts was observed.

In conclusion, our cases show that HIT type II is a life-threatening complication of heparin therapy in children. The presented cases suggest that Org 10172 (Orgaran) is a therapeutic option in these patients.

References

1. Chong BH, Berndt MD (1989) Heparin-induced thrombocytopenia. Blood 58: 53–57
2. Greinacher A (1999) Heparin-induzierte Thrombozytopenie. In: Müller-Berghaus, Pötzsch B (eds) Haemostaseologie. Molekulare und zelluläre Mechanismen, Pathophysiologie und Klinik. Springer, Berlin Heidelberg New York
3. Hach-Wunderle V, Krainer K, Krug B, Müller-Berghaus G, Pötzsch B (1994) Heparin-associated thrombosis despite normal platelet counts. Lancet 344: 469–70
4. Magnani HN (1993) Heparin-induced thrombocytopenia (HIT): an overview of 230 Patients treated with Orgaran (Org 10172). Thomb Haemost 70: 554–61
5. Melanson SW, Silver B, Heller MB (1996) Deep vein thrombosis, pulmonary embolism, and the white clot syndrome. Am J Emerg Med 14: 558–60.

Heparin Concentration, Activated Clotting Time, and Markers of Coagulation Activation During Pediatric Heart Catheterization

B. Roschitz, A. Beitzke, A. Gamillschek, B. Leschnik,
M. Köstenberger, W. Muntean

Background

Arterial thrombosis is the most frequent complication of percutaneous catheterization in children [1]. Several mechanisms of arterial thrombosis following cardiac catheterization are described. These include formation and propagation of a thrombus initiated by intimal injury at the site of introduction of the arterial needle, guide wire and catheter, sometimes in association with subintimal dissection and intimal flap formation [2]. Platelets may become deposited on the catheter and may result in partial or total occlusion of an artery when the catheter is withdrawn [3]. Also, artery spasm may occur when the catheter is introduced into the artery and contributes to thrombus formation [2,4]. However, few data, especially from children, address appropriate dosages of heparin during cardiac catheterization.

Freed et al. concluded that heparin in a 100 IU kg^{-1} body weight dosage administered during percutaneous catheterization is effective in preventing arterial thrombosis in children 10 years of age or younger [5]. Girod et al. investigated 1316 catheterized infants and children prospectively for femoral artery thrombosis following cardiac catheterization and suggested that a very low incidence of arterial thrombosis could be achieved with systemic heparinization [6]. Saxena et al. have shown that administration of either a 50 IU kg^{-1} or a 100 IU kg^{-1} body weight dosage of heparin was equally efficacious [7]. Investigations of the coagulation status, however, were not included in these studies.

Vielhaber et al. evaluated markers of coagulation activation in children undergoing cardiac catheterization with intermittent flush heparin [8]. Grady et al. measured fibrinopeptide A and activated clotting time (ACT) in 36 children who were either flushed with heparin saline or had an administration of 50 IU or 100 IU heparin/kg body weight. They concluded that administration of a heparin bolus to maintain an ACT >200 s prevents a significant increase in thrombin activity [9]. However, in many other clinical situations such as cardiopulmonary bypass or extracorporeal membrane oxygenation no correlation between heparin levels and ACT could be shown [10,11].

Thus, in our study we compared heparin concentrations, ACT, and markers of coagulation activation during cardiac catheterization in infants and children.

I. Scharrer/W. Schramm (Ed.)
30th Hemophilia Symposium Hamburg 1999
© Springer-Verlag Berlin Heidelberg 2001

Table 1.

Heart disease	TGA	PDA	TI, AI	ASD II	PST	Fallot	PFO	AIST	PA, VSD
n=20	2	2	1	2	2	5	1	1	4

Patients and Methods

The study group consisted of 20 patients.

The mean age was 8 years (range 1 month to 17 years).

The diagnoses of all patients are shown in Table 1.

A diagnostic, hemodynamic catheterization was performed in all 20 patients; 6 patients had an additional interventional procedure.

A heparin bolus of 100 IU/kg body weight was administered directly after arterial puncture. Blood samples for coagulation studies were obtained before, 5 min after, and 30 min after arterial puncture and at the end of heart catheterization.

The blood samples were drawn into 5 ml tubes containing 0.5 ml 3.8% sodium citrate (in children below an age of 3 years only 2 ml blood was obtained). Simultaneously, blood samples for ACT measurement were collected in non-heparinized syringes and added to test tubes containing celite as activator and placed immediately in the Hemochron Jr. Microcoagulation System.

Heparin content was determined with an anti-Xa chromogenic assay, Coacute Heparin from Chromogenix. F1+2 and D-dimer formation were analyzed by using an ELISA obtained by Coachrom.

Results

The mean value of the ACT obtained at baseline was 144 s (131–185 s).

The 100 IU kg^{-1} body weight heparin bolus did significantly elevate the baseline ACT; 15 min after heparin administration the mean ACT was 310 s.

Anti-Xa heparin contents showed a strong overall correlation to the ACT as seen in Figure 1.

Although an equal dosage of 100 IU kg^{-1} body weight was administered to each patient, heparin concentrations varied over a wide range (Fig. 2).

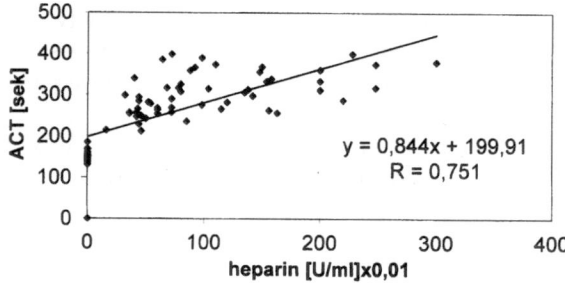

Fig. 1. ACT vs. heparin levels

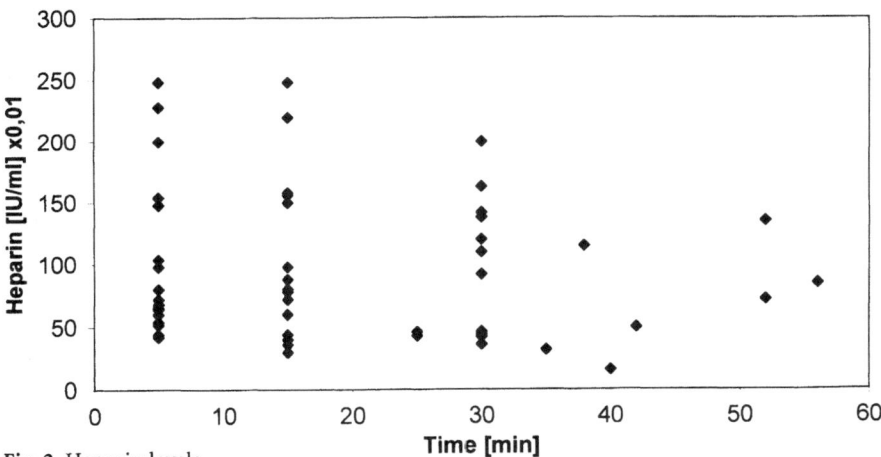

Fig. 2. Heparin levels

Table 2.

Age (a)	Procedure	Duration (min)	F1+F2 (nmol l^{-1})	D-dimer (ng l^{-1})
1 7/12	Diagnostic	13	1.80	–
1/12	Diagnostic	54	1.3	–
7	ASD occlusion	20	1.4	–
15	PFO occlusion	15	1.3	–
13	Diagnostic	30	12.5	706

There were no significant differences in ACT or markers of coagulation activation between patients undergoing diagnostic versus interventional procedures.

Thrombin generation (F1+2) showed a coagulation activation in five patients, but no concomitant clinical thrombosis was observed and none of the patients experienced a pulse loss after the procedure (Table 2). No post-catheterization bleeding was found either, but two children developed a hematoma.

Conclusions

Administration of heparin (100 IU kg^{-1} body weight) resulted in therapeutic heparin levels, but some children showed highly increased contents of heparin. Thus, immediate assessment of the coagulation status is important during cardiac catheterization. With a strong overall correlation between ACT and anti-Xa-heparin levels the ACT appears to be a useful tool for this bedside determination of the accurate coagulation status.

However, this study also indicates that a general dosage of 100 IU kg^{-1} body weight does not provide adequate heparin levels shown by coagulation activation in

25%, and the development of a hematoma in 10% of the patients. Further investigations with larger study groups will be necessary to define optimal heparin concentrations during heart catheterization in children.

References

1. Lang EK (1963) A survey of the complications of percutaneous retrograde arteriography. Radiology 81: 257–263
2. Mortensson W, Hallbook T, Lundstrom NR (1975) Percutaneous catheterization of the femoral vessels in children. II. Thrombotic occlusion of the catheterized artery: frequency and causes. Pediat. Radiol. 4: 1–9
3. Formanek G, Frech RS, Amplatz K (1970) Arterial thrombosis formation during percutaneous catheterization. Circulation 41: 833–839
4. Bergstrom K, Jorulf H (1976) Reaction of femoral and common carotid arteries in infants after puncture or percutaneous catheterization. Acta Radiol 17: 577–580
5. Freed MD, Keane FK, Rosenthal A (1974) The use of heparinization to prevent arterial thrombosis after percutaneous cardiac catheterization in children. Circulation 50: 565–569
6. Girod DA, Roger AH, Randall LC (1982) Heparinization for prevention of thrombosis following pediatric percutaneous arterial catheterization. Pediatr Cardiol 3: 175–180
7. Saxena A, Gupta R, Kumar RK, Kothari SS, Wasir HS (1997) Predictors of arterial thrombosis after diagnostic cardiac catheterization in infants and children randomized to two heparin dosages. Cathet-Cardiovasc-Diagn 41 (4): 400–403
8. Vielhaber H, Kohlhase B, Kehl H, Fliedner M, Kececioglu D, Veltmann H, Vogt J, Nowak-Göttl U (1996) Flush heparin during cardiac catheterisation prevents long-term coagulation activation in children without APC-resistance- preliminary results. ThrombRes 81 (6): 651–656
9. Grady M, Eisenberg P, Bridges N (1995) Rational approach to use of heparin during cardiac catheterization in children. JACC 25 (3): 725–729
10. Chan AK, Leaker M, Burrows FA, Williams WG, Gruenwald CE, Whyre L, Adams M, Brooker LA, Adams H, Mitchell L, Andrew M (1997) Coagulation and fibrinolytic profile of pediatric patients undergoing cardiopulmonary bypass. Thromb Haemost 77 (2): 270–277
11. O'Neill AI, Mc Allister C, Corke CF, Parkin JD (1991) A comparison of five devices for the bedside monitoring of heparin therapy. Anaesth Intensive Care 19 (4): 592–596

Therapeutic Options in Immune Thrombocytopenic Purpura in Childhood

M. Serban, V. Borla, P. Tepeneu, D. Mihailov, C. Jinca, D. Lighezan, W. Schramm

Introduction

Immune thrombocytopenic purpura (ITP) is a disorder that has distinct clinical manifestation and outcome in children and adults. During childhood, ITP is mainly self-limited in its natural course, with a better long-term prognosis even in its chronic form [3,6,7].

However, because of its potential severity, several medical options have been used prior to splenectomy, or when this procedure has either failed or been refused by the patient. In children, these options have been reported mainly in the chronic form of ITP, a form for which the therapy is characterized by controversy [1,2,4,5].

Our concerns regarding a more efficient therapeutic regimen in children justified this retrospective study.

Patients and Methods

We retrospectively compared the outcomes of 91 consecutive patients with ITP, 46 males and 45 females aged between 1 year and 16 years, treated in the 3rd Pediatric Clinic and its outpatient department in the period 1989–1999. The distribution of the cases at admission into the clinic, based on the evaluation form, was: 57 cases (62.63%) with acute ITP and 34 cases (37.37%) with chronic ITP; 27 cases presented the mild form (stage I), 34 cases the moderate form (stage II), and 30 cases the severe form (stage III).

The criteria for inclusion in the study were the following: platelets (PLT) $< 100 \times 10^9$ l^{-1}; normal/increased number of megakaryocytes; positive platelet-associated Ig (IgG/IgM).

The exclusion criteria were: Evans syndrome, secondary ITP and ITP associated with HIV infection.

The therapeutic protocols consisted of »front-line« therapy or alternative therapy.
1. »Front-line« therapy:
   - Symptomatic therapy
   - Intravenous immunoglobulins (IV Ig): 0.4 g kg^{-1} day^{-1}, 3–5 days, or 0.8–1 g kg^{-1} day^{-1}, 1–2 days, repeated after 2–4 weeks
   - Corticotherapy: conventional regimen: prednisone/prednisolone p.o.: 1–2 mg kg^{-1} day^{-1}, 2–3 weeks, then rapid tapering off to final withdrawal; »pulse corticotherapy«: i.v. dexamethasone, 20–30 mg kg^{-1} day^{-1}, 3–4 days

I. Scharrer/W. Schramm (Ed.)
30th Hemophilia Symposium Hamburg 1999
© Springer-Verlag Berlin Heidelberg 2001

Table 1. Evaluation criteria

Criteria		Therapeutic response		
		Complete remission	Partial remission	Failure
Clinical	Petechiaes	–	+/–	+
	Other hemorrhages	–	+	+
Biological	Platelet count	>100 x 10^9 l^{-1}	50–100 x 10^9 l^{-1}	<50 x 10^9 l^{-1}

Table 2. Evaluation of the ITP course based on a score system

Clinical parameters:	Points	Biological parameters:	Points
Without symptoms	0	PLT >100 x 10^9 l^{-1}	0
Ecchymosis/hematoma	1	PLT 50 x 10^9 l^{-1}	1
Generalized petechiae	2	PLT 10 x 10^9 to $50x10^9$ l^{-1}	2
Bleeding of the oral mucosa,	3	PLT 5 x 10^9 to $10x10^9$ l^{-1}	3
or abdominal petechiae,		PLT <5 x 10^9 l^{-1}	4
or subconjunctival hemorrhages,			
or gastrointestinal bleeding,			
or hematuria			

Interpretation of score:
  Complete remission (CR) = 0 points
  Partial remission (PR) ≤4 points
  Failure = 4–10 points

2. Alternative therapy:
  – Danazol: p.o. 4–7 mg kg^{-1} day^{-1}, 2–3 months
  – $IFN_{\alpha2b}$ s.c., $3x3x10^6$ IU/week, 6–8 months
  – Splenectomy

The biological parameters considered for monitoring were:
– Hematological: platelet count, bleeding time, clot retraction time, prothrombin consumption, bone marrow smear with megakaryogram
– Immunological: platelet-associated Ig, rheumatoid factor, LE cells, Coombs test, anti-DNA antibodies, cryoglobulins

The assessment was estimated on the same parameters (Table 1), with an attempt at quantitative evaluation on a score system (Table 2).

Results

In acute ITP we had three medical options: symptomatic therapy (15 cases), i.v. polyvalent Ig (6 corticorefractory cases) and corticotherapy (42 cases). The patients who did not receive specific treatment (only symptomatic drugs) had a sponta-

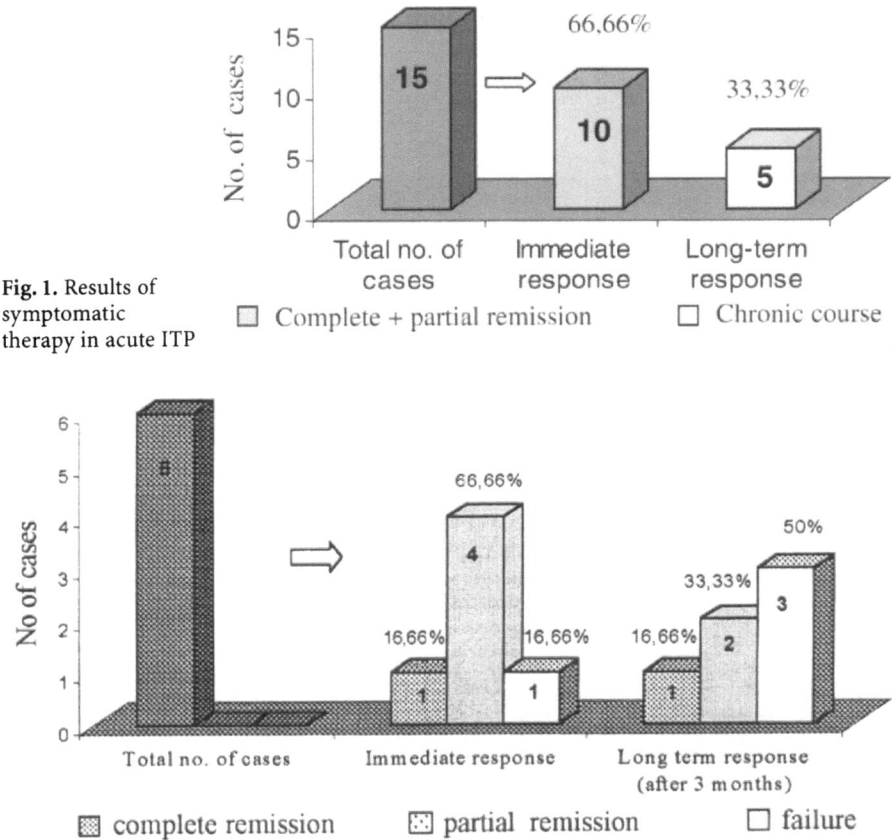

Fig. 1. Results of symptomatic therapy in acute ITP

Fig. 2. Results of therapy with i.v. Ig in acute ITP

neous remission in 66.66% of cases (Fig. 1). The group treated with i.v. Ig showed an immediate favorable outcome (complete + partial remission) in 83.33% of cases (5/6), but they relapsed within 3 months in 50% of cases (3/6) (Fig. 2). In the group treated with corticosteroids we obtained remission in 83.33% of cases and 16.66% of cases developed a chronic condition (Fig. 3). Pulse corticosteroid therapy, used in 2 patients, achieved complete remission in 1 case.

In chronic ITP we used the following protocols: i.v. Ig (8 cases), conventional corticotherapy (34 cases), »pulse corticotherapy« (3 cases), danazol (7 cases), IFN (5 cases), splenectomy (5 cases).

The group treated with i.v. Ig showed an immediate favorable response in 75% of cases (6/8), but followed by relapse in the long-term in 62.50% of cases (5/8) (Fig. 4). Using continuous oral corticotherapy, we obtained remission in 44.11% of cases and relapse in the long-term in 55.89% of cases (Fig. 5); »pulse corticotherapy« used in 3 patients failed, without improving the platelet response. The patients who received danazol showed a favorable response in the long-term in 28.57% of cases. Four

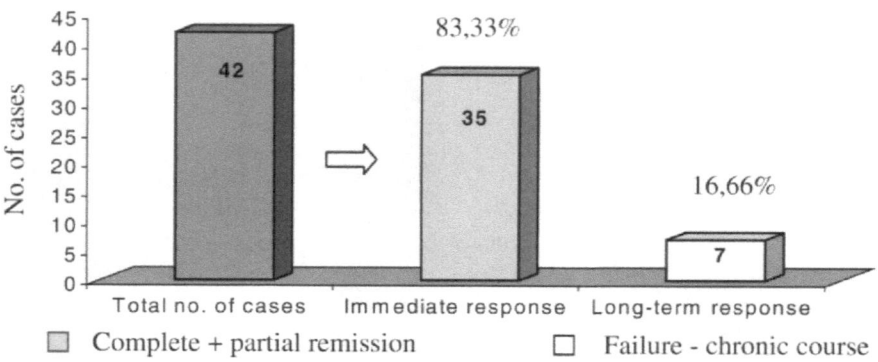

Fig. 3. Results of conventional corticosteroid therapy in acute ITP

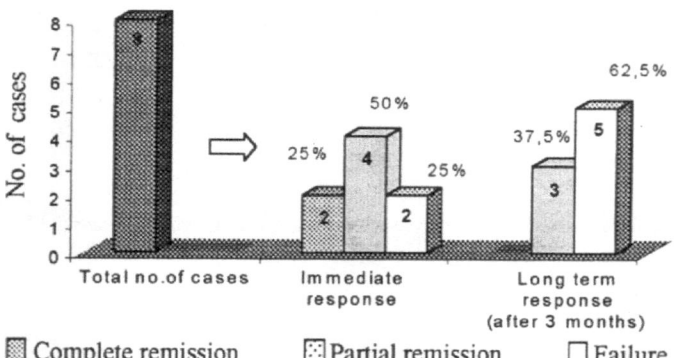

Fig. 4. Results of therapy with i.v. Ig in chronic ITP

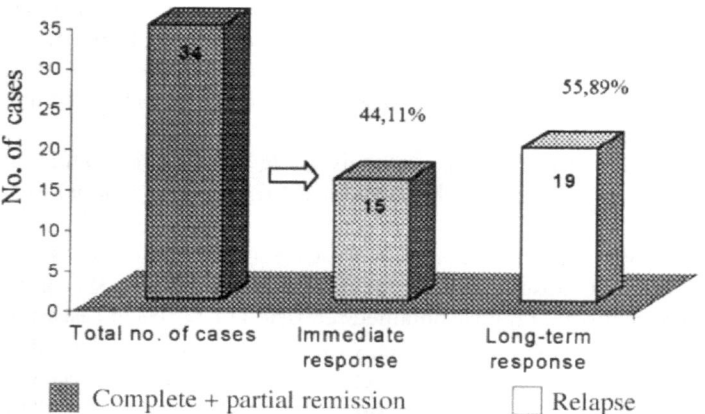

Fig. 5. Results of conventional corticotherapy in chronic ITP

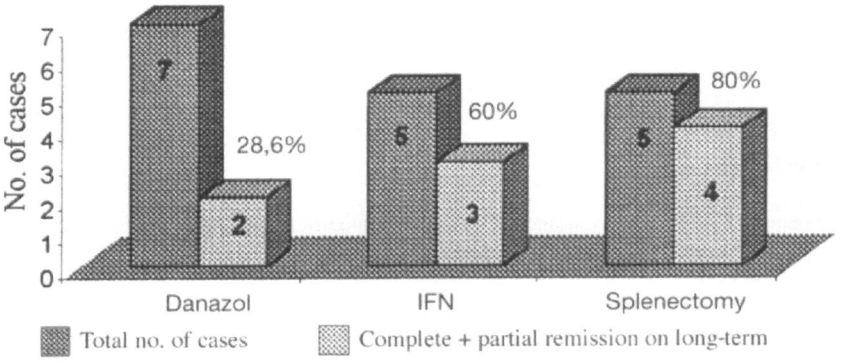

Fig. 6. Results of alternative therapy in chronic ITP

(80%) of the 5 patients who underwent splenectomy experienced remission (Fig. 6). Interferon, used initially for viral-associated infection (VHB), proved its efficiency on improving the platelet counts in 60% of cases.

Discussion and Conclusions

In both children and adults, there are important unsolved issues in diagnosis and management of ITP, that have major cost implications. That is particularly true for the pediatric ITP, in that it is mostly symptomatic, requiring a therapeutic intervention, and because the indication of splenectomy, taking into account the natural history of the disease at this age, is not a therapy of first choice.

As in other studies, our clinical experience with ITP treatment, aiming at maintenance of the platelet count at a level sufficient to provide adequate hemostasis (PLT $\geq 30-50 \times 10^9$ l^{-1}), to prevent life-threatening complications and perhaps enable patients to postpone or avoid splenectomy, is inconclusive.

Treatment decisions therefore remain controversial: i.v. Ig may be preferable to corticosteroids (conventional or pulse high-dose regimen) as initial treatment for children with ITP. They have the advantage of their prompt response, leading to a rapid rise in platelet count, without a decisive improvement of the long-term outcome. Corticosteroids have comparable effects to i.v. Ig, but despite their low cost they remain drugs of second option because of their slow platelet response and their potentially severe side effects and long-term consequences on the immune system.

We can report astonishingly good results with the use of IFN α2b; even without achieving a seroconversion of HBV infection, it succeeded in controlling the evolution in 3/5 patients with the severe form of ITP, who failed on corticosteroids and i.v. Ig. Our indication for splenectomy was rather restrictive, but was followed in 80% of cases by good control of the evolution.

In conclusion, we feel justified in establishing a regional registry of chronic ITP and in including the patients in a prospective study in order to obtain results more useful for statistical evaluation.

References

1. Baronci C., Petrone A., Miano C., et al.: Treatment of acute idiopathic thrombocytopenic purpura in children. A retrospective evaluation of 120 cases. Ann Ist Super Sanita 1998, 34 (4): 457–461.
2. Bocher A., Hagmann F.G., Kreiter H.: Die chronische idiopathische thrombozytopenische Purpura. Aktuelles Therapiekonzept und Einführung in Pathophysiologie, Klinik und Diagnostik. Med. Klin 1998, 93 (12): 707–18.
3. BlanchetteV., Freedman J.,Garvey B.: Management of chronic immune thrombocytopenic purpura in children and adults. Semin. Hematol. 1998, 35 (1 Suppl 1): 36–51.
4. Corrigan J.J.Jr.: Treatment dilemma in childhood idiopathic thrombocytopenic purpura (comment). Lancet 1997, 350 (9078): 602–3.
5. George J.N., Woolf S.H., Raskob G.E: Idiopathic thrombocytopenic purpura: a guideline for diagnosis and management of children and adults. Ann. Med 1998, 30 (1): 38–44.
6. Kuhne T., Imbach P.: Chronic immune thrombocytopenic purpura in childhood. Semin Thromb Hemost 1998, 24 (6): 549–53.
7. Tarantino M.D., Goldsmith G.: Treatment of acute immune thrombocytopenic purpura. Semin Hematol 1998, 35 (1 Suppl 1): 28–35.

Camps for Children and Young Adults with Hemophilia in Germany, Austria, and Switzerland

W. Effenberger, H. Hartl, W. Kalnins, R. Kobelt, R. Bachhuber

Upon the initiatives of different institutions and private individuals various camps for children and young adults are organized in the German-speaking countries. These camps offer a variety of recreational activities and are based on different concepts regarding their medical, educational and sporting/physiotherapeutic designs.

The common goal is to transmit the fundamentals of a normal life. Hemophilia is to be mastered by the individual, rather than dominating his every-day life. The adolescent with hemophilia should learn how to control his disease as far as possible without his parents and doctors. Therefore, children and young adults are trained in self-infusion at most holiday camps. If they are already skilled in self-infusion, their technique will merely be supervised, as errors may occasionally have been adopted that need to be corrected. Holiday camps of this kind are only feasible within a financially tolerable frame, because numerous associations, institutions and the pharmaceutical industry are granting financial support.

Specific features and differences between the various holiday camps are discussed below.

Participation of Foreign Guests

The DHG (Vöhl by Lake Eder) and ÖHG (Fath by Lake Waldschacher) both invite children and adolescents coming from their official twinning partners (Latvia and Romania). During their stay at the holiday camp guest children are supplied with blood coagulation concentrate, which is generously donated by pharmaceutical companies, and are trained in self-infusion.

Attendants

These are older persons with hemophilia or pedagogically trained lay people at the holiday camps organized by the DHG, ABB-IGH, BBB, or SHG. In the ÖHG camp attendants are specially trained educators who are at the same time undergoing their practical training within the framework of their studies. The BBB employs psychologists and is the only organization which also invites parents as attendants.

At all holiday camps visits by parents are restricted, although possible.

I. Scharrer/W. Schramm (Ed.)
30th Hemophilia Symposium Hamburg 1999
© Springer-Verlag Berlin Heidelberg 2001

Medical Care

In the holiday camps organized by the DHG, ABB-IGH, ÖHG, or SHG a doctor is permanently on duty. Only in the BBB camp medical care is provided on demand in a nearby hospital or by a doctor who is experienced in the treatment of hemophilia and who comes to the holiday camps once or twice a week. Additionally, medical checkups are done by nurses or male nurse assistants at the DHG, ABB-IGH and ÖHG camps. In all camps doctors, nurses and assistants, and physical therapists work together as a team.

Physical Activities

The ÖHG camp describes itself as a rehabilitation camp. Here, intensive physical therapy is provided as individual or group therapy by several physical therapists. Such therapy, however, which does not neglect the play components and offers opportunity for free creation, extends over the whole morning. In the afternoon a sports program, including swimming, sailing, wind surfing and tennis is offered. The ABB-IGH and the SHG camps each employ a physical therapist.

At the DHG holiday camp an additional sports program is supervised by trained coaches and includes canoeing, sailing, and wind surfing. Moreover, its medical staff considers it very important to familiarize the children and adolescents with regular physical and sports activities. At the camp at Lake Werbellin physical therapy is provided on demand. Here, the emphasis is on playing physical activities. The camps in Switzerland employ sport therapists, who are providing children and adolescents with hemophilia with reasonable borderline experiences.

Locations

The DHG holiday camp is organized on the premises of a youth hostel (single houses for very small groups) in Vöhl by Lake Eder, so that the children with hemophilia can also meet other groups and tourists staying at the youth hostel.

The ABB-IGH camp takes place in Altenhof by Lake Werbellin, and, 1 or 2 of the approximately 12 housing blocks of this holiday camp facility are entirely occupied by this group, the rest being reserved for other groups. It is a special feature of this holiday camp that it offers living together with other disabled persons (integrated holiday camp). The BBB camp is located in a youth village and also enables contact with other young adults.

The ÖHG rehabilitation camp uses the premises of a boarding house at Lake Waldschacher. Contacts with other adolescents can be made on the neighboring campsite, at the restaurant and on the meadow for sunbathing. The SHG camps either use alpine huts or bungalows.

Table 1. The camps

Location	What?	Date	Organization	Contact person	Fees	Accommodation	Friends etc.	Doctor
Vöhl, Lake Eder	Summer camp (8–14 years)	27 July–5 August (German summer holidays, except Bavaria and Bad.-Württ.)	DHG	A. Kreienbring (Tel.: +49-208-8999844)	DM 500; DM 36/day	Youth hostel, log cabins	Welcome, especially girls	24 h at the camp
Altenhof, Lake Werbellin	Summer camp (7–15 years)	22 July–5 August and 5–14 August	ABB-IGH	W. Effenberger (Tel.: +49-228-2875188)	DM 450; DM 30/day	Youth village, houses	Welcome; also girls	24 h at the camp
Bad Tölz youth village	Summer camp (7–18 years)	8 days, summer holidays, Bavaria	BBB	R. Bachhuber (Tel.: +49-89-5160530)	DM 190; DM 27/day	Youth village	No	Twice a week – in emergencies: regional hospital
Fath, Lake Wald-schacher	Rehabilitation summer camp (6–25 years)	15 July–6 August	ÖHG	H. Hartl (Tel.: +43-2231-61320/ +43-676-5303500)	DM 850; DM 40/day	Boarding house; standard as youth hostel	No girls	24 h
Aeschiried, Lake Thun	Summer camp	29 July–5 August	Dr. Kobelt	R. Kobelt (Tel.: +41-31-9616115)	DM 240	Alpine hut	No	24 h
Ibiza, Spain	Adventure camp (13–20 years)	7 days, spring	Dr. Kobelt	R. Kobelt (Fax: +41-31-9616051)	DM 240; DM 30/day	Bungalows	No; children with VWD yes	24 h

Participants

At the BBB and the SHG camps only people with hemophilia are accepted. Friends of youngsters with hemophilia may attend the DHG, ABB-IGH and ÖHG camps, while the DHG and ABB-IGH camps also accept girls (the holiday projects suffer from an acute lack of girls, a fact which is especially criticized by the young adults).

Fees

Fees are dependent on the total costs and the financial support granted. A sports program with sailing and wind surfing or an intensive physical therapy program are, of course, adding to the costs. Only for the Austrian camp the health insurance covers part of the fees, as this camp is a rehabilitation camp. The lowest fees of 27 DM per day are those of the BBB camp, the highest fees of 36 DM per day are due for the DHG holiday camp. For the ÖHG holiday camp a daily lump-sum fee of 40 DM is charged. However, the Austrian health insurance pays between 20% at minimum and 80% at maximum for insured members. All organizations offer financial support in needy cases.

Information about the camps discussed is presented in Table 1.

Clinical Experience with the PFA-100 System in Children and Adolescents

J. WENDISCH, N. MÜNCHOW, G. SIEGERT, R. KNÖFLER, S. HOFMANN

Introduction

The in *vitro* platelet function system, PFA-100 System (Dade Behring), has been developed to assess platelet-dependent primary hemostasis in citrated whole blood [7]. The method is also reported to be suitable for a quantitative measurement of vWF platelet-dependent function.

Materials and Methods

Blood samples are aspirated under constant suction through a capillary and a 0.45-µm aperture in a membrane coated with fibrillary type 1 equine tendon collagen and either epinephrine (CEPI) or adenosine 5'-diphosphate (CADP). These stimuli and the high shear rates used result in platelet adhesion and aggregation. This leads to the formation of a platelet plug in the aperture. The time required to obtain full occlusion of the aperture is defined as the closure time (CT).

There are already many published results about applications of this diagnostic method [2, 3, 6, 8, 9]. For example, the PFA-100 System has been suggested as a screening test to identify disorders associated with primary hemostasis [4, 5].

Our investigations were performed to examine the PFA-100 System in pediatric applications and the suitability of the method as preoperative screening.

Subjects

Altogether 204 measurements of the CT were made in 164 children and adolescents, ranging from 3 years to 18 years of age:
i)   Before elective ENT surgery, if the patient's history includes bleeding symptoms
ii) In patients manifesting acute bleeding events without a known reason
iii) In patients with immunothrombocytopenia (ITP)
iv) In patients with established von Willebrand disease (vWD)
v)   In the framework of therapy with ASA or Minirin

Reference values had been established in 76 children in earlier investigations.

I. Scharrer/W. Schramm (Ed.)
30th Hemophilia Symposium Hamburg 1999
© Springer-Verlag Berlin Heidelberg 2001

Laboratory Investigations

All persons investigated in the diagnostic group were subjected to the following tests using citrated plasma for clotting analysis and buffered citrated whole blood for PFA-100:

1. Compulsory: CT with CADP and CEPI, aPTT, platelet count, hematocrit, fibrinogen
2. Optional: F VIII:C, vWF:Ag, vWF:RCof, vWF:CBA, multimeric analysis, platelet vWF, platelet aggregation in platelet-rich plasma or whole blood, blood group, bleeding time (BT)

All children with assumed vWD were investigated for vWF on at least three occasions. The lowest values obtained were included in the calculations used for test evaluation and patient diagnosis. The PFA-100 System CT and the BT were measured one to two times. Medications which could affect coagulation and hemostasis were considered.

Diagnostic criteria for mild vWD type 1 were: vWF:CBA- and vWF:Ag-values in the range 35–60% and personal bleeding symptoms or family history of bleedings.

Results

In 141 children measurement of CT was performed to exclude a primary hemostasis disorder:

69 had a prolonged CT	5 without any obvious reason
	55 with type 1/2/3 vWD
	9 with thrombocytopenia/platelet disease
72 had a normal CT	55 had normal primary hemostasis
	5 patients with type 1 vWD
	12 patients with suspected type 1 vWD

In 23 patients the CT was measured while they were taking ASA or Minirin. Only 8 out of 13 had a prolonged CT with CEPI during ASA treatment (Fig. 1).

All previously prolonged CT in patients with vWD returned to normal after Minirin treatment (0.3 μg kg^{-1} bw). In 5 children who had different CTs measured on a number of occasions, the results were not reproducible in later measurements.

Summary

All type 2/3 vWD were identified but not all patients with type 1 vWD were recognized. In the case of suspected vWD, further investigations were always required (vWF, multimeric analysis). The measurement of CT did not add any further information in a possible type 1 vWD. As far as the diagnosis of vWD is concerned, all relevant clinical and laboratory results are required.

All patients with platelet diseases were identified.

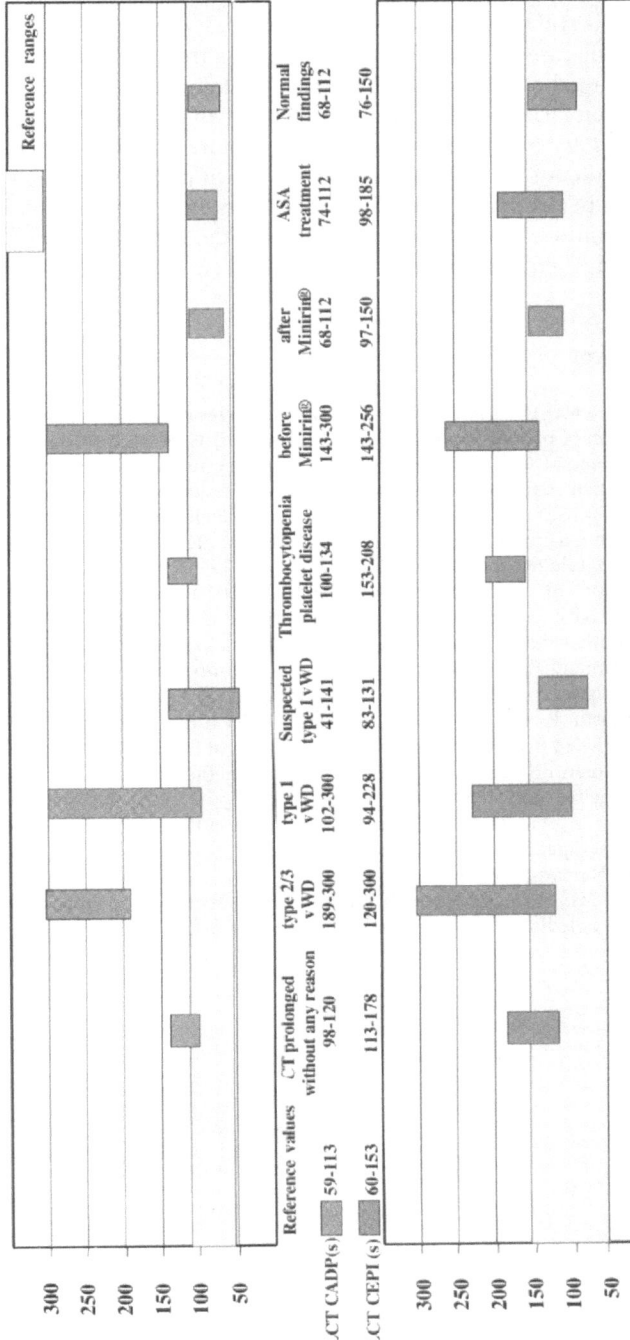

Fig. 1. The measured values (range) of CT with CADP and CEPI in the different groups

Not all patients receiving ASA treatment had a prolonged CT with CEPI; the reason is still unknown.

In the cases of known vWD and Minirin treatment, the measurement of CT was a good method to monitor the efficacy of Minirin.

When false results were obtained or when results were not reproducible, extensive and expensive additional tests are required.

We do not recommend measuring CT with PFA-100 System as a general screening test before surgery because to many results were doubtful. This leads to further uncertainties. However, we conclude that the measurement of the CT is a suitable method when platelet disease is suspected and for monitoring Minirin treatment.

References

1. Carcao MD, et al. The Platelet Function Analyzer (PFA-100): a novel in-vitro system for evaluation of primary hemostasis in children. Br J Haematol. 101 (1998) 70-3.
2. Cattaneo M, et al. Evaluation of the PFA-100 system in the diagnosis and therapeutic monitoring of patients with von Willebrand disease. Thromb Haemost. 82 (1999) 35-9.
3. Escolar G, et al. Evaluation of acquired platelet dysfunctions in uremic and cirrhotic patients using the platelet function analyzer (PFA-100): influence of hematocrit elevation. Haematologica 84 (1999) 614-9.
4. Favaloro EJ, et al. Use of a novel platelet function analyzer (PFA-100 trade mark) with high sensitivity to disturbances in von Willebrand factor to screen for von Willebrand's disease and other disorders. Am J Hematol. 62 (1999) 165-174.
5. Fressinaud E, et al. Screening for von Willebrand disease with a new analyzer using high shear stress: a study of 60 cases. Blood 91 (1998) 1325-31.
6. Harrison P, et al. Performance of the platelet function analyser PFA-100 in testing abnormalities of primary haemostasis. Blood Coagul Fibrinolysis 10 (1999) 25-31.
7. Mammen EF, et al. PFA-100 system: a new method for assessment of platelet dysfunction. Semin Thromb Hemost. 24 (1998) 195-202.
8. Meskal A, et al. The platelet function analyzer (PFA-100) may not be suitable for monitoring the therapeutic efficiency of von Willebrand concentrate in type III von Willebrand disease. Ann Hematol. 78 (1999) 426-30.
9. Rand ML, et al. Use of the PFA-100 in the assessment of primary, platelet-related hemostasis in a pediatric setting. Semin Thromb Hemost. 24 (1998) 523-9.

Endothelial Activation Markers in Health and Disease – Big Endothelin-1 and Endothelin-1 in Children

S. HOFMANN, R. KNÖFLER, E. KUHLISCH, G. WEISSBACH

Introduction

Three pharmacologically distinct isopeptides of endothelin derived from three distinct genes have been identified and described [16,24,34,39].

Endothelin-1 consists of 21 amino acids and is released mainly from endothelium but also from epithelium, leukocytes, macrophages, tumor-, kidney-, and smooth muscle cells. The release from activated endothelium is mediated by thrombin, adrenaline, cytokines, endotoxin, vasopressin and angiotensin II. Endothelin-1 is the most potent vasoconstrictor so far discovered and it also stimulates the proliferation of vascular musculature [6,25,39]. The short half-life in human plasma of 1.5 min [13] is due to a rapid clearance by endothelium in lung and kidney [24].

Big endothelin-1 is the precursor of endothelin-1 and consists of 38 amino acids. The vasoconstrictive activity of big endothelin-1 is about 100-fold lower than that of endothelin-1 [34]. The peptide is converted into endothelin-1 by an endopeptidase named the endothelin converting enzyme [35]. The half-life of big endothelin-1 in human plasma is approximately 30 min [13] and therefore significantly longer compared to that of endothelin-1. According to the literature [2,36], in human plasma big endothelin-1 and endothelin-1 are present in nearly equimolar concentrations. However, the endothelin-1 plasma concentration may be influenced by the rapid clearance of endothelin-1 from plasma.

Only few reports exist about the behavior of endothelial activation markers in children. Measuring the endothelin-1 plasma concentration with an enzyme immunoassay, we have not found statistically significant differences between healthy newborns, infants and schoolchildren as well as between a pediatric control group and children suffering from different diseases [18,19,20]. Our results did not correspond with the data reported in the literature which were obtained using radioimmunoassays. This prompted us to determine big endothelin-1 and endothelin-1 in plasma samples from healthy children and adults as well as from pediatric patients suffering from different diseases. Thrombomodulin and von Willebrand factor as established endothelial activation markers were determined additionally.

I. Scharrer/W. Schramm (Ed.)
30th Hemophilia Symposium Hamburg 1999
© Springer-Verlag Berlin Heidelberg 2001

Patients and Methods

Probands

The control group (CONTROL) consisted of 49 healthy infants and schoolchildren (mean age: 12.7 years, range: 4–20 years). Furthermore, the parameters were determined in 46 healthy newborns (43 full-term and three pre-term – birth in the 30th, 31st and 34th week of pregnancy) and 17 healthy adults.

Forty pediatric patients were divided into the following groups:
- 11 with serious infections (purulent meningitis, osteomyelitis) – SEPSIS
- 10 with tumors before treatment (5 acute leukemias, 5 solid tumors) – TUMOR
- 10 with febrile, uncomplicated diseases – FEVER
- 7 with autoimmune vasculitis (Schoenlein-Henoch purpura) – PURPURA
- 2 with hemolytic-uremic syndrome – HUS

Blood Sampling

Blood was collected from peripheral veins into EDTA-containing tubes (Sarstedt, Germany). From all children blood was obtained only in case of routine blood sampling for the determination of other parameters. The samples were centrifuged within 30 min after blood collection and stored at –70°C until measurement.

Laboratory Methods

Endothelial activation markers were measured using enzyme immunoassays (ELISA). The test kits for determination of big endothelin-1 and endothelin-1 were purchased from Biomedica (Vienna, Austria). According to the manual of the big endothelin-1 test, the specificity is 100% for big endothelin-1 and lower than 1% for the C-terminal fragment and for the three endothelin isoforms. The endothelin-1 test sensitively measures the endothelin isoforms 1 and 2 but not endothelin-3 and big endothelin. The tests for thrombomodulin and von Willebrand factor were purchased from Stago (Asniéres, France).

The tests were carried out according to the manufacturers' recommendations.

Statistical Analysis

The one-way variance analysis and the chi-square test were used to analyze differences between the groups. A value of $p < 0.05$ was considered to be significant. Relations between the parameters were tested including all values measured by determination of correlation coefficients according to Spearman.

Results

Comparison of Control Group with Groups of Adults and Newborns

The calculated mean values and standard deviations for the groups tested are shown in Table 1.

Table 1. Plasma concentrations of endothelial activation markers in the groups studied

	Big ET-1 (fmol ml⁻¹)	ET-1 (fmol ml⁻¹)	TM (ng ml⁻¹)	vWF (%)
Control group	0.95 ± 0.68	0.24 ± 0.22	8.31 ± 6.48	58.69 ± 37.36
Newborns	$1.23 \pm 0.44^{*}$	0.54 ± 0.92	$78.24 \pm 51.73^{**}$	65.28 ± 30.44
Adults	1.02 ± 0.67	0.36 ± 0.46	5.21 ± 3.73	73.93 ± 28.42

Big ET-1 (big endothelin-1); ET-1, (endothelin-1); TM, (thrombomodulin); vWF, (von Willebrand factor)
Values are given as means ± SD (standard deviation)
Asterisks (newborns group) indicate statistically higher concentrations compared to the other two groups
(significance level: $^{*}p<0.05$, $^{**}p<0.01$)

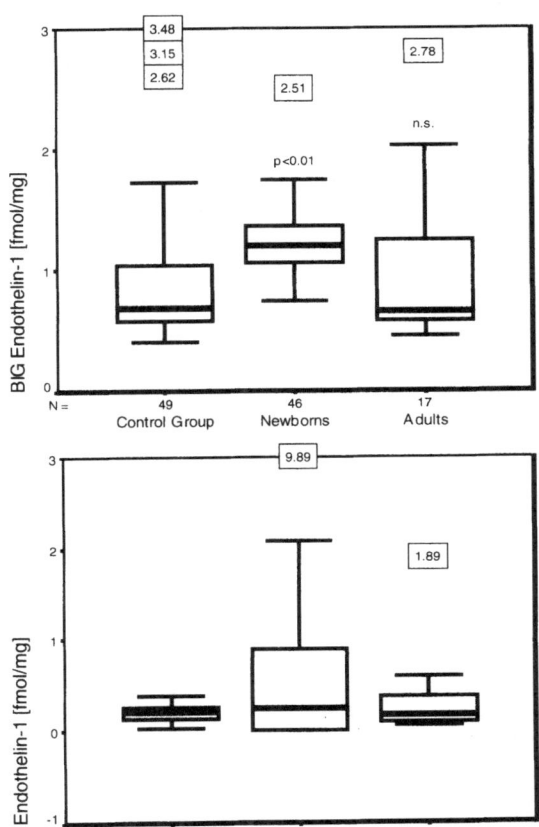

Fig. 1. Box plots for the markers big endothelin-1 and endothelin-1 in the control group, newborns and adults. The upper and lower border of box indicate the 75th and 25th percentile, respectively. The line in the box represents the median. Data above the box plots describe extreme values. The newborns showed significantly higher big endothelin-1 values than the control group and adults. No differences between the groups were found for endothelin-1

The group of healthy newborns showed statistically significant higher big endothelin-1 values compared to the control group and to the group of adults (Figure 1). The mean value for endothelin-1 in the control group was lower compared to newborns and to adults, but the difference did not reach statistical significance. A wide distribution of values was observed in the group of newborns (Figure 1).

In contrast to endothelin-1, the thrombomodulin plasma concentration was markedly increased in newborns, and the differences to the other two groups were highly significant.

The von Willebrand factor concentrations were not significantly different between the three groups.

Comparison of Control Group with Groups of Patients

The calculated mean values and standard deviations for all groups tested are shown in Table 2.

As shown in Figure 2, in patients suffering from serious infections and tumors a wide distribution of big endothelin-1 concentrations was observed. The mean values of all patients' groups were upper the mean of the control group, but statistically significant higher big endothelin-1 plasma concentrations were observed only in the ten patients with tumors and in the two patients with HUS.

In all patients' groups the mean thrombomodulin concentrations were above the mean of the control group. In accordance to big endothelin-1, a statistical significant difference was detected only for patients with tumors and with HUS. For thrombomodulin, statistically significant differences were detected for all patients' groups. An extremely high thrombomodulin concentration (213.5 ng ml^{-1}) was measured in a patient suffering from acute myelogenous leukemia who died due to multi-organ failure a few days after start of chemotherapy.

Compared to the control group, the von Willebrand factor concentration was significantly different in the groups of patients with serious infections and with febrile, uncomplicated diseases.

Table 2. Plasma concentrations of endothelial activation markers of the control group and the patient groups

	Big ET-1 (fmol ml^{-1})	ET-1 (fmol ml^{-1})	TM (ng ml^{-1})	vWF (%)
Control group	0.95±0.68	0.21±0.10	5.29±0.97	58.69±37.36
Sepsis	1.33±0.65	0.49±0.64	21.41±13.08	126.63±57.34***
Tumor	1.98±1.22**	2.63±4.34	45.72±60.32***	41.71±18.72
Fever	1.31±0.55	0.47±0.74	18.61±7.16	129.97±70.69***
Purpura	1.18±0.57	0.17±0.26	11.96±4.73	52.90±34.01
HUS	4.20±0.28***	1.87±1.91	73.39±8.96**	95.56±53.03

Big ET-1, big endothelin-1; ET-1, endothelin-1; TM, thrombomodulin; vWF, von Willebrand factor
Values are given as means ± SD (standard deviation)
Asterisks indicate statistically higher concentrations than the other groups (*$p<0.05$, **$p<0.01$, ***$p<0.001$)

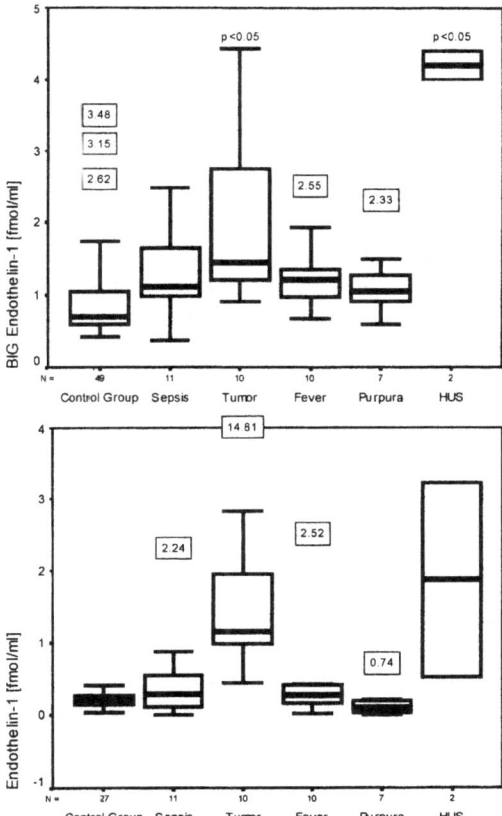

Fig. 2. Big endothelin-1 and endothelin-1 plasma concentrations in the control group and in patients. Patients with malignant tumors before treatment and patients with HUS showed significantly higher big endothelin-1-values than the control group. No statistically significant differences between this groups were found for endothelin-1

Correlation Analysis of Endothelial Activation Markers

The results of correlation analysis are given in Table 3. Correlations were found between big endothelin-1 and endothelin-1 ($r=+0.341$) as well as between big endo-

Table 3. Correlation analysis of endothelial activation markers by determination of correlation coefficients according to Spearman

	Big ET-1	ET-1
Big endothelin-1 (Big ET-1)	–	
Endothelin-1 (ET-1)	+0.341 $p<0.001$ $n=130$	–
Thrombomodulin	+0.409 $p<0.001$ $n=131$	n.s.
von Willebrand factor	n.s.	n.s.

All values measured were included. (n.s., not significant)

thelin-1 and thrombomodulin ($r=+0.409$). Endothelin-1 was neither correlated with thrombomodulin nor with the von Willebrand factor.

Discussion

In our previous investigations we had observed that newborns and children with different diseases showed no differences in plasma endothelin-1 concentrations compared to a control group consisting of healthy infants and schoolchildren [18,19,20]. These results did not correspond to the data reported in the literature, but we had used a different test system – a recently developed enzyme immunoassay. At that time no data obtained from samples of pediatric patients measured by this test were available. In the other studies endothelin-1 was determined by radioimmunoassays, and it was found that in healthy newborns the endothelin-1 plasma levels were significantly higher compared to adults [7,8,11,12,15,21,32]. Furthermore, in clinical studies markedly increased endothelin-1 plasma levels were detected in newborns suffering from respiratory distress syndrome [1,8,17,21,22,28,32], children with chronic renal diseases [5,33] and with Kawasaki syndrome [26]. Data are also available for endothelin-1 concentrations in adults. Increased plasma levels have been described in serious infections [3,37], DIC [38], pulmonary hypertension [23] and in systemic autoimmune diseases [14,27]. The discrepancies between our results and the data reported in the literature could be explained by methodological problems. The measurement of samples by radioimmunoassays requires special preparation methods such as extraction and chromatographic enrichment. It has been reported that these procedures influence the results [4,31]. In contrast, using the ELISA technique endothelin-1 can be measured directly in plasma. Furthermore, the different cross-reactivities to the endothelin isoforms and big endothelins which influence the specificity have to be considered [36]. Another problem results from the short endothelin-1 half-life of only a few minutes in the circulating blood. This is due to a fast tissue distribution and a binding to high-affinity endothelin receptors [13,30]. Recently, the question was discussed if the determination of big endothelin-1 should be preferred to the measurement of endothelin-1 [13,36]. Big endothelin-1 has a half-life of approximately 30 min, and therefore increased plasma levels of big endothelin-1 may be detectable also in the systemic circulation and not only locally [9,10]. In this way the big endothelin-1 plasma concentration could indirectly, but more exactly than the determination of endothelin-1, reflect the physiological effects of endothelin-1. The aim of our study was to test this hypothesis. In samples from healthy children and adults as well as from pediatric patients suffering from different diseases, endothelin-1 and big endothelin-1 plasma concentrations were determined using the ELISA technique.

Statistically higher big endothelin-1 plasma concentrations were found in the group of newborns (1.23 ± 0.44 fmol ml^{-1}) compared to the groups of healthy children (0.95 ± 0.68 fmol ml^{-1}) and adults (1.02 ± 0.67 fmol ml^{-1}). With regard to the endothelin-1 concentration, the mean value of the newborn group (0.54 fmol ml^{-1}) was double as high than that of the control group (0.24 fmol ml^{-1}), but this was due to high endothelin-1 values in a few newborns. Because of the high standard deviation in the newborn group (0.92 fmol ml^{-1}), the difference was statistically not significant. Thrombomodulin was markedly increased in the group of newborns. This result is supported by data of Orbe et al. [29] who reported that thrombomodulin concentrations in cord blood from healthy newborns are elevated compared to thrombomodulin plasma concentrations of older children outside the perinatal period and of adults.

The increased plasma levels of big endothelin-1 and thrombomodulin in newborns may indicate a perinatal activation of endothelial cells. The fact that a marked increase of endothelin-1 plasma concentrations was observed only in few newborns supports the hypothesis that an increase of the endothelin-1 concentration occurs mainly locally in the vascular system.

The mean big endothelin-1 values in the group of healthy children (0.95 ± 0.68 fmol ml^{-1}) and of adults (1.02 ± 0.67 fmol ml^{-1}) were higher than the reference value (≤0.7 fmol ml^{-1}) given by the manufacturer of test. In contrast, the mean endothelin-1 values of the control group (0.24 ± 0.22 fmol ml^{-1}) and of adults (0.36 ± 0.46 fmol ml^{-1}) were within the given reference range (0.2–0.7 fmol ml^{-1}). Therefore, our results do not support the data of Aubin [2] and Suzuki et al. [36] who found nearly equimolar concentrations of endothelin-1 and big endothelin-1 in human plasma.

The mean big endothelin-1 values of all patients' groups were higher than the mean of the control group but statistically significant differences were found only for patients suffering from tumors and from hemolytic uremic syndrome. No statistically significant differences were found for endothelin-1 but in some patients very high endothelin-1 values were measured. The highest value (14.81 fmol ml^{-1}) was detected in a child suffering from a malignant neurogenic tumor which occupied almost the whole abdomen. Surprisingly, this patient showed only a slightly increased big endothelin-1 concentration of 1.55 fmol ml^{-1}.

In accordance with big-endothelin-1, thrombomodulin was markedly increased in patients with tumors and hemolytic uremic syndrome. In contrast, an increase of the von Willebrand factor was found in patients with serious infections and febrile, uncomplicated diseases.

Taking the hypothesis into consideration that big endothelin may be increased in the systemic circulation, whereas endothelin-1 is increased mainly locally, an absent or slight correlation between the two parameters could be expected. Accordingly, we found a correlation coefficient of +0.341 obtained from the values of 130 samples. Big endothelin-1 and thrombomodulin (+0.409) were more closely correlated but lower than expected. No correlation was found between von Willebrand factor and big endothelin-1, suggesting a different release mechanism from endothelial cells.

Conclusion

Taking the small number of patients and the heterogenicity of diseases included in our study into consideration, it could be hypothesized that in children an increase of big endothelin-1 plasma concentration indicates an endothelial cell activation. The sensitivity of this marker is comparable to that of thrombomodulin. The determination of endothelin-1 seems not to be useful for the detection of an endothelial cell activation in pediatric patients. However, a markedly increased endothelin-1 plasma concentration may indicate a systemic endothelial cell activation or severe local damage of endothelium. For final conclusions more clinical data are needed.

References

1. Allen SW, Chatfield BA, Koppenhafer A, Schaffer MS, Wolfe RR, Abman SH. Circulating immunoreactive endothelin-1 in children with pulmonary hypertension. Am Rev Respir Dis 1993; 148: 519–522
2. Aubin P, Le Brun G, Moldovan F, Villette JM, Creminon C, Dumas J, Homyrda L, Soliman H, Azizi M, Fiet J. Sandwich-type enzyme immunoassay for big endothelin-1 in plasma: concentrations in healthy human subjects unaffected by sex or posture. Clin Chem 1997; 43,1: 65–70
3. Battistini B, Forget MA, Laight D. Potential roles in systemic inflammatory response syndrome with a particular relationship to cytokines. Shock 1996; 16: 95–98
4. Battistini B, Dorleans-Juste P, Sirois P. Endothelins: Circulating plasma levels and presence in other biologic fluids. Lab Invest 1993; 68: 600–627
5. Blazy J, Dechaux M, Charbit M, Brocart D, Souberbielle J-C, Gagnadoux MF, Guillot F, Sachs C. Endothelin-1 in children with chronic renal failure. Pediatr Nephrol 1994; 8: 40–44
6. Brunner F, Stessel H, Watzinger N, Loeffler BM, Opie LH. Binding of endothelin to plasma proteins and tissue receptors: Effects on endothelin determination, vasoactivity, and tissue kinetics. FEBS Lett 1995; 373: 97–101
7. Clerico A, del Chicca MG, Zucchelli GC et al. Critical evaluation of endothelin assay. Int J Tiss Reac 1994; 14: 79–87
8. Coceani F, Armstrong C, Kelsey L. Endothelin is a potent constrictor of the lamb ductus arteriosus. Can J Physiol Pharmacol 1989; 67: 902–904
9. De Nucci G, Thomas R, Dorleans-Juste P, Antunes E, Walder C, Warner TD, Vane JR. Pressor effects of circulating endothelin are limited by its removal in the pulmonary circulation and by the release of prostacyclin and endothelium-derived relaxing factor. Proc Natl Acad Sci USA 1988; 85 (24): 9797–9800
10. D'Orleans-Juste P, Lidbury PS, Warner TD, Vane JR. Intravascular big endothelin increases circulating levels of endothelin-1 and prostanoids in the rabbit. Biochem Pharmacol 1990; 39 (9): 21–22
11. Ekbald H, Arjamaa O, Vuolteenaho O, Kääpä P, Kero P. Plasma endothelin-1 concentrations at different ages during infancy and childhood. Acta Paediatr 1993; 82: 302–303
12. Hakkinen LM, Vuolteenaho OJ, Leppaluoto JP, Laatikainen TJ. Endothelin in maternal and umbilical cord blood in spontaneous labor and at elective cesarean delivery. Obstet Gynecol 1992; 80: 72–75
13. Hemsen A, Ahlborg G, Ottosson-Seeberger A, Lundberg JM. Metabolism of big endothelin-1 (1–38) and (22–38) in the human circulation in relation to production of endothelin-1 (1–21). Regul Peptides 1995; 55: 287–297
14. Hergesell O, Andrassy K, Nawroth P. Elevated levels of markers of endothelial cell damage and markers of activated coagulation in patients with systemic necrotizing vasculitis. Thromb Haemost 1996; 75: 287–297
15. Ihara Y, Sagawa N, Hasegawa M, Okagaki A, Li XM, Inamori K, Itoh H, Mori T, Saito Y, Shirakami G. Concentrations of endothelin-1 in maternal and umbilical cord blood at various stages of pregnancy. J Cardiovasc Pharmacol 1991; 17 (Suppl. 7): 443–445

16. Inoue A, Yanagisawa M, Kimura S, Kasuya Y, Miyauchi T, Goto K, Masaki T. The human endothelin family: three structurally and pharmacologically distinct isopeptides predicted by three separate genes. Proc Natl Acad Sci U S A 1989; 86: 2863-2867
17. Kääpä P, Kero P, Ekblad H, Erkkola R, Arjamaa O. Plasma endothelin-1 in the neonatal respiratory distress syndrome. Ann Chir Gyn 1994; 83: 110-112
18. Knöfler R, Hofmann S, Weissbach G, Neef B, Hirsch T. Erste Ergebnisse der Endothelin-bestimmung bei Kindern. In: 27. Hämophilie-Symposion Hamburg 1996. Scharrer I, Schramm W, Hrsg. Berlin, Heidelberg, New York, Tokyo: Springer 1998; 458-466
19. Knöfler R, Hofmann S, Weissbach G, Kuhlisch E, Neef B, Otte M, Pargac N, Nachtrodt G. Molecular markers of the endothelium, the coagulation and the fibrinolytic systems in healthy newborns. Semin Thromb Hemost 1998; 24,5: 453-461
20. Knöfler R, Hofmann S, Weissbach G, Kuhlisch E, Neef B, Lauterbach I. Aktivierungsmarker des Endothels und der Hämostase bei Erkrankungen im Kindesalter. In: 41. Hamburger Symposion über Blutgerinnung 1998. Matthias FR, Rasche H, Hrsg. Stuttgart-Schattauer, Basel,Grenzach-Wyhlen: Ed. Roche 1999; 301-314
21. Kobayashi H, Puri P. Plasma endothelin levels in congenital diaphragmatic hernia. J Pediat Surg 1994; 29: 1258-1261
22. Kojima T, Isozaki-Fukuda Y, Takedatsu M, Ono A, Hirata Y, Kobayashi Y. Plasma endothelin-1 like immunoreactivity levels in neonates. Eur J Pediat 1992; 151: 913-915
23. Komai H, Adatia JT, Elliot MJ, De Leval MR, Haworth SG. Increased plasma levels of endothelin-1 after cardiopulmonary bypass in patients with pulmonary hypertension and congenital heart disease. J Thorac Cardiovasc Surg 1993; 106: 473-478
24. Levin ER. Endothelins. N Engl J Med 1995; 333: 356-363
25. Mathew V, Lerman A. Clinical implications of a sandwich enzyme immunoassay for big endothelin-1. Clin Chem 1997; 43,1: 9-10
26. Ogawa S, Zhang J, Yuge K, Watanabe M, Fukazawa R, Kamisago M, Seki T, Hirayama T. Increased plasma endothelin-1 concentration in Kawasaki disease. J Cardiovasc Pharmacol 1993; 22 Suppl. 8: 364-366
27. Ohdama S, Takano S, Miyake S, Kubota T, Sato K, Aoki N. Plasma thrombomodulin as a marker of vascular injuries in collagen vascular diseases. Am J Clin Pathol 1994; 101: 101-113
28. Ohno Y, Mizutani S, Kuranchi O, Nishida Y, Arii Y, Tomoda Y. Umbilical plasma concentration of endothelin-1 in intrapartum fetal stress: Effect of fetal heart rate abnormalities. Obstet Gynecol 1995; 86: 822-825
29. Orbe I, Paramo JA, Pinacho A, Hermida J, Rocha E. Plasma thrombomodulin is increased in cord blood of healthy newborns. Thromb Haemost 1995; 73: 326
30. Plumpton C, Haynes WG, Webb DJ, Davenport AP. Measurement of C-terminal fragment of big endothelin-1: A novel method for assessing the generation of endothelin-1 in humans. J Cardiol Pharmacol 1995; 26 (Suppl 3): 34-36
31. Rolinski B, Sadri I, Bogner J, Goebel FD. Determination of endothelin-1 immunoreactivity in plasma, cerebrospinal fluid and urine. Res Exp Med Berl 1994; 194: 9-24
32. Rosenberg AA, Kennaugh J, Koppenhafer SL, Loomis M, Chatfield BA, Abman SH. Elevated immunoreactive endothelin-1 levels in newborn infants with persistent pulmonary hypertension. J Pediat 1993; 123: 109-114
33. Ross RD, Kalidindi V, Vincent JA, Kassab J, Dabbagh S, Hsu JM, Pinsky WW. Acute changes in endothelin-1 after hemodialysis for chronic renal failure. J Pediat 1993; 122: 74-76
34. Rubanyi GM, Parker Botelho LH. Endothelins. FASEB J 1991; 5: 2713-2720
35. Schiffrin EL, Touyz RM. Vascular biology of endothelin. J Cardiovasc Pharmacol 1998; 32 (Suppl 3): 2-13
36. Suzuki N, Matsumoto H, Miyauchi T, Kitada C, Tsuda M, Goto K et al. Sandwich-enzyme immunoassays for endothelin family peptides. J Cardiovasc Pharmacol 1991; 17 (Suppl 7): 420-422
37. Takakuwa T, Endo S, Nakae H, Kikichi M, Suzuki T, Inada K, Yoshida M. Plasma levels of TNF-alpha, endothelin-1 and thrombomodulin in patients with sepsis. Res Commun Chem Pathol Pharmacol 1994; 84: 261-269

38. Wada H, Minamikawa K, Wakita Y, Nakasae T, Kaneko T, Ohiwa M, Tamaki S, Deguchi K, Shirakawa S, Hayashi T, Suzuki K. Increased vascular endothelial cell markers in patients with disseminated intravascular coagulation. Am J Hematol 1993; 44: 85–88
39. Yanagisawa M, Kurihara H, Kimura S, Tomobe Y, Kobayashi M, Mitsui Y, Yazaki Y, Goto K, Masaki T. A novel potent vasoconstrictor peptide produced by vascular endothelial cells. Nature 1988; 332: 411–415
40. Yoshibayashi M, Nishioka K, Nakao K, Saito Y, Matsumura M, Ueda T, Temma S, Shirakami G, Imura H, Mikawa H. Plasma endothelin concentrations in patients with pulmonary hypertension associated with congenital heart defects. Circulation 1991; 84: 2280–2285

IX.e Poster: Case Reports

Dramatic Intra-Abdominal Bleeding –
First Symptom of Hemophilia B in a Neonate

J. WENDISCH, K. GROSSER, G. SIEGERT

Introduction

At the present time, hemophilia is diagnosed in 50–60% of patients immediately after birth because of a positive family history. A further 30% of patients are identified by bleeding during medical procedures or by monitoring blood coagulation parameters.

However, in a small minority of patients the diagnosis is made only after symptoms of bleeding occur. This usually happens when a baby begins to become more active. By this time the child has often reached its first birthday. Bleeding complications during the neonatal period are rare.

Case History

We here report the case of a full-term neonate with a negative family history of bleeding disorders. The patient was the second child of healthy parents. There were no complications during pregnancy. A normal birth took place in a district hospital. At birth, the babies weight was 3330 g. The first examination of the child revealed nothing unusual. The child's development was normal and trauma during the period immediately before birth could not be confirmed later. The APGAR score remained unchanged at 10. Vitamin K was given orally.

However, on the 3rd day after birth the child had a swollen, bluish scrotum. Surgery was carried out because testicular torsion was suspected but this could not be confirmed. Instead there were approx. 30–40 ml blood in the scrotum. The general condition of the baby initially improved post-operatively. However, 15 h after surgery the child presented symptoms of shock and an increasingly distended abdomen. An ultrasound scan revealed a large amount of fluid in the abdominal cavity. Postoperatively and with the onset of shock symptoms, 50 ml of virus-inactivated fresh frozen plasma (Octaplas) were administered.

On the 3rd day after birth the baby arrived at our clinic. At that time, the following laboratory parameters were obtained: Hb 3.9 mmol l^{-1}; Hc 0.19; platelet count 84 GPT l^{-1}; PTT 49 s; TPT 49%; fibrinogen 0.97 g l^{-1}. The hemorrhagic shock was treated by transfusions of erythrocytes and platelets. After his vital signs had stabilized, an explorative laparotomy was carried out by the pediatric surgeons.

About 200 ml fresh blood and a 200-ml clot were removed from the abdominal cavity. Inspection of the abdominal organs revealed a 2 cm x 2 cm area of sub-cap-

I. Scharrer/W. Schramm (Ed.)
30th Hemophilia Symposium Hamburg 1999
© Springer-Verlag Berlin Heidelberg 2001

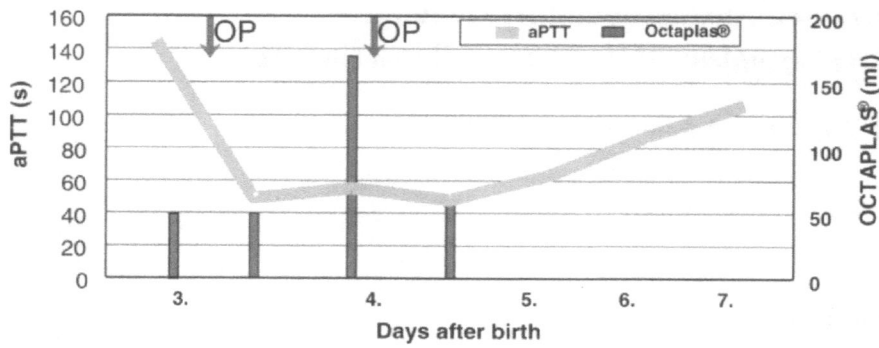

Fig. 1. aPTT levels during Octaplas substitution in a patient with hemophilia B

sular bleeding on the left lobe of the liver and an approximately 5-cm capsule lace-ration on the latero-dorsal surface of the spleen. There was diffuse bleeding from the exposed parenchymal surface of the spleen (5 cm x 2 cm). It was difficult to stop the bleeding. The spleen was »wrapped« in a modified vicryl net bag. Periopera-tively, the size of the hematoma on the liver capsule increased so that it had to be opened. After the bleeding from the two organs closed, and no further source of intra-abdominal bleeding was found. During and after surgery a total of 230 ml Octaplas was infused.

During the first 36 h after surgery, the PTT value was between 55 s and 63 s. At 48 h after plasma infusion, the PTT was found to be 87 s and rose to 106 s at 72 h (Figure 1). Analysis of individual factors was carried out and showed that factor IX activity was 1%, no factor IX inhibitor was detectable, and factor VIII activity was 87%.

There were no further complications and no more symptoms of bleeding.

Discussion and Conclusions

A ruptured spleen and a hematoma of the liver capsule led to a severe intra-abdominal bleeding in a full-term neonate with hemophilia B. The baby had severe symptoms of a hemorrhagic shock. A cause for the organ bleeding could not be found retrospectively. It was not possible to establish that the baby had suffered any trauma.

Ruptures of the spleen have also been reported in healthy neonates [3,8]. An occult spleen rupture was described [4]. In neonates with hemophilia B initial symptoms of spontaneous bleeding were mainly skin bleeding, extracranial bleed-ing (ECH) and intracranial bleeding (ICH) [2,5,9]. Kulkarni and Lusher [6] publish-ed a review of the literature from 1966 to 1996. About 40 reports on 102 patients with bleeding symptoms were analyzed. Over 60% of the patients had an ICH. Other spontaneous bleeding events were reported sporadically, e.g., a history of gastro-intestinal bleeding [1], a bleeding from the spleen [5], as well as adrenal and liver hematomas [7] without any cause of the spontaneous bleeding.

Before the first surgery the baby had a markedly prolonged aPTT (144 s). This result was explained as an effect of the emergency. Determination of factor VIII and IX would have led to a correct diagnosis.

The aPTT is a reliable parameter for diagnosing severe hemophilia. In cases of a doubt aPTT of factor VIII and IX needs to be measured.

During the hemorrhagic shock situation the identification of hemophilia in our patient was difficult. Since, on the 3rd and 4th days after birth, Octaplas were administered, the aPTT values were within the normal range for neonates (Fig. 1). The factor-IX concentration in Octaplas is given as ca. 0.5 U ml^{-1}. On the 3rd day after birth, the patient received 100 ml and, on the 4th day 230 ml. This is equivalent to quantities of factor IX of 50 U and 115 U. »Normalization« of the aPTT by this replacement is conceivable. The hemophilia was diagnosed when administration of Octaplas had stopped.

This case demonstrates that selective coagulation analysis is necessary if there are bleeding symptoms of unknown etiology.

Bleeding from parenchymatous organs is very rare in hemophilic neonates. We were unable to obtain any information about any trauma being sustained during the delivery of our patient. The cause of the hemorrhage in this case remains unclear.

References

1. Conway JH, Hilgartner MW: Initial presentations of pediatric hemophiliacs. Arch Pediatr Adolesc Med 6 (1994) 589–94
2. Baujard C, Gouyet L, Murat I Diagnosis and anaesthesia management of haemophilia during the neonatal period. Paediatr Anaesth 1998; 8 (3): 245–7
3. Delta BG, Eisenstein EM, Rothenberg AM: Rupture of a normal spleen in the newborn: report of a survival and review of the literature. Clin Pediatr (Phila) 6 (1968) 373–6.
4. Herlocher JE, Foley W, Thompson NW, Campbell DA: Occult rupture of the spleen. Rev Surg 5 (1969) 370–1
5. Johnson-Robbins LA, Porter JC, Horgan MJ: Splenic rupture in a newborn with hemophilia A: case report and review of the literature. Clin Pediatr (Phila) 38 (1999)117–96.
6. Kulkarni R, Lusher JM: Intracranial and extracranial hemorrhages in newborns with hemophilia: a review of the literature. J Pediatr Hematol Oncol 21 (1999) 289–9
7. Le Pommelet C, Durand P, Laurian Y, Devictor D: Haemophilia A: two cases showing unusual features at birth Haemophilia 1998 Mar;4(2) 122–5
8. Matsuyama S, Suzuki N, Nagamachi Y: Rupture of the spleen in the newborn: treatment without splenectomy. J Pediatr Surg 1 (1976) 115–6
9. Ries M, Klinge J, Rauch R, Chen C, Deeg KH: Spontaneous subdural hematoma in a 18-day-old male newborn infant with severe hemophilia A.Klin Padiatr 210 (1998) 120–4

Postoperative Bleeding in a Sufficiently Substituted Patient with Severe Hemophilia A: Successful Therapy with Administration of Recombinant Factor VIIa

H.J. Siemens, S. Brückner, J. Gille, A. Martinez-Schramm, M. Ruslies, H.A. Katus

Introduction

It has been known for a while that hemostasis is initiated by the formation of a complex consisting of tissue factor and circulating factor VIIa [4]. After the application of high doses of recombinant factor VIIa (NovoSeven) highly effective hemostasis can be achieved even in inhibitor-hemophiliacs with life-threatening bleeding episodes who are resistant to any other kind of standard therapy [10,11]. Recombinant factor VIIa becomes active only after the formation of a complex with tissue factor, which is released from the deeper layers of the vessel wall after tissue damage. Recently, recombinant factor VIIa has been successfully used in various hemorrhages of other origin, such as factor VII-deficiency [2], inhibitors against von-Willebrand factor in von-Willebrand's disease type III [5], thrombopenias [9], thrombopathies [12], and acquired hemophilia [8]. There are numerous other hemorrhagic diatheses which can be diagnosed in the coagulation laboratory and thus, the use of factor VIIa is currently extended to patients with acute bleeding problems who would not primarily be considered for substitution therapy. The preliminary data, presented at the 5th NovoNordisk Symposium (Copenhagen, May 1999) come from investigations in patients, in whom, due to the kind of surgery involved, blood transfusions are common (e.g., cardiac valve prosthesis). Other patients included were those with bleeding episodes while on oral anticoagulation or those who need relapse prophylaxis after subarachnoid hemorrhage. Another potential indication is seen in patients undergoing prostatectomy even for benign reasons in order to reduce perioperative blood loss in these mostly elderly patients. Taking this into account, we are only a few steps away from the trial use of factor VIIa in all patients, who according to all laboratory criteria have a normal coagulation status, yet bleeding occurs or continues nonetheless. So far, sufficient data to prove that NovoSeven is effective in (postoperatively) bleeding patients with normal coagulation tests is not available. Based on these considerations, we decided to use NovoSeven in one of our patients with longstanding recurrent hemorrhage and »normal coagulation test results«.

I. Scharrer/W. Schramm (Ed.)
30th Hemophilia Symposium Hamburg 1999
© Springer-Verlag Berlin Heidelberg 2001

Case Report

The patient is a 50-year-old white Caucasian male with severe hemophilia A. Factor activity was repeatedly measured to be less than 1%. The underlying defect is probably a novel gene mutation since our patient is the only member of the family with the disease. After having been substituted during his childhood, the patient developed antibodies against hepatitis B, which eventually resolved and also against hepatitis C which took a chronic course. The patient has elevated liver enzymes and a relatively high virus load of >150,000 copies μl^{-1}. Since 1986 an infection with HIV 1 has been present with a virus load close to the detection limit and a CD4 helper cell count of 400 pl^{-1} (normal range >530 pl^{-1}). The patient is currently not receiving any therapy against hepatitis C or the HIV infection.

After a motorcycle accident in 1971, the right leg had to be amputated above the knee because of a completely crushed knee joint. The patient received a leg prosthesis, but had been unable to use it for the past several years due to recurrent painful swelling of the stump. He is therefore dependent on a wheel chair. The remaining femur was obviously resected during the years since 1971. The patient had refused continuous prophylaxis and had received on-demand substitution of approximately 20,000 IU of a recombinant factor VIII preparation per year. Under this regimen, he had only occasionally suffered from hemorrhages into the left knee joint and both elbow joints.

During the summer of 1999, the patient presented to the emergency room with a monstrous, painful swelling of the stump, which had increased over the preceding 6 months and had now reached a circumference of 75 cm (normal approx. 42 cm). As already mentioned, the patient had suffered from recurrent painful stump swellings over the past 10 years. Now he could hardly sit in his wheel chair. The CT and MRI scans showed numerous fluid retentions which corresponded to recent and older partly calcified hematomas. A malignant process could be excluded.

The patient was referred to the department of orthopedics. Originally, it was only planned to tap the hematomas. Because of the fact that several membranous »chambers« had formed, it was not possible to sufficiently reduce their contents. Therefore, a surgical intervention became necessary. A total of 3 l of fluid could be removed. The stump was afterwards described as thin and slender by the surgeon.

First Operation: Perioperative Substitution Therapy

Direct preoperatively, a bolus of 1000 IU of factor VIII concentrate (plasma product) was given. On the day of surgery as well as during the following 3 weeks, factor VIII concentrate was administered as a continuous infusion (see Fig. 1). Factor VIII:C activity was always well above 70%, sometimes measured twice or three times a day. Despite adequate substitution and factor VIII activity, several hemorrhages into the stump occurred during the days after surgery. This led to a stump situation almost as severe as the initial finding. The patient developed a fever and an *Staphylococcus epidermidis* infection was diagnosed. CRP and fibrinogen

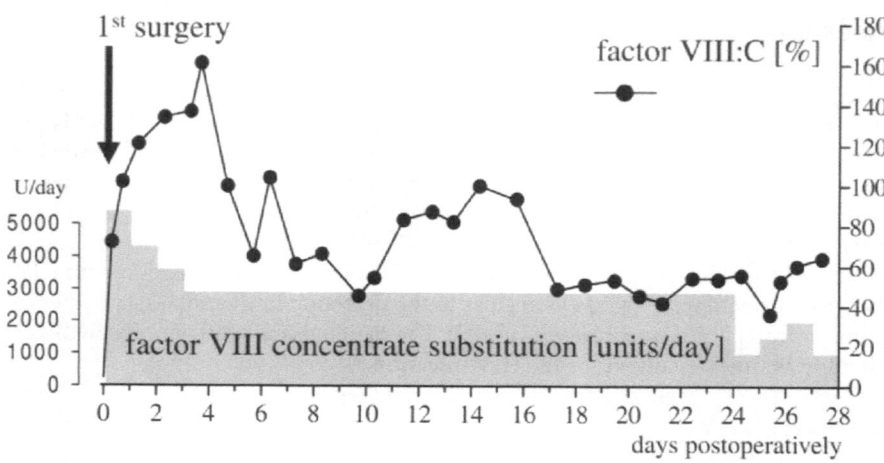

Fig. 1. Factor VIII:C substitution and level (%) following the first operation

concentrations were elevated. Further surgical interventions could therefore not be performed.

Second Operation: Successful Treatment

Four weeks after the initial surgery, the newly formed hematomas had to be removed again. Factor VIII concentrate was given continuously in the usual manner in order to »normalize« coagulation tests (see Fig. 2). This time, a recombinant prepa-

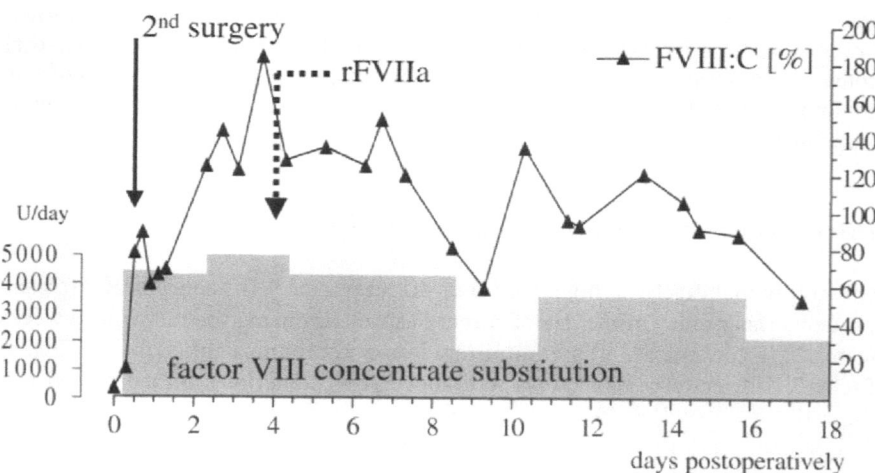

Fig. 2. Factor VIII:C substitution and level (%) following the second operation

ration was administered. Factor VIII:C activity always lay above the level considered safe and sufficient.

Hemorrhagic Shock Due to Drainage Bleed

During the night of the 2nd postoperative day a massive hemorrhage with shock symptoms occurred and the patient was transferred to the anesthesiology intensive care unit. The measurement of coagulation markers including factor XIII and factor VIII activities as well as platelet count did not give any hint at a systemic bleeding disorder. An inhibitor was not present (<0.3 BU ml^{-1}) and a systemic hyperfibrinolysis was excluded. Another bleed into the stump was imminent and we therefore decided to administer NovoSeven twice at a dosage of 240 KIU (approx. 4.5 KIU kg^{-1} bw) with an interval of 4 h. Shortly after the first bolus, the bleeding from the drains was markedly reduced and ceased completely after the second bolus. The patient's further course on a regular ward was unremarkable, the stump has been thin and slender to this day and further controls did not show any signs of newly formed hematomas. After 3 weeks of in hospital treatment, the patient was discharged in good condition.

Discussion and Conclusion

Recombinant factor VIIa (rFVIIa) has meanwhile become an important instrument in the therapy of acute bleeding episodes in inhibitor-hemophiliacs [11]. Other causes of bleeding disorders are treated with rFVIIa in some very small studies [1]. So far, the data are not sufficient to generate valid and reliable results. In our patient, we believe that despite so-called »normal laboratory« results, the administration of rFVIIa has initiated a stable postoperative hemostasis after bleeding complications could not successfully be treated with the usual measures. It remains to be investigated in further randomized studies, whether this approach to uncontrollable bleeding episodes in patients with normal or normalized coagulation tests is a promising alternative for the future.

An impediment for the use of rFVIIa as an »universal hemostatic agent« in patients without an inhibitor may be the lack of prospective randomized trials, and overall in this particular respect little clinical experience with this drug. Furthermore, there have been occasional reports of a prothrombotic effect of the preparation similar to the one observed with PPSB concentrates. However, according to in vitro observations this risk seems to be small [7].

Another potential field for the use of rFVIIa are patients with reduced factor VII activity due to coumarin or possibly liver cirrhosis. In healthy volunteers on coumadin [6] and volunteers with liver cirrhosis [3], reduced factor VII activity could be antagonized by rFVIIa in a dose-dependent manner between 12 h and 24 h. Since the price for this product has remained high, the manufacturer is challenged to support adequate trials. Unfortunately, this demand has not yet found a positive answer. It seems that, as usual, all interesting new developments in medicine and the related questions, will not be dealt within the German medical and scientific community.

Summary

Hemostasis is initiated by the formation of a complex of tissue factor and circulation factor VIIa. Recombinant factor VIIa (NovoSeven), which becomes active only after forming a complex with tissue factor, can initiate highly effective hemostasis even in inhibitor-hemophiliacs with life-threatening episodes. We here report the case of a 50-year-old white Caucasian male with severe hemophilia A (factor activity less than 1%) who presented to the emergency room with a monstrous painful swelling of his right leg stump.

After the exclusion of a malignant process, the numerous recent and older, partly calcified hematomas had to be surgically removed. Continuous peri- and postoperative factor VIII substitution (plasma product) with a constant factor VIII:C activity of well above 70% was unable to control the situation and postoperative hemorrhage into the stump recurred. A *Staphylococcus epidermidis* infection complicated the case and a second operation 4 weeks after the initial surgery became necessary. Peri- and postoperatively, a recombinant factor VIII preparation was administered. During the night of the 2nd postoperative day, massive hemorrhage and shock occurred and the patient was transferred to the ICU. There was no laboratory clue as to the underlying cause of the bleeding. All factor activities lay within normal limits, an inhibitor was not present. Since further hemorrhage was imminent, recombinant factor VIIa concentrate (NovoSeven) was administered twice at a dose of 240 KIU with an interval of 4 h. After the first bolus, bleeding decreased markedly and ceased completely after the second bolus. The patient's further course was uneventful.

There have been several case reports so far, in which factor VIIa was used as a safe and reliable agent in uncontrollable hemorrhages of various origin other than inhibitor patients. The case presented here supports this finding and as yet the adverse-effect profile of the preparation seems to be low. Adequate prospective randomized trials should be initiated so as to make the drug available (i.e., cheaper) to a larger group of potential patients who might profit from its fast and safe way of action.

References

1. Anonymous. New Aspects of Hemophilia Treatment. Proceedings of the 3rd symposium. Copenhagen, Denmark, September 21–23, 1995. Haemostasis 26 Suppl 1: 1–166, 1996
2. Bauer KA: Treatment of factor VII deficiency with recombinant factor VIIa. Haemostasis 26 Suppl 1: 155–158, 1996
3. Bernstein DE, Jeffers L, Erhardtsen E, Reddy KR, Glazer S, Squiban P, Bech R, Hedner U, Schiff ER: Recombinant factor VIIa corrects prothrombin time in cirrhotic patients: a preliminary study. Gastroenterology 113: 1930–1937, 1997
4. Broze GJ, Jr.: Tissue factor pathway inhibitor and the current concept of blood coagulation. Blood Coagul.Fibrinolysis 6 Suppl 1: S7–13, 1995

5. Ciavarella N, Schiavoni M, Valenzano E, Mangini F, Inchingolo F: Use of recombinant factor VIIa (NovoSeven) in the treatment of two patients with type III von Willebrand's disease and an inhibitor against von Willebrand factor. Haemostasis 26 Suppl 1: 150–154, 1996

6. Erhardtsen E, Nony P, Dechavanne M, French P, Boissel JP, Hedner U: The effect of recombinant factor VIIa (NovoSeven) in healthy volunteers receiving acenocoumarol to an International Normalized Ratio above 2.0. Blood Coagul.Fibrinolysis 9: 741–748, 1998

7. Gallistl S, Cvirn G, Muntean W: Recombinant factor VIIa does not induce hypercoagulability in vitro. Thromb.Haemost. 81: 245–249, 1999

8. Hay CR: Acquired haemophilia. Baillieres. Clin.Haematol. 11: 287–303, 1998

9. Kristensen J, Killander A, Hippe E, Helleberg C, Ellegard J, Holm M, Kutti J, Mellqvist UH, Johansson JE, Glazer S, Hedner U: Clinical experience with recombinant factor VIIa in patients with thrombocytopenia. Haemostasis 26 Suppl 1: 159–164, 1996

10. Lusher J, Ingerslev J, Roberts H, Hedner U: Clinical experience with recombinant factor VIIa. Blood Coagul.Fibrinolysis 9: 119–128, 1998

11. Lusher JM: Recombinant factor VIIa (NovoSeven) in the treatment of internal bleeding in patients with factor VIII and IX inhibitors. Haemostasis 26 Suppl 1: 124–130, 1996

12. Peters M, Heijboer H: Treatment of a patient with Bernard-Soulier syndrome and recurrent nosebleeds with recombinant factor VIIa [letter]. Thromb.Haemost. 80: 352, 1998

Continuous Infusion of Recombinant FIX (BeneFIX) During Herniotomy in an Infant

J. Wendisch, G. Siegert

Introduction

Perioperative prophylaxis or treatment of severe bleedings in patients with hemophilia A or B and von Willebrand disease requires substitution of coagulation factors for a longer period of time. Recently continuous infusion (CI) has been used as an alternative to bolus injections to avoid fluctuations in factor plasma levels [1,7]. This mode of replacement therapy was found to decrease the consumption of factor concentrates by between 20% and 50% resulting in a reduction of treatment costs. So far, data with FIX concentrates and CI are available for plasma-derived FIX (pdFIX) only [1,6,7,8]. Here we report on an infant with severe hemophilia B undergoing herniotomy. CI of recombinant FIX (BeneFIX, Baxter, Hyland Immuno Division) was performed to cover surgery.

Patient Data

The patient was 3 months old and weighed 5.6 kg. FIX activity was <1%. A decision to herniotomy was made, because an inguinal hernia on the right side could not be repositioned. Because of severe postnatal bleedings the patient had received infusions with FFP and transfusions as well. Until then FIX had not been substituted. The patient was negative in terms of antibodies against HIV 1+2, HBV (except anti-HBs), HCV and Parvovirus B19. HAV-IgG and anti-HB antibodies could be demonstrated, presumably a placental transfer from his mother.

Diagnostic Procedures

Preoperatively, a FIX inhibitor was excluded and FIX levels (one-stage procedure) and aPTT were determined. On the day of surgery FIX and aPTT were measured five times, during the 1st postoperative day three times, and later once daily up to the 5th postoperative day.

Continuous Infusion

Recombinant FIX (BeneFIX, Baxter, Hyland Immuno Division) was used for this child perioperatively for the first time. BeneFIX is the first recombinant FIX prepa-

I. Scharrer/W. Schramm (Ed.)
30th Hemophilia Symposium Hamburg 1999
© Springer-Verlag Berlin Heidelberg 2001

ration and was launched in Germany in January 1999. No substances derived from blood or plasma are used in the manufacturing process. Virus elimination during production results in an overall reduction of >11 log. After reconstitution BeneFIX is stable for more than 24 h at 25°C [5]. Compared to plasma-derived FIX concentrates recovery of BeneFIX is about 28% lower, which is presumably due to minor structural variations in the FIX molecule leading to a change in clearance [4].

BeneFIX was resuspended according to instructions given (250 IU per 5 ml aqua ad inj) and infused via an infusion pump (IVAC 770, 20-ml syringe) at a rate of 0.4 ml h^{-1} and 0.5 ml h^{-1}, respectively. Because of the low infusion volume isotonic NaCl solution was infused in the bypass at 15 ml h^{-1}. Heparin was *not* added to the solutions used.

Results and Discussion

A bolus of 90 U kg^{-1} (500 U) was given preoperatively. The decision for such a high dose was made because a lower recovery compared to pdFIX was anticipated (see above). We aimed at a perioperative FIX level of about 60%. CI was not started immediately after bolus injection to allow a measurement of in vivo recovery. Thirty minutes after bolus injection FIX activity was at 58%, corresponding to a recovery of 33%.

CI was started following blood sampling for the determination of recovery. The initial FIX dosage was 3.6 U kg^{-1} h^{-1}. There were no bleeding complications during surgery which lasted 30 min. Because of a decrease in FIX level down to 38% immediately after surgery, the child received another bolus of 250 U and CI was continued at 4.5 U kg^{-1} h^{-1}. On the day of surgery, FIX plasma levels were between 41% and 47%. Dosage for CI was kept constant up to the 5th postoperative day, FIX levels residing at 28–37% (Figure 1).

Total consumption of BeneFIX was 3500 U. Using only bolus injections 4500–5000 U would have been needed. A decrease of FIX dosage during treatment as reported for plasma derived preparations [1] was not possible. This also seems to be due to an alteration in clearance. During CI no phlebitis occurred at the site of

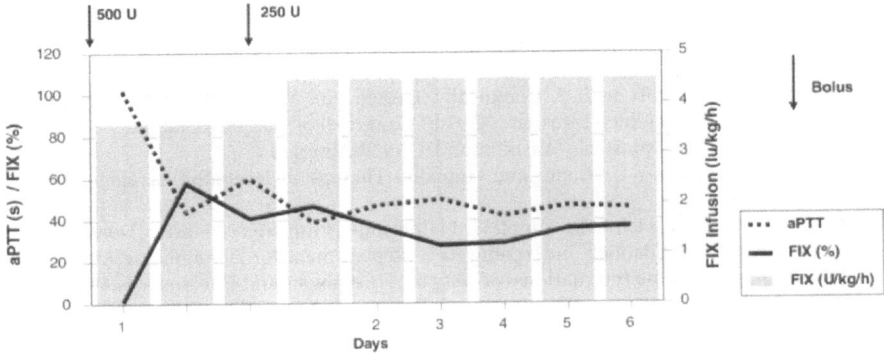

Fig. 1. FIX level and aPTT in the patient before and during continuous infusion of BeneFIX

injection. The stability of the dissolved product at room temperature had been shown by various authors before [3,5].

Wound healing in our patient took place without any complications. The child was dismissed on day 8 post-surgery; further treatments with BeneFIX have not so far been necessary. Findings in virus serology were essentially unchanged 3 months after therapy; HAV IgG decreased. There were no signs of FIX inhibitor development.

Conclusion

Clinical efficacy of BeneFIX given to an infant as CI during herniotomy could be demonstrated. Constant FIX levels were obtained, bleeding complications did not occur. Due to an apparently altered clearance of this preparation compared to plasma-derived FIX concentrates higher doses of bolus injections are required. There appears to be a demand for higher dosage during CI as well. No adverse events were observed. Compared to treatment with bolus injections the total factor IX requirement was 23% lower. CI was easy to perform and to control. Peri- and postoperative continuous infusion of BeneFIX was safe and efficacious in our patient.

References

1. Auerswald G., Auberger K., Kreuz W.: Kontinuierliche Infusion von Faktor VIII- und IX-Konzentraten als alternative Therapie, insbesondere auch bei v.Willebrand-Syndrom Typ 3. 28. Hämophilie-Symposion, Hamburg 1997, Abstract p. 94
2. Von Depka Prondzinski M., Eisert R., Barthels M., Ganser A.: Peri- und postoperative kontinuierliche Infusion rekombinanter Faktor VIII-Konzentrate bei Hämophilie A. Scharrer I., Schramm W. (Hrsg.), 28. Hämophilie-Symposion, Hamburg 1997, (1999) 182–6
3. Von Depka Prondzinski M., Aschermann G., Biewener A., Barthels M., Ganser A.: Aktivitätsmessungen von rekombinantem Faktor IX-Konzentrat und seine Eignung für die kontinuierliche Infusion. 29. Hämophilie-Symposion, Hamburg 1998, Abstract p. 124
4. Gilbert C.W. 2nd, Beebe I.A., Nielsen B.: Recombinant Factor IX. Thrombosis and Haemostasis 78 (1997) 261–65
5. Miescher P.A. and Jaffe E.R. (Eds.): Recombinant Factor IX for the treatment of Hemophilia B. Seminars in Hematology 35 (1998) Suppl. 2
6. Schulman S., Smith O., Wallensten R., Berntorp E., Lethagen S., Tjonnfjord G.: Surgery in Hemophilia B Patients with A Chemically Treated and Virus Filtered FIX-Concentrate (Nanotiv) in Continuous Infusion. XVIIth Congress of the International Society on Thrombosis and Haemostasis, Washington DC 1999, Abstract
7. Varon D., Martinowitz U.: Continuous Infusion Therapy in Haemophilia. Haemophilia 4 (1998) 431–35
8. Wolf H.-H., Voigt W., Hein W., Schmoll H.-J.: Continuous Infusion of Plasma-Derived Factor IX Concentrate in a Patient Undergoing Knee Replacement for Hemophiliac Arthropathy. XVIIth Congress of the International Society on Thrombosis and Haemostasis, Washington DC 1999, Abstract

Clinical Course of Intramuscular Bleeds in a Patient with Factor XIII Deficiency

S. GOTTSTEIN, R. KLAMROTH, C. HEINRICHS

Presentation

A 16-year-old female with suspected von Willebrand's disease was referred to our Hemophilia Treatment Center. She suffered from persisting pain and swelling in her left hip, which was increasing with movement and had developed after a fall during a trekking trip. X-ray studies of the hip joint had been performed without evidence of a fracture. No improvement of the symptoms had been achieved by several i.v. applications of Haemate HS.

Previous Medical History

Since birth the patient had experienced several bleeding episodes. After delivery, an umbilical bleeding was noticed. Mucosal bleedings and bruises followed in early childhood.

At the age of 1 year von Willebrand's disease was diagnosed. In childhood, intestinal bleeding was the predominating symptom. Menarche at the age of 12 years and menstruation were normal. There is no family history of bleeding disease.

Clinical Presentation

We saw a 16-year-old student in good general health condition, body mass index normal. Medical examination showed no abnormalities except for a swelling cranial from the left trochanter major. There was no visible hematoma or palpable induration, fluctuation or warming. Posture and gait were adversely affected and range of motion in the left hip was decreased. Several hematomas in different stages of resorption were found on the lower legs.

Diagnosis

MRI of the left hip was performed and showed a hematoma in the left small gluteus muscle.

Extended hemostasiologic laboratory analysis revealed a factor XIII deficiency of 13% residual activity. No evidence of von Willebrand's disease was found: factor

I. Scharrer/W. Schramm (Ed.)
30th Hemophilia Symposium Hamburg 1999
© Springer-Verlag Berlin Heidelberg 2001

VIII, Ristocetin cofactor and von Willebrand factor were normal. The multimers of the von Willebrand factor showed a normal pattern.

Therapy

At the next appointment in the Hemophilia Center the patient presented with a painful and fresh hematoma of the right hand. There was a decrease in range of motion in the thumb. The patient reported no trauma of the hand. At this point, substitution therapy with factor XIII concentrate (Fibrogammin) was initiated. We started with daily application of 1000 IU Fibrogammin i.v. and the hematoma resolved within a week.

As the patient then complained about left-sided hip pain again, substitution was continued with 1250 IU on every 3rd or 4th day for 3 months and could then be reduced to one application every 2 weeks, maintaining an intermediate level of factor XIII activity of over 20%. MRI showed significant improvement 16 months after the injury and after 7 months of therapy with Fibrogammin.

After 6 months of treatment there was no change in immune status (CD4/CD ratio, CD4 count) or sign of fresh infection through herpes virus, parvovirus, CMV or EBV. Immunization against hepatitis A and B was performed and followed by antibody formation. Tests for HCV-RNA and antibodies against hepatitis C virus remained negative.

Clinical Outcome

The patient is currently well and without complaints and regained full range of motion in her left hip. She has learned to perform i.v. self-injection and is able to travel and to take part in sports, e.g., trekking and tennis. No further bleeding complications have so far occurred.

Comment

Minimal hemostatic activity of factor XIII is indicated to be 7% in the literature [1].

This case of a young patient with factor XIII deficiency illustrates that bleeding complications also occur with »borderline« levels of factor XIII activity.

The demanded dose and frequency of substitution appeared to be relatively variable, indicating the necessity of laboratory controls during substitution treatment. Substitution therapy was apparently well tolerated and safe, and showed a convincing effect on hematomas in different stages of resorption.

References

1. Egbring R, Kröninger A, Seitz R. Factor XIII Deficiency: Pathogenetic Mechanisms and Clinical Significance. Semin Thromb Haemost 1996, 22(5): 419–425

Immunthrombocytopenia and Lupus Antibodies in a Patient with Hemophilia A

C. Wermes, F. Bergmann, K. Welte, K.-W. Sykora

Background

Childhood lupus antibodies (LA) are often seen in the context of infections of the upper respiratory tract. They normally disappear spontaneously. In most cases the children do not suffer bleedings or thromboses [2,3].

Case Report

The 16-year-old boy carried a diagnosis of mild hemophilia A (FVIII activity 19%) that was made at the age of 1 year.

When he was 2 years old he developed alopecia areata of unknown origin, with later spontaneous regression. At the same time he had his first major joint bleeding of the ankle. An extended examination to exclude rheumatic diseases was not done.

At the age of 9 years, lupus antibodies were diagnosed for the first time. Once again, he had an increased bleeding tendency to bleed into joints and muscles.

When the boy was 15 years old we recognized again an alopecia areata, an increased bleeding tendency, and elevated cardiolipin-antibodies (CLA). The bleeding-time was prolonged and also the aPTT was longer than before (51 s versus 45 s). The mixing test showed pathological results (6–9 s difference). The patient developed an immune-thrombocytopenia (ITP), the platelet count was decreased to 5000 μl^{-1}. At the same time auto-antibodies against the platelet glycoprotein-receptor Gp IIb/IIIa were found. The patient had bleedings of the skin and the mucous membranes in contrast to the bleeding signs he showed the years before, when he mainly suffered from bleedings of the joints and muscles, as is typically seen in patients with hemophilia A. After treatment with prednisone (250 mg daily) over 6 weeks with decreased doses at the end of the treatment, the clinical symptoms and the laboratory parameters normalized rapidly. Only CLA remained elevated. However, the boy suffered from the side-effects of steroids including a cushingoid facies, striae distensae, steroid-induced acne, and he felt weak and tired. The course of laboratory parameters in the patient during treatment are shown in Figure 1.

Five months later he relapsed with alopecia, ITP and increased LA. Therefore, he was treated with dexamethasone-pulses (40 mg m^2 day^{-1} for 4 days). He received a total of five courses of dexamethasone in 4-week intervals. The daily dose was

I. Scharrer/W. Schramm (Ed.)
30th Hemophilia Symposium Hamburg 1999
© Springer-Verlag Berlin Heidelberg 2001

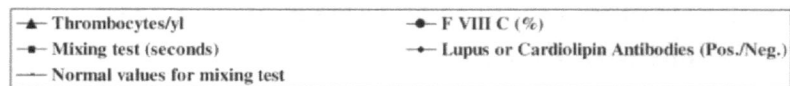

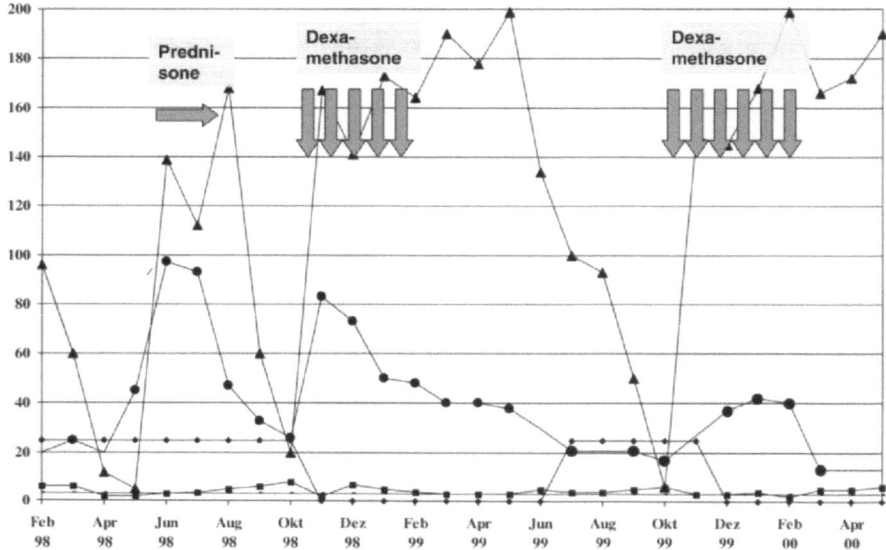

Fig. 1. Course of laboratory parameters in the patient during treatment

40 mg m² body surface. After the first course, the platelet count increased to normal values, LA disappeared, and the bleeding tendency normalized rapidly.

After 11 months of remission, a second relapse occurred. Once more, a positive LA titer and a decrease of platelet count was observed. Treatment with dexamethasone was again immediately successful. LA disappeared 2 weeks later, the platelet counts normalized, and the clinical bleeding tendency disappeared. The patient is now in remission at 6 months follow-up. Dexamethasone therapy was tolerated well and the patient had, besides some tiredness 2 or 3 days after the treatment course, no side effects. Extended laboratory investigation showed no evidence of systemic lupus erythematosus or another collagen-vascular disease.

Discussion

Bleeding tendency as well as ITP in context with childhood lupus-antibodies are uncommon. Several mechanisms underlying the disease in this case are possible.

Orlando et al. [4] showed a reduced platelet adhesion with a prolonged bleeding time consecutively in patients with CLA. The interference of CLA with platelet function is a possible explanation for the enhanced bleeding tendency of the patient during the first time, when platelet count was in the normal range, e.g., at the age of 9 years. The antibodies directed against the glycoprotein Gp IIb/IIIa receptor may have interfered with collagen binding and platelet aggregation, resulting in an acquired form of Glanzman's disease. In addition, we found elevated titers of LA and CLA during our patient's episodes of ITP. At the same time, an auto-antibody against the platelet receptor Gp IIb/IIIa was detected serologically.

As Fanelli et al. [1] have shown, platelets can be activated by CLA (increased CD62 expression). This also could lead to enhanced platelet consumption and thrombocytopenia.

A fourth possibility is the binding of the LA to phospholipids on the platelet surface resulting in increased capturing of the platelets in the spleen. It is possible that more than one of the mechanisms described here is responsible for the clinical signs in our patient.

Conclusion

We report a patient with hemophilia A, who developed childhood LA and an immune-mediated thrombocytopenia at the same time. Therapy with dexamethasone pulses was a well tolerated and effective treatment in our patient.

Children with hemophilia who increase their bleeding tendency may be suspected of having developed childhood LA. They should be investigated carefully, especially when they develop an aPTT that is more prolonged than previously.

References

1. Fanelli A, Bergamini C, Rapi S, Caldini A, Spinelli A, Buggiani A, Emmi L. Flow cytometric detection of circulating activated platelets in primary antiphospholipid syndrome. Correlation with thrombocytopenia and anticardiolipin antibodies. Lupus 1997; 6(3): 261–7
2. Male C, Lechner K, Eichinger S, Kyrle PA, Kapiotis S, Wank H, Kaider A, Pabinger I. Clinical significance of lupus anticoagulants in children. J Pediatr 1999; 134(2):199–205
3. Mingers A, Sutor AH. Lupusinhibitoren im Kindesalter. Hämostaseologie 1992; 12:101–6
4. Orlando E, Cortelazzo S, Marchetti M, Sanfratello R, Barbui T. Prolonged bleeding time in patients with lupus anticoagulant. Thromb Haemost 1992; 68(5):495–9

Cerebral Sinus Thrombosis after Asparaginase Therapy

H.-H. Wolf, O. Dorligschaw, W. Voigt, H.-J. Schmoll

In patients suffering from acute lymphoblastic leukemia (ALL), hepatic or hemostaseologic complications are seen due to lymphoblastic infiltration of the liver.

L-asparaginase is an essential antineoplastic agent in therapy of acute lymphoblastic leukemia [1], but L-asparaginase is known to induce anaphylactoid, pancreatic, hepatotoxic, thrombotic, as well as hemorrhagic complications [2–4]. In patients with thrombophilic diathesis, therefore, thrombotic complications could be most severe.

Pharmacology

Lymphoblastic proliferation in ALL depends on the availability of the amino acid asparagine. Unlike normal human tissue, lymphoblasts lack sufficient activity of the enzyme asparagine synthetase [5].

The pharmacologic effect of L-asparaginase treatment is to minimize plasma concentrations of asparagine.

Both *Erwinia*- and *E. coli*-derived L-asparaginase therefore are a major constituent of most antileukemic protocols around the world [6]. Depression of asparagine plasma concentrations is measurable for one to several days after administration of these drugs. Depending on pharmacologic criteria, application of L-asparaginase has to be administered during induction chemotherapy every day or every other day respectively [7, 8].

In 87.6% of plasma probes of ALL patients, the new polyethylene glycolated (PEG-) asparaginase induces complete depletion of asparaginase after intravenous administration of 1000 IU/m². Plasma half-life of PEG-asparaginase is prolonged twice or three times compared to *Erwinia*- or *E. coli*-derived preparations, and asparagine plasma concentrations are reduced for up to 14 days [5, 9,10]. Therefore, only one single application of PEG-asparaginase is scheduled during induction chemotherapy according to the German Multicenter ALL protocol [11].

Hemostaseologic Effects of L-Asparaginase

In children treated with 10,000 IU/m² *E. coli*-derived L-asparaginase, depletion of plasma concentrations of fibrinogen, plasminogen, and α2-antiplasmin as well

I. Scharrer/W. Schramm (Ed.)
30th Hemophilia Symposium Hamburg 1999
© Springer-Verlag Berlin Heidelberg 2001

as elevation of t-PA and D-dimer plasma concentrations were seen on days 12, 15, 18, 21, 24, 27, 30, and 33. There was a strong correlation between L-asparaginase plasma activity and occurrence of the abnormal hemostaseologic parameters [12–14].

There are only a few experiences with L-asparaginase in patients with hemostaseologic disorders. In patients with thrombophilic risk factors, hemostaseologic complications are assumed to be more severe if asparaginase with prolonged serum activity is administered [15–17].

Patient's Characteristics

We report on a 28-year-old male patient with T-lymphoblastic leukemia and large mediastinal lymphoma (Table 1). At time of admission to the hospital there was a supraclavicular and cervical swelling due to a partial thrombosis of the left subclavian and jugular veins. Heparin therapy was administered for 7 days in order to prolong aPTT (80 s), but was stopped when thrombocytopenia (<50 Gpt/l) occurred. There was no thrombophilic diathesis known in the patient's history. Thrombophilic risk factors had not been tested so far.

Table 1. Laboratory data

Time point	Leukocytes	Platelets	Partial thrombo-plastin time	aPTT	Fibrinogen	AT	d-Dimer
	(Gpt/l)	(Gpt/l)	(%)	(s)	(g/l)	(%)	(mg/l)
Admission	23.2	132	89	23	3.3	114	
Day 12	4.6	154	89	37	1.1	64	0.27
Day 14	2.5	95	79	82	1.0	46	
Day 16	1.3	33	46	64	0.5	51	0.57
Day 17	0.9	35	86	31	0.9	61	0.54
Day 24	5.2	130	87	49	3.9		3.24

On day 11, a central venous catheter was placed via the right subclavian vein. Chemotherapy with cyclophosphamide, high-dose steroids, doxorubicin, and vincristine was performed on days 1–15. The patient presented with severe granulocytopenia (<1 Gpt/l) and thrombocytopenia (<20 Gpt/l) on day 17. PEG-asparaginase 1000 IE/m² was administered intravenously on day 11.

The patient presented with epileptiform convulsion on day 16. Computer tomography revealed huge intracerebral hemorrhage and complete thrombosis of the cavernous sinus. Heparin adjusted to aPTT was administered, but another profuse intraventricular bleeding and cerebral edema occurred on day 22. There was complete thrombosis of all basal cerebral veins. Cerebral compression could be reduced only by several neurosurgical interventions, partial resection of the calotte, and implantation of a ventriculoperitoneal drainage.

Hemostaseologic Parameters

Hemostaseologic tests were done after surgery. Besides an APC ratio of 1:4, several other thrombophilic risk factors were found. A heterozygotic G1691A mutation of the factor V gene was recognized, but no mutation of the prothrombin gene was found.

There were elevated serum concentrations of homocysteine and a homozygotic C677T mutation of the methylene-tetrahydrofolate-reductase gene. Lipoprotein(a) was within the normal range. During induction chemotherapy of ALL, low plasma concentrations of antithrombin (51%), protein C (36%), protein S activity (40%), as well as F XII (70%) and fibrinogen (<1 g/l) were seen. Thrombocytopenia (<10 Gpt/l) and reduction of plasma concentrations of almost all coagulation factors were induced by chemotherapy.

Hemostaseologic Therapy

Intravenous therapy of 6 IE/kg per hour low-molecular-weight (LMW) heparin, in order to adjust 0.4–0.5 U/ml anti-Xa plasma concentration, was administered for 65 days. Within a further 7 months, LMW heparin was administered sub-cutaneously.

After a 6-week therapy with LMW heparin, intracerebral pressure normalized and ventriculoperitoneal drainage could be implanted. Thrombosis of the sinus cavernosus, subclavian, and cervical veins slowly resolved. Neurologic sequelae were left hemiplegia and paralysis of the motor speech area.

Conclusions

Asparaginase therapy may induce severe hemostaseologic, hepatic, and pancreatic disorders. Therefore, thrombotic and hemorrhagic complications are seen in many leukemia patients [16, 18, 19]. To prevent severe thrombotic complications, we recommend pretherapeutic screening of the major thrombophilic risk factors – APC ratio, FV Leiden and prothrombin mutation, lipoprotein(a) and homocysteine, protein C and protein S – especially if L-asparaginase with prolonged serum half-life is to be administered.

References

1. Capizzi, R.L., Asparaginase revisited. Leuk Lymphoma, 1993. 10: p. 147–150.
2. Asselin, B.L. The three Asparaginases: Comparative pharmacology and optimal use in childhood leukemia. in Drug Resistance in Leukemia. 1998. Amsterdam.
3. Weiss, R.B., Hypersensitivity reactions. Semin Oncol, 1992. 19: p. 458–477.
4. Lee, A.Y.Y. and Levine M.N., The thrombophilic state induced by therapeutic agents in the cancer patient. Semin Thromb Haemostasis, 1999. 25(2): p. 137–145.
5. Müller, H.J. and Boos J., Use of L-asparaginase in childhood ALL. Critical Reviews in Oncology/Hematology, 1998. 28: p. 97–113.

6. Hoelzer, D., Treatment of acute lymphoblastic leukemia. Semin Haematol, 1994. 31: p. 1–15.

7. Ahlke, E.e.a., Dose reduction of asparaginase under pharmacokinetic and pharmacodynamic control during induction therapy in children with acute lymphoblastic leukemia. British J Haematology, 1997. 96: p. 675–681.

8. Boos, J., et al., Monitoring of asparaginase activity and asparaginase levels in children on different asparaginase preparations. Europ J Cancer, 1996. 32A(9): p. 1544–1550.

9. Douer, L.J.e.a. PEG L-Asparaginase (PEG-ASP): Phamacokinetics (PK) and clinical response in newly diagnosed adults with acute lymphoblastic leukemia (ALL) treated with multiagent chemotherapy. in Int Symp on Asparaginase. 1998. Los Angeles.

10. Ho, D.H.e.a., Clinical pharmacology of polyethylen glycol L-asparaginase. Drug Metab Dispos, 1986. 14: p. 349–352.

11. Freund, M. and D. Hoelzer, Akute Lymphatische Leukämie (ALL), in Kompendium Internistische Onkologie, H.-J. Schmoll, K. Höffken, and P. K., Editors. 1999, Springer: Berlin-Heidelberg-New York. p. 36–70.

12. Nowak-Göttl, U.e.a., Changes in coagulation and fibrinolysis in childhood acute lymphoblastic leukemia re-induction therapy using three different asparaginase preparations. Eur J Paediatr, 1997. 156: p. 848–850.

13. Mauz-Körholz, C., et al., Low rate of severe venous thromboses in children with ALL treatment according to COALL-92 and -97 protocol. Klin Pädiatr, 1999. 211(4): p. 215–217.

14. Eckhof-Donovan, S., et al., Thrombosen bei Kindern mit akuter lymphoblastischer Leukämie unter dem COALL-Protokoll. Klin Pädiatr, 1994. 206: p. 327–330.

15. Kirschke, R., et al., Coagulation and fibrinolysis in children with acute lymphoblastic leukemia treated according to the COALLL-05-92-protocol. Klin Pädiatr, 1998. 210: p. 285–290.

16. Alberts, S.R., et al., Thrombosis related to the use of L-asparaginase in adults with acute lymphoblastic leukemia: a need to consider coagulation monitoring and clotting factor replacement. Leuk Lymphoma, 1999. 32(5–6): p. 489–496.

17. Castaman, G., R. F., and E. Dini, Thrombotic complications during L-asparaginase treatment for acute lymphocytic leukemia. Hametologica, 1990. 75: p. 567–569.

18. Schulz, U., et al., Sinusvenethrombose unter L-Asparaginase-Therapie. Klin Pädiatr, 1994. 206: p. 342–345.

19. Reddingius, R.E., et al., Dural sinus thrombosis in children with cancer. Med Pediatr Ocol, 1997. 29: p. 296–302.

Severe Neonatal Thrombosis in a Patient with Factor V Q:506 Mutation and the G20210A Prothrombin Mutation

C. Wermes, J. Strehlau, M. von Depka Prondzinski, K. Welte, K.-W. Sykora

Background

In childhood, thromboses are most common in neonates and adolescents. Well-known hereditary risk factors are the factor V Q:506 mutation manifesting itself as APC resistance, and a reduced level of protein C, protein S, and antithrombin and dysfibrinogenemia. Also, the forming of abnormal plasminogen and disturbances in the release of fibrinolytic substances from the endothelium are discussed as risk factors for the development of thrombosis. Further prothrombotic newly described risk factors are the prothrombin G20210A mutation, an increased level for lipoprotein(a), and the MTHFR mutation (methylenetetrahydrofolate reductase), as well as the intron 16 ACE polymorphism (angiotensin-converting enzyme).

Case Report

History

A boy was born by cesarean section in the 41st week of an uneventful pregnancy. The Apgar score was 9/10/10, the umbilical arterial pH was 7.26. The boy weighed 4400 g (90th percentile), his length was 54 cm (75th percentile). The mother had no gestational diabetes. On the second day of life, the patient showed proteinuria, thrombocytopenia, and a palpable right kidney, and was suspected of having renal vascular thrombosis.

Diagnostics

Duplex ultrasound during the first days of life led to the diagnosis of venous thromboses of both renal veins and the vena cava inferior (Fig. 1).

Coagulation investigations were performed. The patient was heterozygous for the factor V Q:506 mutation, the G20210A mutation in the prothrombin gene, and the C677T MTHFR mutation (Table 1). All other diagnostic tests showed normal values (Tables 1, 2).

Routinely performed additional examinations showed normal results. Newborn screening (metabolic diseases) was negative. Examination of the amino acids in the

I. Scharrer/W. Schramm (Ed.)
30th Hemophilia Symposium Hamburg 1999
© Springer-Verlag Berlin Heidelberg 2001

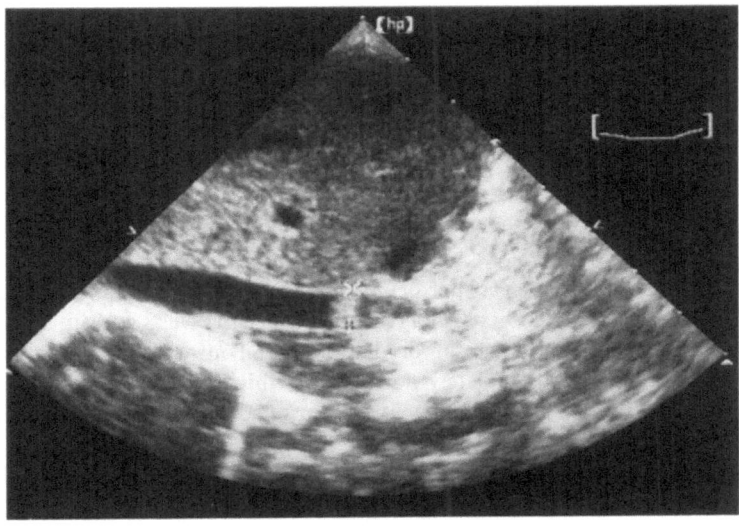

Fig. 1. Thrombosis of the vena cava (picture A. Bökenkamp)

Table 1. Diagnostics for thrombophilia – gene mutations

Gene mutation	Result
Factor V Q:506 mutation	Heterozygous
Prothrombin G20210A mutation	Heterozygous
C677T MTHFR mutation	Heterozygous
ACE polymorphism intron 16	Insertion

Table 2. Diagnostics for thrombophilia – coagulation investigations

Parameter	Result	Age-dependant normal range (at time of diagnosis)
Quick	108%	>40%
aPTT	38 s	42.6±8,6 s
Factor II	120%	63±15%
Factor V	100%	95±25%
Factor XII	104%	50–120%
APC resistance	1.4	>2.0
Protein C chromogenic substrate	38%	42±11%
Protein S free	85%	50±14%
Antithrombin	68%	67±13%
Lipoprotein(a)	<0.05 g/l	<0.30 g/l
Plasminogen activity	73%	70–120%
Plasminogen activator-inhibitor	8.0 AU/ml	</=20 AU/ml
Fibrinogen	2.7 g/l	3.12±0.75 g/l
Homocysteine	3.1 μmol/l	5.0–15.0 μmol/l
D-Dimers	>20,000 μg/l	<500 μg/l

blood and urine was normal. The blood group was A, rhesus positive. Antibody tests and the direct Coombs tests were negative.

The ECG showed normal tracings, no malformations and no intracardial thromboses were seen on echocardiography. An ultrasound of the brain showed no signs of bleeding or thrombosis.

Therapy

Fibrinolytic therapy was performed with rt-PA (Actilyse) in combination with low-dose unfractionated heparin. Fresh frozen plasma was given in addition on day 1 of treatment, and antithrombin on days 1 and 2. Four days later the flow in the thrombotic vessels was completely normalized, which could be confirmed by ultrasound (Fig. 2). Anticoagulant treatment was continued with a low-molecular-weight heparin (LMWH) for 3 months. During the first year of life, no additional thromboses occurred. The patient received primary prophylactic treatment with LMWH in risk situations. Such risk situations were episodes with infections or diarrhea with dehydration. During the first year of the patient's life, prophylactic treatment with LMWH was necessary three times for several days. D-dimers were elevated during these episodes, confirming the higher coagulability of the patient's blood in these situations.

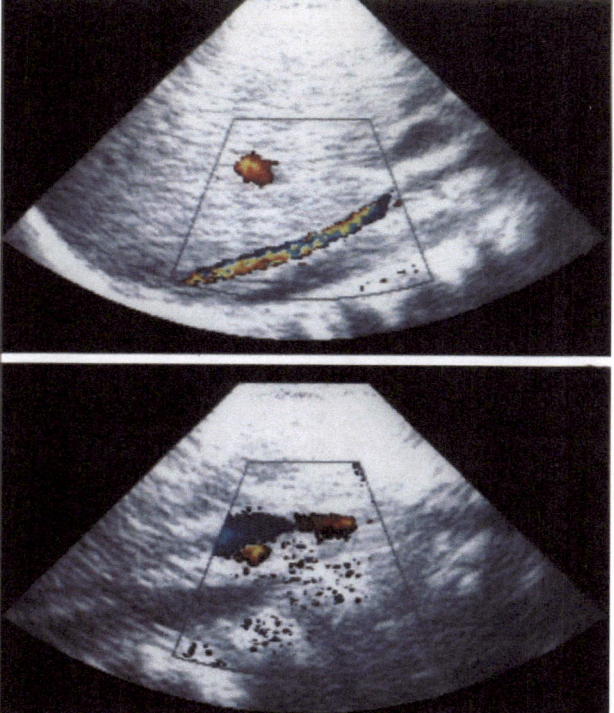

Fig. 2. Recanalization of the vena cava thrombosis (picture A. Bökenkamp)

Discussion

The reason for the severe thrombophilia of this child is a combination defect of the factor V Q:506 mutation and the prothrombin G20210A mutation. These mutations are established risk factors for thrombophilia. In addition, the patient is heterozygous for the MTHFR mutation. The importance of the MTHFR mutation as a risk factor for thrombosis is controversially discussed in the literature.

Adult patients with a combination of heterozygous factor V Q:506 and the prothrombin mutation often suffer from thromboses earlier in life, and thromboses are located at atypical sites and often manifested spontaneously, as shown by Ehrenforth et al. [1] and de Stefano et al. [4]. A study by Nowak-Göttl et al. [2] in children suffering from acute lymphoblastic leukemia (ALL) demonstrated that combination defects resulted in an increased risk of thrombosis. On the other hand, these children also had cancer and additional exogenous risk factors such as chemotherapy, central venous lines, and others. They also had different combination defects than the child reported here. Recently, the case of a 6 year-old girl with the combination of heterozygous factor V Q:506 mutation and the heterozygous prothrombin G20210A mutation suffering from Budd-Chiari syndrome was reported. This is also an unusually located thrombosis with manifestation early in life [3].

Conclusion

To our knowledge, this is the first case report of a spontaneous manifestation of thrombosis in a newborn with a combination defect of the heterozygous factor V Q:506 and the heterozygous prothrombin G20210A mutation. Adult patients with combination defects show atypically located and often spontaneous thromboses that occur early in life. This case illustrates that this experience may also extend to infants.

References

1. Ehrenforth S, von Depka Prondzinski M, Aygören-Pürsün E, Nowak-Göttl U, Scharrer I, Ganser A: Study of the Prothrombin Gene 20210 GA Variant in FV:Q506 Carriers in Relationship to the Presence or Absence of Juvenile Venous Thromboembolism. Arterio Scler Thromb Vasc Biol 1999; 19: 276–280
2. Nowak-Göttl U, Wermes C, Junker R, Koch HG, Schobess R, Fleischhack G, Schwabe D, Ehrenforth S: Prospective Evaluation of the Thrombotic Risk in Children with Acute Lymphoblastic Leukemia Carrying the MTHFR TT 677 Genotype, the Prothrombin G20210 A Variant, and Further Prothrombotic Risk Factors. Blood 1999; 93(5): 1595–99
3. Oner AF, Arslan S, Caksen H, Ceylan A: Budd-Chiari syndrome in a patient heterozygous for both factor V Leiden and the G20210 A mutation on the prothrombin gene. Thromb Haemost 1999; 82:1366–7
4. de Stefano V, Martinelli I, Mannucci PM, Paciaroni K, Chiusolo P, Casorelli I, Rossi E, Leone G: The risk of recurrent deep venous thrombosis among heterozygous carriers of both Factor V Leiden and the G20210 A Prothrombin mutation. N Engl J Med 1999; 341:801–6

Elevated Lp(a) Level and Heterozygous Factor V Mutation FV 1691 AG in a 26-Year-Old Female with Ischemic Colitis

E. Aygören-Pürsün, W. Gross, I. Scharrer

Introduction

Elevated levels of human plasma lipoprotein(a) [Lp(a)] are known to be a geneti-cally determined risk factor for coronary heart disease, cerebrovascular disease, and peripheral arterial and venous obstruction. They may also play a role in the patho-genesis of venous thromboembolism.

Lp(a) plasma levels are genetically determined and remain very constant during the life of the individual, although there is marked variation within the population, with an inverse correlation between the size of the Apo(a) protein and the Lp(a) plasma levels. As well as a slight effect of hormonal and dietary factors, levels can be effectively influenced via LDL apheresis.

The importance of Lp(a) in atherothrombosis is known from immunoreactive studies showing Lp(a) in atherosclerotic plaques: this is explained by binding of Lp(a) to fibrin and an accumulation of fibrin in these areas. It is very probable that the struc-tural similarity between Lp(a) and plasminogen causes local hypofibrinolysis, thus having a role in the clinical manifestation of arterial thromboembolism.

The relationship between elevated Lp(a) levels (>30 mg/dl) and atheromatous disease has been documented best in coronary heart disease (CHD) where cross-sec-tional studies have shown that plasma Lp(a) levels of patients with CHD are significantly higher than in normal populations. Lp(a) is an independent risk factor, and there is a correlation between the extent of CHD and the restenosis rate of venous bypasses. The correlation is less clear in prospective studies, results of which show that Lp(a) is not predictive of the occurrence of a coronary event or the progression of CHD. Nevertheless, long-term studies have shown that Lp(a) levels are significantly higher in those who later suffered coronary events. More recent findings show eleva-ted Lp(a) levels in troponin T-positive patients with unstable angina pectoris.

Case Study

Clinical Description

A 26-year-old female patient with a 2-year history of angina abdominalis was admitted as an emergency complaining of diarrhea, abdominal cramping, and vomiting. Colonoscopy revealed ischemic colitis, subsequently confirmed by histo-

I. Scharrer/W. Schramm (Ed.)
30th Hemophilia Symposium Hamburg 1999
© Springer-Verlag Berlin Heidelberg 2001

logy, of the region between the descending and sigma colon. Angiographic studies of the inferior mesenteric artery showed ischemia with absence of a vascular arcade at the affected level of colon.

Low-dose thrombosis prophylaxis with heparin led to an improvement in symptoms, and the patient was later discharged on no medication. However, she was seen again as an outpatient in Frankfurt with recurrent symptoms and was treated with Fraxiparin 2x0.4 ml/day. This led to an improvement in symptoms, which have now cleared completely since changing to acetyl acetic acid 100 mg/day.

The patient's family history showed premature arterial events. Her father died of myocardial infarction at 25 years of age, and at postmortem examination showed evidence of hypoxic heart muscle damage of variable duration, and an obstructive thrombus in the ramus interventricularis anterior. Her father's twin brother was still alive, but had had two myocardial infarctions at the age of 44 and by 45 had needed cardiac bypass surgery (five vessels).

Risk Factors

Exclusion of a source of cardiac emboli and classical atherosclerotic risk factors was followed by thrombophilic screening of the patient. This showed a heterozygous FV mutation FV 1691 AG with APC resistance and a very high Lp(a) level of 79–80 mg/dl. Although the FV 1691 AG mutation is not normally associated with arterial thromboembolism, it may have had a precipitating role in the presence of the elevated Lp(a) level.

The twin brother of the deceased father also had a heterozygous FV mutation FV 1691 AG with APC resistance and an Lp(a) level at the upper limit of normal (31 mg/dl), in addition to the classic risk factors for CHD, which were diabetes, arterial hypertension, elevated cholesterol, and tobacco abuse.

Summary

Measurement of Lp(a) should be included in the routine testing of clotting investigations in cases of premature onset of arterial thromboembolism and atherosclerotic diseases. Even though Lp(a) levels are genetically determined, there are therapeutic possibilities for treatment. It remains unclear whether the lowering of an elevated Lp(a) level leads to a reduced risk of atherosclerosis.

References

1. Dahlen G, Guyton JR, Attar M et al. Association of levels of lipoprotein Lp(a), plasma lipids, and other lipoproteins with coronary artery disease documented by angiography. Circulation 1986; 4: 758–765
2. Jauhiainen M, Koskinen P, Ehnholm C et al. Lipoprotein (a) and coronary heart disease risk: a nested case-control study of the Helsinki Heart Study participants. Atherosclerosis 1991; 89: 59–67

3. Kostner GM, Avogaro P Gazzolato G et al. Lipoprotein (a) and the risk for myocardial infarction. Atherosclerosis 1981; 38: 51–61
4. Marburger C, Hambrecht R, Niebauer J et al. Association between lipoprotein (a) and progression of coronary artery disease in middle-aged men. Am J Cardiol 1994; 73: 742–746
5. Nowak-Göttl U et al. Increased lipoprotein (a) is an important risk factor for venous thrombosis in childhood. Circulation 1999; 100: 743–748
6. Perski A, Olsson G, Landou C et al. Minimum heart rate and coronary atherosclerosis: independent relations to global severity and rate of progression of angiographic lesions in men with myocardial infarction at a young age. Am Heart J 1992; 123: 609–616
7. Ridker PM, Hennekens CH, Stampfer MJ. A prospective study of lipoprotein (a) and the risk of myocardial infarction. JAMA 1993; 270: 2195–2199.
8. Rosengren A, Wilhelmsen L, Eriksson E et al. Lipoprotein (a) and coronary heart disease: a prospective case-control study in a general population sample of middle aged men. Br Med J 1990; 301: 1248–1251
9. Stubbs P, Seed M, Moseley D et al. A prospective study of the role of lipoprotein (a) in the pathogenesis of unstable angina. Eur Heart J 1997; 18:603–607

Acquired Hemophilia in Women Postpartum

M. Mohren, A. Jakob, L. Kanz, K. Jaschonek

Introduction

Factor VIII inhibitors occur in 15–25% of patients with severe hemophilia A while being substituted with factor VIII concentrates, as well as spontaneously in non-hemophiliac individuals. The latter usually are young women, who develop a factor VIII inhibitor either during pregnancy or more likely postpartum, or elderly patients with a predisposing concomitant disease such as rheumatoid arthritis, systemic lupus erythematosus, or non-Hodgkin's lymphoma [1]. Non-hemophiliac patients with acquired factor VIII inhibitors often show a more severe bleeding tendency than hemophiliacs, with a lethality rate of 22% [1]. Intra-articular bleedings are rare in this patient group.

Patient

A 25-year-old patient with a spontaneous hematoma of the left quadriceps muscle and intra-articular bleeding into the left ankle and knee was admitted to our hospital 2 weeks after normal delivery of her first child. The following laboratory results were obtained: hemoglobin 7.1 g/dl; aPTT 75 s; Quick 112%; factor VIII:C <1%; and presence of a factor VIII inhibitor with 4 Bethesda units. A normal DRVVT and platelet neutralization procedure ruled out the presence of a lupus anticoagulant.

High-dose immunoglobulins were given over 7 days, treatment with 2000 IU t.i.d. FEIBA was initiated for 3 days. While on this regimen, the patient's hemoglobin stabilized, the muscle hematoma and the intra-articular bleedings resolved. During the following months there remained a decreased factor VIII activity of 3–7% without any further bleeding tendency. Within 1 year after this bleeding episode, factor VIII activity normalized (factor VIII:C 100%) without any specific treatment. The patient remained asymptomatic and showed normal factor VIII activity for a follow-up of 3 years.

Discussion

Due to its low incidence, there is no clear concept on how to treat factor VIII inhibitors in non-hemophiliac patients, based on randomized trials [2, 4]. Inhibitors arising postpartum particularly show a very high spontaneous remission rate of almost 100% within 2.5 years. Immunosuppression with azathioprine or cyclophosphamide seems to shorten the inhibitor activity, while corticosteroids do not

I. Scharrer/W. Schramm (Ed.)
30th Hemophilia Symposium Hamburg 1999
© Springer-Verlag Berlin Heidelberg 2001

show any beneficial effect [2]. However, one study with a small number of patients failed to confirm these results [3].

FEIBA as well as recombinant FVIIa are effective in treating severe bleeding complications [5, 6]. Since our patient showed no further bleeding activity after a 3-day course of FEIBA (recombinant FVIIa was not commercially available at that time), we decided not to initiate immunosuppressive therapy.

References

1. D. Green, K. Lechner A survey of 215 non-hemophilic patients with inhibitors to factor VIII. Thrombosis and Haemostasis 1981; 45: 200–03
2. I. Hauser, B. Schneider, K. Lechner. Post-Partum Factor VIII Inhibitors. Thrombosis and Haemostasis 1995; 73 (1): 1–5
3. R. Lottenberg, T. Kentro, C. Kitchens. Acquired Hemophilia. Arch Intern Med-Vol 147, 1987
4. E.O. Meili, H. Dazzi, A. von Felten. Rekombinanter aktivierter Faktor VII zur Blutstillung bei erworbener Hemmkörper-Hämophilie. Schweiz Med Wochenschr 1995; 125: 405–11
5. J.J. Michiels et al. Acquired haemophilia A in women postpartum : management of bleeding episodes and natural history of the factor VIII inhibitor. Eur J Haemotol 1997: 59: 105–109
6. B. Neidhardt, O. Bartels, B. Hahn. Hemmkörperhämophilie A post partum. DMW 1985, 110. Jg., Nr.20

IX.f Poster: Hemorrhagic Disorders

Modulation of Antigens of Neutrophil Granulocytes by Extracorporal Apheresis

M. MAERZ, K. GUTENSOHN, P. KUEHNL

Introduction

Today, transfusions of platelet products are important blood components for the management of patients suffering from congenital or acquired platelet or hemostatic disorders. Platelet products may be prepared by apheresis. Production of platelet concentrates by this method is usually performed in an extracorporal circuit. Due to the influence of the extracorporal system, different interactions may occur between the blood and artificial components of the apheresis device [1, 2]. These effects are provoked mainly by the contact between the donor's blood and biomaterials as well as shear stress.

In this study, the influence of platelet-pheresis on antigen alterations of platelets and leukocytes was analyzed. For this purpose, flow cytometry was applied.

Materials and Methods

Platelet-pheresis was performed on a COBE Spectra cell separator (COBE Laboratories, Lakewood, USA) in 10 healthy and drug-free volunteer donors (5 females, mean age 39.8 years; 5 males, mean age 32.8 years). ACD was used as anticoagulant at a ratio of 1:6. The procedure time was 60 min on average.

During apheresis, blood samples were obtained via a sample connector (pvb medizintechnik, Kirchseeon, Germany) from the outlet line, before starting the procedure, at 15, 30, and 60 min. For flow cytometry of platelet and leukocyte antigens, aliquots of whole blood were immediately fixed and stabilized with 40% glyoxale (Merck), 10% paraformaldehyde (Serva, Heidelberg, Germany), and 0.15 M phosphate buffer (Merck), thereafter diluted with phosphate buffer containing 0.2% w/v of glycine (Serva) and stored at +4°C. Direct labeling was performed with monoclonal antibodies against CD41a and CD62p (Coulter-Immunotech, Hamburg, Germany) for platelets. Neutrophil granulocytes were detected by CD45 for identification; additionally, CD11a, CD11b, CD11c, and CD18 were applied (Coulter-Immunotech).

Flow cytometric analysis was performed on a FACScan cytometer (Becton Dickinson, Mountain View, USA). In each sample, 5000 events were analyzed. Thereafter, analyses of flow cytometric data were performed using CELLQuest software (Becton Dickinson). Data with a P value of less than 0.05 were regarded as significant.

I. Scharrer/W. Schramm (Ed.)
30th Hemophilia Symposium Hamburg 1999
© Springer-Verlag Berlin Heidelberg 2001

Results

During apheresis, significant changes could be detected for the structural antigen CD41a (GPIIb-IIIa; $P<0.01$). Standardized mean channel fluorescence intensity (MCFI) increased for CD41a from 0.77 ± 0.31 to 1.21 ± 0.62 MCFI. The activation-dependent antigen CD62p (P-selectin) increased moderately from 0.67 ± 0.36 to 1.37 ± 0.59 MCFI ($P<0.01$) (Figs. 1, 2).

Also, an increase of the selectins CD11b (0.64 ± 0.43 to 1.48 ± 0.91 MCFI; $P<0.01$) and CD11c (0.82 ± 0.34 to 1.26 ± 0.55 MCFI; $P<0.01$) could be detected on neutrophil granulocytes. A significant decrease could be detected for the selectin CD11a on neutrophil granulocytes (1.07 ± 0.09 to 0.89 ± 0.23 MCFI; $P<0.01$). The expression of CD18 on neutrophil granulocytes did not change significantly ($P>0.05$).

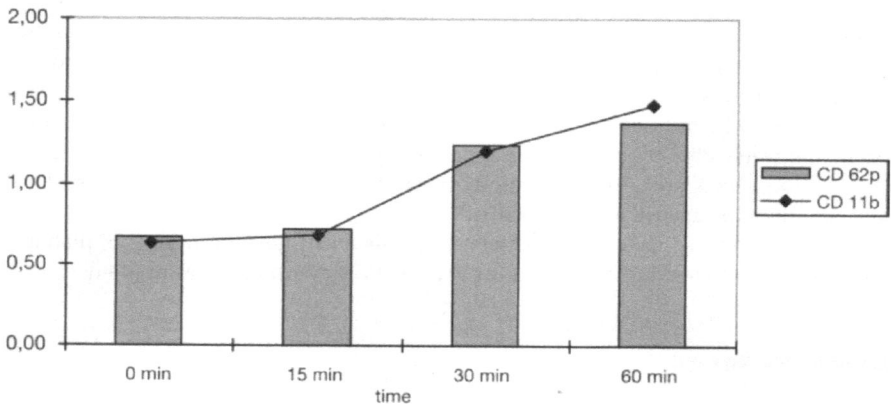

Fig. 1. Increase of CD62p MCFI (P-selectin) on platelets and of CD11b MCFI (integrin) on neutrophil granulocytes during apheresis

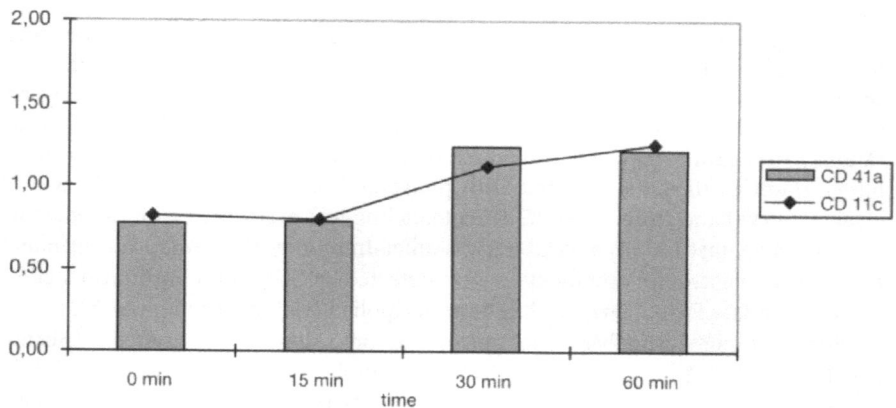

Fig. 2. Increase of CD41a MCFI on platelets and of CD11c MCFI (integrin) on neutrophil granulocytes during apheresis

Discussion

When platelets are removed from the circulation of the donor and are exposed to biomaterials of the extracorporal system during apheresis, various cellular changes occur. These changes are also reflected by alterations of membrane glycoproteins. Up- and downregulation, conformational changes of antigens, and formation of neoepitopes may occur. Some of these changes demonstrate the activated state of platelets, and as shown in previous studies with other extracorporal devices, platelet activation can reach high levels during apheresis [1].

In this study, we could demonstrate that platelets become activated during apheresis. The expression of P-selectin (CD62p) and the binding of fibrinogen to platelets progressively increased over the course. P-selectin plays an important role in the binding process of platelets with leukocytes. This glycoprotein on the surface of activated platelets represents a rapidly inducible receptor for white blood cells and mediates platelet–leukocyte binding. Predominantly sialylated, fucosylated lactosaminoglycans and P-selectin glycoprotein ligand-1 are involved in this process [3].

Also, antigens of white blood cells were altered. The fluorescence expression of the integrins CD11b and CD11c of neutrophil granulocytes increased during the procedure. For these integrins, intracellular storage pools exist in neutrophil granulocytes which may be upregulated upon activation. These transmembrane proteins are able to bind to cytoskeletal proteins and are involved in extracellular signal communication [4]. Increased expression of these adhesion receptors has been noted after neutrophil activation and adhesion [5].

Earlier observations in extracorporal devices also demonstrated a CD11b and CD11c upregulation [6, 7]. Of further interest is the kinetic of the integrin expression, which is dependent on the intensity of shear forces, biomaterials, and the subtype of white blood cells [8]. In addition, a large amount of experimental data indicate that platelet activation elicits neutrophil granulocyte responses and that neutrophil granulocytes in turn modulate platelets [6, 7, 8]. The parallel antigenic alterations of platelets and neutrophil granulocytes in this study may promote platelet–leukocyte interactions [8, 9, 10].

Conclusion

1. During apheresis with the COBE Spectra cell separator, significant changes in platelet and leukocyte antigens can be detected.
2. These aspects may be considered as activation of platelets and neutrophil granulocytes.
3. Cell–cell contact, shear forces, and interaction with the biomaterial possibly induce platelet activation and upregulation of integrins on neutrophil granulocytes.
4. The parallel alteration of platelet and neutrophil granulocyte antigens may promote platelet–leukocyte interactions.

References

1. Gutensohn K, Maerz M, Kuehnl P. Hematother 6; 1997: 315–321
2. Muehrke D, McCarthy P, Kottke-Marchant K, et al. J Thorac Cardiovasc Surg 112; 1996: 472–483
3. McEver RP, Martin MN. J Biol Chem 259; 1984: 9799–9804
4. Carlos T, Harlan J. Blood 84; 1994: 2068–2101
5. Lawrence M, Springer T. Cell 65; 1991: 859–873
6. Rinder C, Bonan J, Rinder H, et al. Blood 79; 1992: 1201–1205
7. Tielemans C, Delville J-P, Husson C. Clin Nephrol 39; 1993: 158–165
8. Del Mashio, Dejana E, Battoni G. Ann Hematol 67; 1993: 23–31
9. Ruf A, Patscheke H. Br J Haematol 90; 1995: 791–796
10. Diacovo E, Bahr G, Parant M, et al. Blood 88; 1996: 146–157

Glycoprotein IIb/IIIa Receptor Antagonist c7E3 Fab and Anticoagulants Show an Additive Effect on Thrombin-Induced Platelet Aggregation after High Coagulant Challenge in Vitro

M. Köstenberger, S. Gallistl, G. Cvirn, B. Roschitz, W. Muntean

Introduction

In vitro experiments have shown that antibodies to the GP IIb/IIIa receptor have a diminishing effect on free thrombin generation, and these agents have been suggested as anticoagulant drugs [1, 2]. These experiments were performed after activation of platelet-rich plasma (PRP) with low concentrations of tissue thromboplastin, which did not result in fibrinogen polymerization in the absence of platelets. It has been shown that platelet activation plays a major role in the development of thrombosis when the thrombogenic stimulus is mild [3]. On the other hand, the thrombogenic challenge in vivo is difficult to quantify and atherosclerotic plaques might express tissue thromboplastin concentrations that may overcome the anticoagulant effect of direct platelet inhibition. Thus, under high thrombogenic challenge, GP IIb/IIIa inhibition alone might be ineffective in preventing thrombin formation.

Anticoagulant drugs such as recombinant hirudin (rH), low molecular weight heparin (LMWH), and unfractionated heparin (UH) have been demonstrated to inhibit thrombin generation dose-dependently, both in platelet-poor and platelet-rich plasma [4–7]. Anticoagulants not only affect thrombin generation, but also delay thrombin-induced platelet activation [5]. Combined administration of GP IIb/IIIa antagonists, such as the murine/human chimeric antibody fragment c7E3 Fab (abciximab; ReoPro), and anticoagulants might have an additive effect on the inhibition of platelet-mediated thrombin generation, and has proven effective in clinical studies dealing with PTCA and thrombolysis after myocardial infarction in the presence of abciximab and unfractionated heparin [8–10].

We investigated the combined effect of platelet GP IIb/IIIa inhibition and anticoagulant agents on platelet aggregation and thrombin generation induced by endogenously generated thrombin under high coagulant challenge. We, therefore, used a previously described model allowing simultaneous determination of platelet aggregation and thrombin generation [5] in the presence of abciximab and anticoagulants after extrinsic activation of PRP. For high coagulant challenge, clotting was triggered using tissue thromboplastin concentrations that resulted in fibrinogen polymerization independent of platelets.

I. Scharrer/W. Schramm (Ed.)
30th Hemophilia Symposium Hamburg 1999
© Springer-Verlag Berlin Heidelberg 2001

Methods

Platelet Aggregation

Platelet aggregation studies were done using a standard turbidimetric technique in an aggregometer (Bio/Data Corporation, Horsham, Pa., USA). PRP was added to an aggregometer cuvette containing a stir bar. The cuvette was placed in the aggregometer prewarmed to 37°C. Platelet-poor plasma (PPP) was used as the blank. Platelet aggregation was induced by endogenously generated thrombin [5]: After extrinsic activation of plasma containing different concentrations of abçiximab, rH, LMWH, or UH, the anti-aggregating activity of these drugs was expressed as percent inhibition, as described by Herault et al. [2], related to aggregation measured in the absence of inhibitors.

Determination of Thrombin Generation

At timed intervals, 10 µl aliquots of activated PRP were withdrawn and subsampled into 490 µl buffer B containing 255 µM S-2238. The reagents were prewarmed to 37°C. Amidolysis of S-2238 was stopped after 6 min by addition of 250 µl 50% acetic acid. The amount of thrombin generated was quantified by measuring the absorbency by double wavelength (405–690 nm) in the Anthos microplate-reader 2001. The amidolytic activity measured was caused by the simultaneous activity of free thrombin and the α_2-macroglobulin-thrombin complex. The amount of free thrombin was calculated using a method developed by Hemker et al. [11, 12].

Results

Activation of PRP in the absence of abciximab, rH, LMWH, and UH resulted in a sudden onset of thrombin generation after a lag time of 26.5±1.7 s. The peak amount of thrombin concentration was about 150 nM and the calculated thrombin potential in the absence of inhibitors was 280±7 nM/min (Table 1). After activation of PRP by endogenously generated thrombin in the absence of inhibitors, the lag phase until onset of platelet aggregation was 25±2 s. As shown previously [5], onset of platelet aggregation and free thrombin generation occurred simultaneously under our experimental conditions. Results are expressed as means (±SD) of five experiments.

Effect of Abciximab on Platelet Aggregation, Lag Phase
Until the Onset of Platelet Aggregation, and Thrombin Potential

Compared to the aggregation curve monitored in the absence of abciximab, 1 µg/ml abciximab had no anti-aggregating effect. Five, 10, and 20 µg/ml abciximab revealed 44±3%, 74±2%, and 84±2% inhibition of platelet aggregation compared to the control, respectively (Fig. 1). Higher concentrations of abciximab (40, 80 µg/ml) did not result

Table 1. Effects of abciximab, rH, LMWH, and UH on platelet aggregation, lag phase until the onset of platelet aggregation, and thrombin potential compared to control in PRP

	Anti-aggregating activity (%)	Lag phase (s)	TP (nM/min)
PRP	0	25±2	280±7
abciximab (µg/ml)			
5	44±3	34±2	278±11
10	74±2		
20	84±2		
rH (ng/ml)			
300	1.1±0.4	51±3	271±4
600		64±2	256±6
1200		135±5	211±7
LMWH (U/ml)			
0.125	1.1±0.6	25±2	259±5
0.25		27±1	231±7
0.5		30±2	151±16
1		36±3	33±5
UH (U/ml)			
0.125	2.1±0.9	30±3	222±18
0.25		38±5	86±11
0.4		48±3	35±8
0.5		74±6	Traces

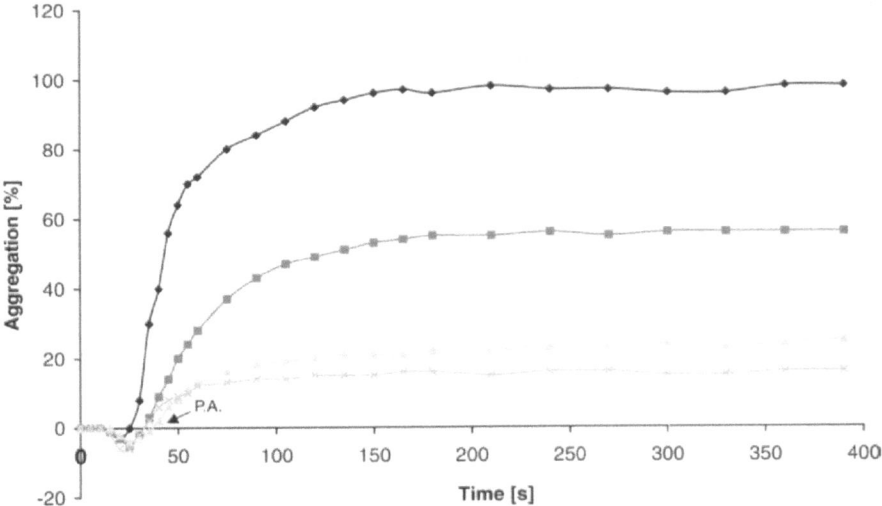

Fig. 1. Platelet aggregation curves in PRP containing 5, 10, or 20 µg/ml abciximab. Lag phase is defined as time until the onset of platelet aggregation occurs (curve crossing the O-line). P.A., onset of platelet aggregation. (◆) Control measurement in the absence of abciximab; (■) 5 µg/ml abciximab (44 ± 3% inhibition of aggregation); (▲) 10 µg/ml abciximab (74 ± 2% inhibition); (✕) 20 µg/ml abciximab (84 ± 2% inhibition). Results are expressed as means (n=5). Standard deviation is not shown for clarity of graph reading

in further inhibition of platelet aggregation (data not shown). In the presence of 5 µg/ml abciximab, the lag phase until the onset of platelet aggregation was prolonged to 34 ± 2 s. Abciximab concentrations higher than 5 µg/ml had no further effect on the lag phase (Table 1). Administration of increasing amounts of abciximab (1, 5, 10, or 20 µg/ml final concentration) had no effect on the thrombin potential (TP).

Effects of Anticoagulants on Platelet Aggregation, Lag Phase Until the Onset of Platelet Aggregation, and Thrombin Potential

Table 1 shows that addition of different amounts of anticoagulants did not result in an anti-aggregating effect compared to non-anticoagulated plasma, but resulted in a dose-dependent prolongation of the lag phase until onset of platelet aggregation. UH, LMWH, and rH decreased the TP dose-dependently.

Combined Effects of Abciximab and rH on Platelet Aggregation, Lag Phase Until the Onset of Platelet Aggregation, and Thrombin Potential

Addition of 300, 600, or 1200 ng/ml rH to PRP containing 5, 10, and 20 µg/ml abciximab had no further inhibitory effect on platelet aggregation but resulted in a prolongation of the lag phase to 63 ± 3, 82 ± 5, and 152 ± 9 s, respectively (Table 2; Fig. 2). The effect of abciximab on the lag phase in hirudinized plasma was independent of the abciximab concentration used.

As shown in Table 2, addition of different concentrations of abciximab to plasma containing 300, 600, or 1200 ng/ml rH had no additive effect on the TP compared to hirudinized plasma in the absence of abciximab.

Table 2. Combined effects of abciximab, rH, LMWH, and UH on the lag phase until the onset of platelet aggregation and thrombin potential measured in PRP

	Lag phase (s)	TP (nM/min)
abciximab (5, 10, or 20 µg/ml) + rH (ng/ml)		
300	63±3	273±5
600	82±5	258±9
1200	152±9	208±6
abciximab (5, 10, or 20 µg/ml) + LMWH (U/ml)		
0.125	35±2	263±7
0.25	39±2	230±15
0.5	45±2	153±12
1	65±6	35±7
abciximab (5, 10, or 20 µg/ml) + UH (U/ml)		
0.125	41±5	225±23
0.25	66±5	84±12
0.4	102±9	36±5
0.5	142±15	Traces

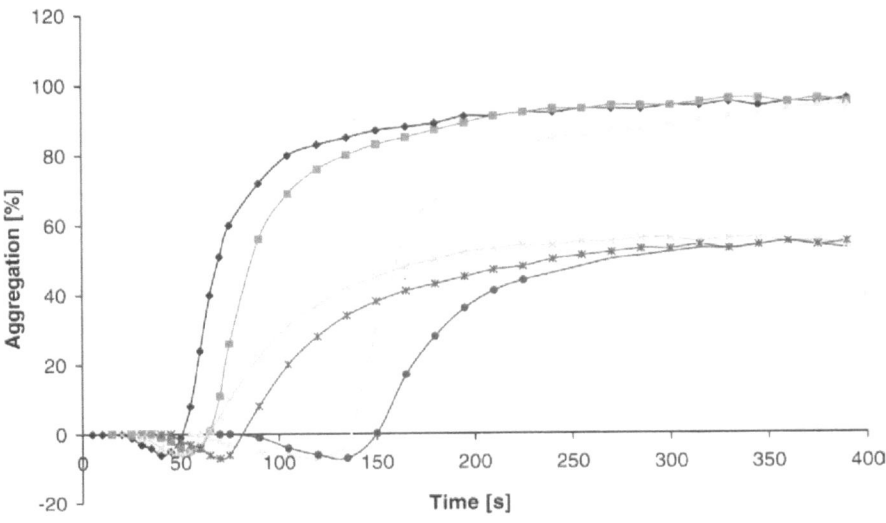

Fig. 2. Platelet aggregation curves in PRP containing 300, 600, or 1200 ng/ml rH in the absence or presence of 5 µg/ml abciximab. Addition of 10 or 20 µg/ml abciximab to plasma containing rH resulted in similar prolongation of the lag phase as for 5 µg/ml abciximab. (◆) 300 ng/ml rH (lag phase until the onset of platelet aggregation of 51 ± 3 s); (■) 600 ng/ml rH (lag phase 64 ± 2 s); (▲) 1200 ng/ml (lag phase 135 ± 5 s); (✕) 300 ng/ml rH and 5 µg/ml abciximab (lag phase 63 ± 3 s); (✳) 600 ng/ml rH and 5 µg/ml abciximab (lag phase 82 ± 5 s); (●) 1200 ng/ml rH and 5 µg/ml abciximab (lag phase 152 ± 9 s). Results are expressed as means (n=5). Standard deviation is not shown for clarity of graph reading

Combined Effects of Abciximab and LMWH on Platelet Aggregation, Lag Phase Until the Onset of Platelet Aggregation, and Thrombin Potential

Addition of 0.125, 0.25, 0.5, or 1 U/ml LMWH to PRP containing 5, 10, and 20 µg/ml abciximab had no further inhibitory effect on platelet aggregation, but resulted in a prolongation of the lag phase to 35 ± 2, 39 ± 2, 45 ± 2, 65 ± 6 s, respectively (Table 2; Fig. 3). Addition of different concentrations of abciximab to PRP containing 0.125, 0.25, 0.5, or 1 U/ml LMWH resulted in a TP of 263 ± 7, 230 ± 15, 153 ± 12, and 35±7 nM/min (Table 2).

Combined Effects of Abciximab and UH on Platelet Aggregation, Lag Phase Until the Onset of Platelet Aggregation, and Thrombin Potential

Addition of 0.125, 0.25, 0.4, and 0.5 U/ml UH to PRP containing 5, 10, or 20 µg/ml abciximab did not result in further inhibition of platelet aggregation compared to PRP containing only abciximab. As observed with rH and LMWH, administration of abciximab (5, 10, or 20 µg/ml) to plasma containing 0.125, 0.25, 0.4, or 0.5 U/ml UH resulted in a prolongation of the lag phase until the onset of platelet aggregation to 41 ± 5, 66 ± 5, 102 ± 9, or 142 ± 15 s, respectively (Table 2; Fig. 4). Addition of

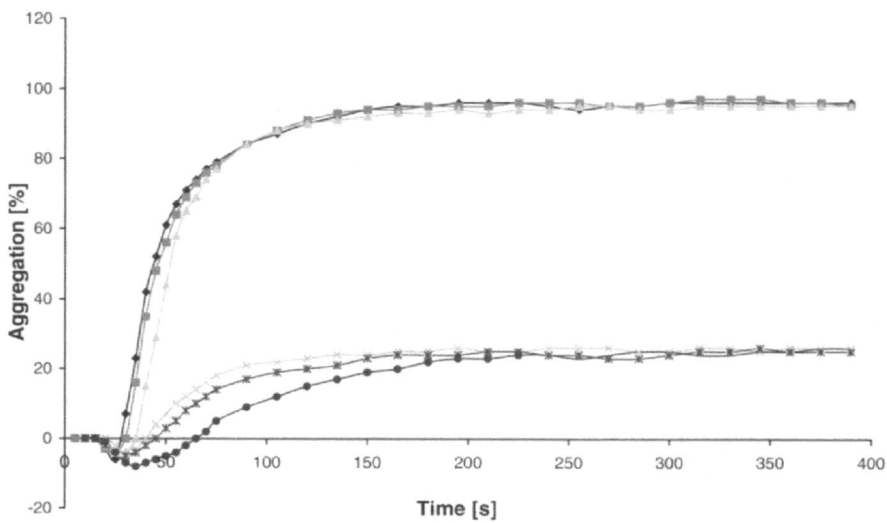

Fig. 3. Platelet aggregation curves in PRP containing 0.25, 0.5, or 1 U/ml LMWH in the absence or presence of 10 µg/ml abciximab. Addition of 5 or 20 µg/ml abciximab resulted in similar prolongation of the lag phase as for 10 µg/ml. (◆) 0.25 U/ml LMWH (lag phase until the onset of platelet aggregation of 27 ± 1 s); (■) 0.5 U/ml LMWH (lag phase 30 ± 2 s); (▲) 1 U/ml LMWH (lag phase 36 ± 3 s); (✕) 0.25 U/ml LMWH and 10 µg/ml abciximab (lag phase 39 ± 2 s); (✳) 0.5 U/ml LMWH and 10 µg/ml abciximab (lag phase 45 ± 2 s); (●) 1 U/ml LMWH and 10 µg/ml abciximab (lag phase 65 ± 6 s). Results are expressed as means ($n = 5$). Standard deviation is not shown for clarity of graph reading

0.125, 0.25, or 0.4 U/ml UH resulted in a TP of 225 ± 23, 84 ± 12, or 36 ± 5 nM/min in the presence of abciximab concentrations (5, 10, and 20 µg/ml), with no significant difference to measurements in the absence of abciximab (Table 2).

Discussion

The GP IIb/IIIa inhibitor abciximab produces an antithrombotic effect by direct inhibition of the binding of natural ligands such as fibrinogen to the GP IIb/IIIa receptor, leading to a dose-dependent inhibition of platelet aggregation [13, 14] and thrombin generation [1]. We investigated the effect of abciximab in an in vitro system which enabled us to determine platelet aggregation and thrombin generation simultaneously. After extrinsic activation of PRP, abciximab exhibited a dose-dependent anti-aggregating effect which reached its maximum at a concentration of 20 µg/ml. This observation is in agreement with the study of Reverter et al. [1], who showed that 15–20 µg abciximab/ml plasma resulted in ~90% blockade of platelet GP IIb/IIIa receptors. In contrast to the study by Reverter et al., who used a 1:4000 dilution of recombinant tissue factor for the activation of PRP, abciximab had no effect on free thrombin generation under our experimen-

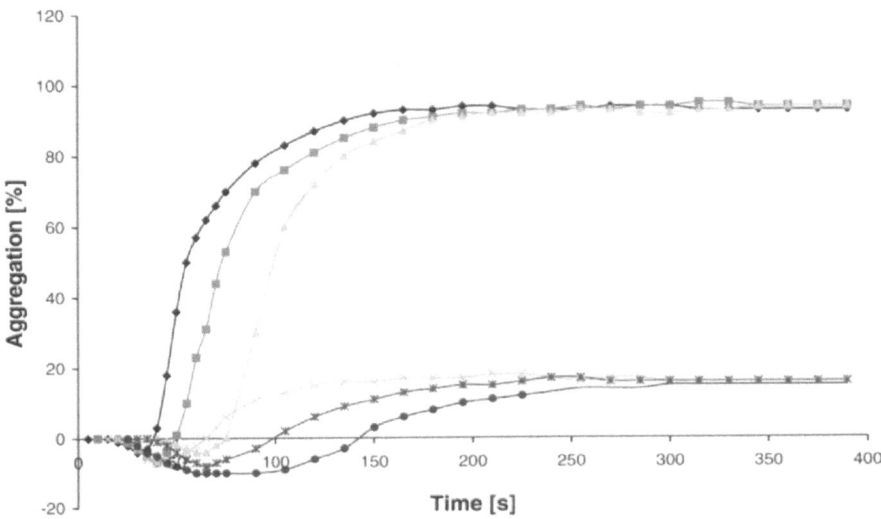

Fig. 4. Platelet aggregation curves in PRP containing 0.25, 0.4, or 0.5 U/ml UH in the absence or presence of 20 μg/ml abciximab. Addition of 5 and 10 μg/ml abciximab resulted in similar prolongation of the lag phase as with 20 μg/ml. (◆) 0.25 U/ml UH (lag phase until the onset of platelet aggregation of 38 ± 5 s); (■) 0.4 U/ml UH (lag phase 48 ± 3 s). (▲) 0.5 U/ml UH (lag phase 74 ± 6 s); (✕) 0.25 U/ml UH and 20 μg/ml abciximab (lag phase 66 ± 5 s); (✱) 0.4 U/ml UH and 20 μg/ml abciximab (lag phase 102 ± 9 s); (●) 0.5 U/ml UH and 20 μg/ml abciximab (lag phase 142 ± 15 s). Results are expressed as means (n=5). Standard deviation is not shown for clarity of graph reading

tal conditions. This observation might be explained by the fact that thrombin generation depends on platelets only in the presence of a low coagulant challenge. It has been shown that low concentrations of thromboplastin that do not stimulate thrombin generation in PPP produce explosive thrombin formation in the presence of platelets, and that at high thromboplastin concentrations the difference between PRP and PPP vanishes [15]. Herbert et al. [3] demonstrated that experimentally induced thrombocytopenia strongly affected thrombus formation under low thrombogenic challenge in experimental venous thrombosis in the rat. In contrast, platelets had no influence on thrombus formation after intravenous administration of a high dose of tissue thromboplastin. They suggested that the antithrombotic activity of anticoagulant compounds may vary depending on the degree of hypercoagulability induced by increasing amounts of tissue factor. GP IIb/IIIa antagonists might be used in clinical situations associated with a possibly high thrombogenic challenge, such as myocardial infarction or stroke which are well known complications of atheromatous plaques. Plaque rupture is thought to be a major precipitant of acute arterial thrombosis [16], exposing circulating blood to thrombogenic plaque proteins [17]. Muhlfelder et al. [18] demonstrated constitutive tissue factor in plaque extracts obtained from patients with obstructive atheromatous disease. The activity of tissue factor was up to one fifth of tissue factor activity of full-strength rabbit thromboplastin, thereby representing a high thrombogenic challenge.

Anticoagulant agents such as rH, LMWH, and UH have been demonstrated to diminish thrombin generation even under high coagulant challenge and have been shown to be effective in the treatment of arterial thrombosis [19]. We, therefore, speculated that the combination of abciximab and anticoagulants would combine antiplatelet and anticoagulant effects. When combining abciximab and anticoagulants under high coagulant challenge we observed a combination of their respective specific effects on inhibition of platelet aggregation and thrombin generation. Thus, since platelet aggregation and thrombin generation occurred simultaneously under our experimental conditions, abciximab prolonged the lag phase until the onset of free thrombin generation in anticoagulated PRP but had no additive effect on the thrombin potential. On the other hand, although platelets had no effect on the amount of thrombin generated under high coagulant challenge, they contributed to alterations of the lag phase until the onset of thrombin generation. The importance of this observation under clinical circumstances is difficult to evaluate, since the major part of the thrombin burst occurs after platelet aggregation has finished and a fibrin plug has been formed [5].

In conclusion, our study demonstrates specific inhibitory effects of abciximab and anticoagulants on platelet aggregation and free thrombin generation under high coagulant challenge. In addition, abciximab showed an additive effect on the lag phase until the onset of platelet aggregation in the presence of the anticoagulants UH, LMWH, and rH. Since a high thrombogenic challenge might occur with rupture of atherosclerotic plaques, our study gives further support to the notion that the combined application of antiplatelet and anticoagulant agents might improve the clinical outcome in atherosclerotic disease.

References

1. Reverter JC, Beguin S, Kessels H, Kumar R, Hemker HC, Coller BS. Inhibition of platelet-mediated, tissue factor-induced thrombin generation by the mouse/human chimeric 7E3 antibody. J Clin Invest 1996; 98: 863–74.
2. Herault JP, Peyrou V, Savi P, Bernat A, Herbert JM. Effect of SR 121566 A, a potent GP IIb-IIIa antagonist on platelet-mediated thrombin generation in vitro and in vivo. Thromb Haemost 1998; 79: 383–8.
3. Herbert JM, Bernat A, Maffrand JP. Importance of platelets in experimental venous thrombosis in the rat. Blood 1992; 80: 2281–6.
4. Gallistl S, Muntean W. Thrombin-hirudin complex formation, thrombin-antithrombin III complex formation, and thrombin generation after intrinsic activation of plasma. Thromb Haemost 1994; 72: 387–92.
5. Gallistl S, Muntean W, Leis HJ. Effects of heparin and hirudin on thrombin generation and platelet aggregation after intrinsic activation of platelet rich plasma. Thromb Haemost 1995; 74: 1163–8.
6. Prasa D, Svendsen L, Stürzebecher J. The ability of thrombin inhibitors to reduce the thrombin activity generated in plasma on extrinsic and intrinsic activation. Thromb Haemost 1997; 77: 498–503.
7. Pieters J, Lindhout T. The limited importance of factor Xa inhibition to the anticoagulant property of heparin in thromboplastin-activated plasma. Blood 1988; 72: 2048–52.

8. The CAPTURE Investigators. Randomised placebo-controlled trial of abciximab before and during coronary intervention in refractory unstable angina: the CAPTURE study. Lancet 1997; 349: 1429-35.
9. The EPILOG Investigators. Platelet glycoprotein IIb/IIIa receptor blockade and low-dose heparin during percutaneous coronary revascularization. N Engl J Med 1997; 336: 1689-96.
10. The EPIC Investigators. Use of a monoclonal antibody directed against the platelet glycoprotein IIb/IIIa receptor in high-risk coronary angioplasty. N Engl J Med 1994; 330: 956-61.
11. Hemker HC, Beguin S. Thrombin generation in plasma: Its assessment via the endogenous thrombin potential. Thromb Haemost 1995; 74: 134-8.
12. Hemker HC, Wielders S, Kessels H, Beguin S. Continuous registration of thrombin generation in plasma, its use for the determination of the thrombin potential. Thromb Haemost 1993; 70: 617-24.
13. Coller BS. GP IIb/IIIa antagonists: Pathophysiologic and therapeutic insights from studies of c7E3 Fab. Thromb Haemost 1997; 78: 730-5.
14. Coller BS, Anderson K, Weisman HF. New antiplatelet agents: Platelet GP IIb/IIIa antagonists. Thromb Haemost 1995; 74: 302-8.
15. Beguin S, Lindhout T, Hemker HC. The effect of trace amounts of tissue factor on thrombin generation in platelet rich plasma, its inhibition by heparin. Thromb Haemost 1989; 61: 25-29.
16. Fuster V, Badimon L, Badimon JJ, Chesebro JH. The pathogenesis of coronary artery disease and the acute coronary syndromes. N Engl J Med 1992; 326: 242-50 and 310-8.
17. Taubman MB, Fallon JT, Schecter AD, Giesen P, Mendlowitz M, Fyfe BS, Marmur JD, Nemerson Y. Tissue factor in the pathogenesis of atherosclerosis. Thromb Haemost 1997; 78: 200-4.
18. Muhlfelder TW, Teodorescu V, Rand J, Rosman A, Niemetz J. Human atheromatous plaque extracts induce tissue factor activity (TFa) in monocytes and also express constitutive Tfa. Thromb Haemost 1999; 81: 146-50.
19. Turpie AG. Clinical potential of antithrombotic drugs in coronary syndromes. Am J Cardiol 1998; 82: 11L-14L.

Between-Drug Comparison of the Effect of Ticlopidine and Acetylsalicylic Acid on Platelets in an In Vitro Circulation Model

M.A. Brockmann, C. Beythien, M.M. Magens, B. Bernien, K. Geidel, A. Alisch, P. Kühnl, K. Gutensohn

Introduction

Different approaches have been made on reducing the risk of acute or subacute reocclusion of stented coronary vessels. To date, no definite solution of these complications has been established. Therefore, we compared the efficaciousness of different dosages of ticlopidine (Tiklyd, Sanofi Winthrop, FRG) and acetylsalicylic acid (ASA, Aspirin, Bayer, Germany), focusing on platelet inhibition by aggregometry and in an in vitro circulating model containing coronary stents.

Methods

For 7 days, volunteers ($n=7$) took one cycle of ASA 100 mg/day, one cycle of ASA 300 mg/day, one cycle of ticlopidine 250 mg/day and one cycle of ticlopidine 500 mg/day in a randomized sequence. Between cycles, medication was paused for a minimum of 14 days for each volunteer. On the morning of the 8th day after starting ingestion of drugs, blood was collected and platelet-rich plasma (PRP) prepared. Platelet count within PRP was standardized to 250x10³/μl. PRP was then filled into an in vitro model, recalcified, and circulation started. Time until stent occlusion (TSO) was measured. Also, aggregometric analysis (APACT, Labor GmbH, Germany) of the standardized PRP was performed using collagen (1 μg/l) and ADP (1 μmol/l) for platelet activation. Maximum aggregation and maximum aggregation ascent were recorded.

Results

Aggregometer analyses with collagen used for platelet activation displayed a significant inhibition of platelet aggregability after ingestion of ASA 100 mg/day and ASA 300 mg/day compared to the aggregability after ingestion of ticlopidine (both dosages) and the control group without drugs ($P<0.05$). Administration of ticlopidine 500 mg/day also resulted in a significant decrease of platelet aggregability compared to the control group. No differences regarding platelet aggregability could be observed between ASA 100 mg/day and ASA 300 mg/day. ADP-activated aggregometry revealed a significant decrease of platelet aggregability after inges-

I. Scharrer/W. Schramm (Ed.)
30th Hemophilia Symposium Hamburg 1999
© Springer-Verlag Berlin Heidelberg 2001

tion of ticlopidine (both dosages) compared to aggregability after administration of ASA (both dosages) and the control group. In addition, ticlopidine 500 mg/day proved to be significantly more efficacious than the minor dosage of ticlopidine. In vitro circulating models showed no differences after use of different antiplatelet drugs.

Conclusion

Taking into consideration gastrointestinal side effects after use of ASA and aggregometric results, administration of the lower dosage of ASA (100 mg/day) should be considered for platelet inhibition after stent implantation.

Rotablation Leads to Significant Platelet Activation: A Flow Cytometric Assessment

J. Bau, C. Beythien, M. Brockmann, P. Kühnl, K. Gutensohn

Introduction

The clinical success of rotablation as one of the modern interventional techniques is limited by possible acute and subacute occlusion of the vessel. Activation of platelets and their consecutive interaction with the rotablated vessel wall play a key role in later ischemic thrombotic complications. We examined the extent of platelet activation during rotablation using flow cytometry.

Materials and Methods

Elective rotablation was performed by use of standard procedures and materials in ten patients with proven coronary heart disease. For anticoagulation, heparin and ASA were used. Blood samples were taken via the arterial sheath before, immediately after, and 30 min after finishing rotablation. Platelet antigens were analyzed by monoclonal antibodies (moab) CD41a, CD42b, CD62p, CD63, and anti-human anti-fibrinogen. After labeling, 10,000 signals were acquired on a cytometer within 4 h of blood collection.

Results

All patients showed significant platelet activation during and after the rotablation compared to baseline values before the intervention. Antigens CD41a and CD42b did not show significant alternations in fluorescence during rotablation (CD41a $P=0.2$; CD42b $P=0.4$). However, significant (*) platelet activation could be detected during and after rotablation measuring the mean channel fluorescence intensity (MCFI) of antigens CD62p, CD63, and fibrinogen binding ($P<0.05$). Thirty minutes after finishing the rotablation there were no further significant changes detectable (ns=**).

I. Scharrer/W. Schramm (Ed.)
30th Hemophilia Symposium Hamburg 1999
© Springer-Verlag Berlin Heidelberg 2001

Rotablation	CD62p	CD63	Fibrinogen
Before	27.1 (±6.2)	21.8 (±4.4)	100.4 (±13.2)
After	47.9 (±11.1)*	33.9 (±11.1)*	152.9 (±28.1)*
30 min after	49.8 (±11.8)**	23.2 (±8.8)**	146.1 (±38.2)**

Conclusion

Rotablation induces significant platelet activation. Flow cytometry is a sensitive and highly specific, multiparametric tool to detect these antigenic changes. The individual platelet activation process is part of a complex cascade of events happening in the rotablated coronary segment leading to complications in some patients. In the future, screening of patients to determine high thrombotic risk seems feasible, and thus the number of patients experiencing threatening complications may be decreased.

Flow Cytometric Comparison of Platelet Activation During PTCA, Stent Implantation, and Rotablation

J. BAU, C. BEYTHIEN, M. BROCKMANN, P. KÜHNL, K. GUTENSOHN

Introduction

Acute occlusion and subacute restenosis of the coronary artery are presently the limiting factors of otherwise successful techniques of interventional cardiology. Platelets and especially activated platelet populations play a key role concerning these typical and sometimes fatal complications. In this study, we used flow cytometry to compare the influences of PTCA, stenting, and rotablation on platelet antigens.

Material and Methods

Thirty patients were included in the study. We recruited 12 patients for the PTCA-only group, 8 for the stent group, and 10 for the rotablator group. To be included, the patients needed to have hemodynamically significant de novo stenosis (>75%). Samples were taken from patients before, directly after and thirty minutes after finishing the procedure directly from the arterial sheath, and an aliquot was immediately stabilized and fixed. Samples were labeled with saturating amounts of monoclonal antibodies against CD41a (GPII-IIIa), CD42b (GPIb-V-IX), CD62p (P-selectin, PADGEM, GMP), and CD63 (GP53). Furthermore, we analyzed the binding of fibrinogen to platelets. Samples were measured using a FACScan cytometer.

Results

CD41a and CD42b did not show significant alternations in mean channel fluorescence intensity (MCFI) directly after and 30 min after finishing PTCA, stenting, and rotablation compared to baseline levels before (PTCA: CD41a $P=0.8$ and 0.9; CD42b $P=0.5$ and 0.2. Stenting: CD41a $P=0.3$ and 0.2; CD42b $P=0.5$ and 0.7. Rotablation: CD41a $P=0.2$; CD42b $P=0.4$ and 0.1). However, platelet activation could be detected directly after PTCA, stenting, and rotablation when measuring the MCFI of CD62p, CD63, and fibrinogen binding (all $P<0.05$). There were again significant changes in MCFI in PTCA and stenting 30 min after finishing the procedures compared to directly after the procedures (CD62p, CD63, and fibrinogen binding, all $P<0.05$), but not in rotablation (CD62p $P=0.1$; CD63 $P=0.9$; fibrinogen binding

I. Scharrer/W. Schramm (Ed.)
30th Hemophilia Symposium Hamburg 1999
© Springer-Verlag Berlin Heidelberg 2001

$P=0.05$). The MCFI for CD62p and fibrinogen binding was highest in rotablation, while the MCFI for CD63 was highest in stenting.

Conclusions

The results of our study show that the three techniques induce significant platelet activation. Activation is higher in stenting than in PTCA, and higher in rotablation than in stenting. Platelet activation keeps rising after PTCA and stenting. On the contrary, platelet activation does not seem to increase after finishing rotablation. Flow cytometry is a specific, multiparametric method to establish platelet activation even in a small subpopulation.

Analysis of Hemostatic Capacity before and after Extracorporal Platelet-Pheresis by the PFA-100 Test System

A. ALISCH, K. GUTENSOHN, M.A. BROCKMANN, P. KÜHNL

Introduction

The PFA-100 test system (Dade Behring, Deerfield, USA) is an in vitro platelet function test which is based on the in vitro bleeding time by Kratzer and Born [1] and characterized by Kundu et al. [2, 3]. It determines the primary hemostasis capacity (PHC) of citrated whole blood expressed by the closure time and shows high sensitivity for platelet dysfunction [4]. The test system monitors the time of occlusion of a collagen-epinephrine- or collagen-ADP-coated membrane under high shear stress conditions. It is easy to handle, only 0.8 ml blood is necessary, and the results are available within 5 min.

During platelet-pheresis, the blood cells are removed from the circulation and exposed to nonphysiological and high shear stress conditions. Various changes occur, collectively referred to as platelet storage lesion [5]. These changes are reflected by alterations of platelet membrane glycoproteins and are dependent on the biomaterials, techniques, and devices applied.

In this study, the PFA-100 test system was used to evaluate the influence of platelet-pheresis on platelet function.

Materials and Methods

PFA-100 Test System

The system consists of an instrument and a disposable test cartridge where primary hemostasis is simulated [3]. In this device, a motor-driven syringe aspirates the blood sample under steady-flow conditions through a 150-μm aperture cut into a collagen-epinephrine- or collagen-ADP-coated membrane. The platelets adhere to the area around the aperture and form a plug (see Fig. 1). The time necessary for the occlusion of the aperture is the closure time (CT) which indicates the platelet function.

Plateletpheresis was performed on the Amicus cell separator (Baxter Healthcare Corp., Deerfield, USA) in 11 healthy and drug-free volunteer donors (5 female, mean age 28.6 years; 6 male, mean age 31.8 years). Blood samples were collected in 3.2% buffered citrate (S-Monovette, Sarstedt, Germany) via a sample connector from the inlet line immediately after starting the procedure and 5 min prior to the end of apheresis.

I. Scharrer/W. Schramm (Ed.)
30th Hemophilia Symposium Hamburg 1999
© Springer-Verlag Berlin Heidelberg 2001

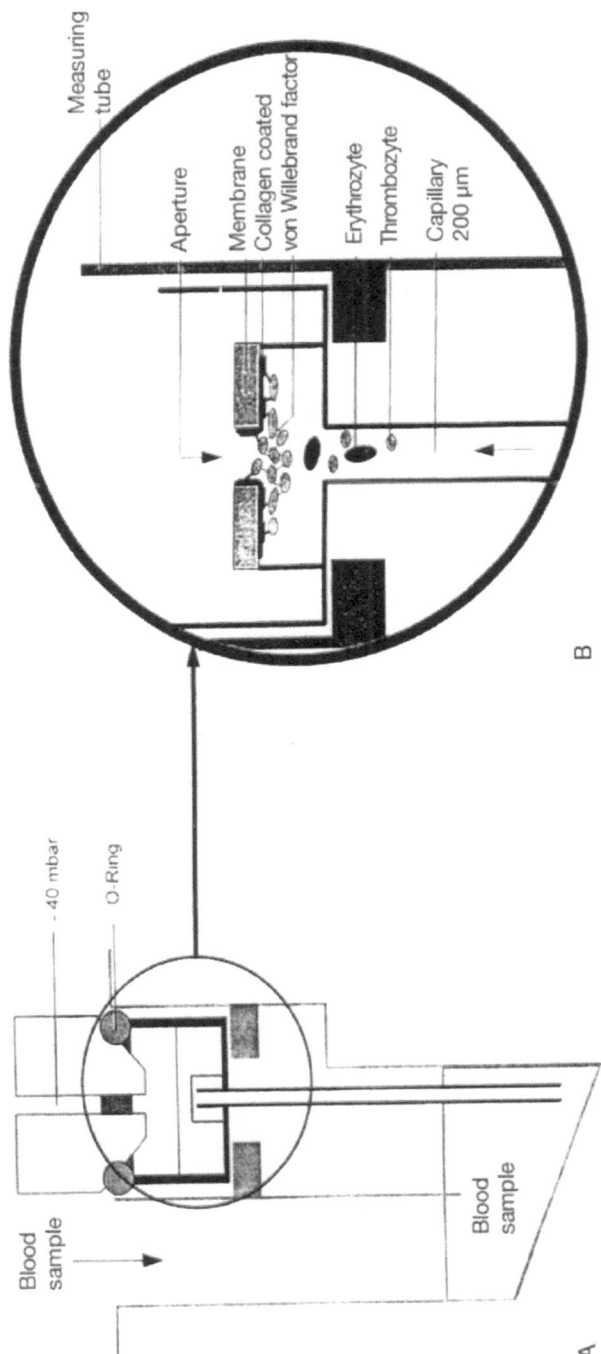

Fig. 1. Process of primary hemostasis in the PFA-100 device

For platelet function analysis, 0.8 ml of the buffered blood sample was used for the measurements, which were immediately performed on the PFA-100 system (software version 1.13) using a collagen-ADP-coated membrane. The measurements were done in duplicate and the results were averaged. Prior to measurements, a daily self-test was performed with the PFA-100 device.

Results

In this study, all 11 platelet-phereses were performed without complications and dropouts. All apheresis kits originated from one single lot (Baxter). The mean collection time was 62 min (range 47–90 min). The mean blood volume processed was 3015 ml (range 2537–3787 ml). The mean platelet count prior to apheresis was 249x10³/µl (range 194–297x10³/µl).

During platelet-pheresis with the Amicus cell separator, no significant changes in the platelet function could be detected by the PFA-100 test system. The platelet ability of forming aggregates showed no loss following the high shear stress conditions of apheresis. The mean closure time of the collagen-ADP-coated membrane at the beginning of platelet-pheresis was 83.7 s (range 67.5–110.0 s) (Fig. 2). It remained stable at 91.1 s (range 75.0–114.0 s) 5 min prior to the end of apheresis (P=0.075).

Discussion

For analysis of primary hemostasis, only a few test systems are available (e.g., aggregometry, bleeding time), often associated with low sensitivity and specificity. In this

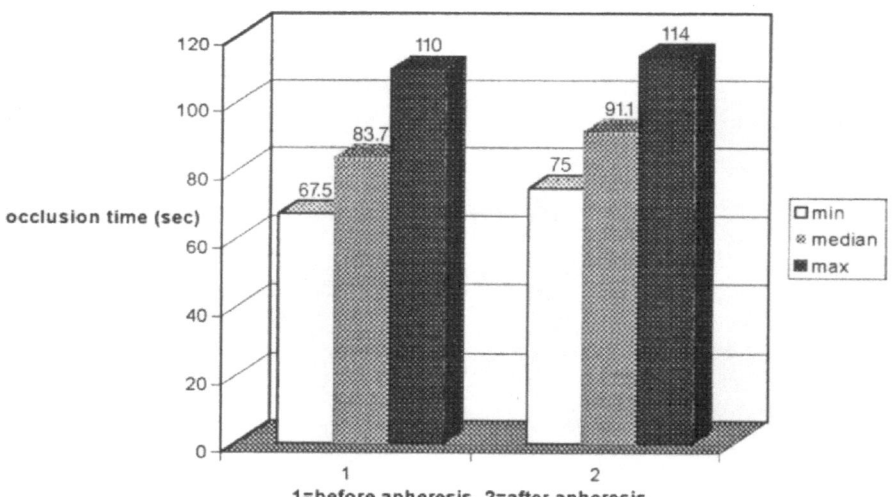

Fig. 2. Occlusion time

study, we applied the PFA-100 test system in platelet-pheresis donors. The test system reflects the hemostatic capacity by measuring the occlusion time of a tubing system coated with collagen-ADP.

We could demonstrate that in the donor population tested in this study, no influence of the hemostatic capacity could be detected by the PFA-100 analyzer. This is surprising, as the nonphysiological ex vivo surrounding interacts with the blood and blood cells. Several reports have shown that predominantly platelets and platelet function are influenced, probably caused by the artificial surfaces and shear forces. This could be shown for hemodialysis [6] and cardiopulmonary bypass [7].

Regarding the results of the study, one must consider that the number of donors was too low to draw a final conclusion. In addition, the possibility that the test system used in this study was not sensitive enough to measure minor changes in platelet function should be kept in mind.

However, we assume that extracorporal circulation does not significantly alter platelet function. Platelet-pheresis seems to be a safe procedure, and the hemostatic capacity of the donors does not seem to be compromised.

Conclusion

During plateletpheresis with the Amicus cell separator, no changes in occlusion time could be detected with the PFA-100. The hemostatic capacity of the donor platelets was not altered.

References

1. Kratzer MAA, et al. Haemostasis 1985; 15: 357–62
2. Kundu SK, et al. Semin Thromb Haemost 1995; 21: 106–12
3. Kundu SK, et al. Clin Appl Thromb Haemost 1996; 2: 241–9
4. Mammen EF, et al. Semin Thromb Haemost 1998; 24: 195–202
5. George JN, et al. Blood Cells 1992; 18: 501–11
6. Gawaz MP, et al. Clin Invest 1994; 72: 424–9
7. Rinder CS, et al. Anesthesiology; 75: 563–70

Heparin Coating of Coronary Stents Increases Time Until Stent Occlusion Due to Delayed Platelet Activation in an In Vitro Circulating Model

M.A. Brockmann, C. Beythien, M.M. Magens, J. Bau, K. Geidel, M. Weilandt, P. Kühnl, K. Gutensohn

Introduction

Acute and subacute reocclusion of stented coronary vessels are still a major risk factor after coronary stent implantation. Implanted stents have been discussed to be a major trigger for platelet activation. Coating of coronary stents has been found to improve clinical outcome after stent implantation due to decreased platelet activation. Therefore, in this study we monitored the time until stent occlusion (TSO) in an in vitro circulation model, filled with platelet-rich plasma (PRP) and containing uncoated or heparin coated stents (Hepamed, Medtronic, Germany). Furthermore, the extent of platelet activation within PRP during circulation in the in vitro model was measured using flow cytometry.

Methods

PRP from seven volunteers was standardized to a platelet count of $250 \times 10^3/\mu l$ and then filled into an in vitro model. Thereafter, recalcification was performed and circulation was started. Samples were drawn every 5 min until occlusion of the system and TSO (min) was measured. Platelet antigens were analyzed by flow cytometry (FACScan, Becton Dickinson, USA) using monoclonal antibodies (CD41a, CD42b, CD62p, CD63 (all Coulter-Immunotech, Germany) and anti-fibrinogen (Biopool, Sweden).

Results

In vitro circular systems containing no stents (control) occluded after 16 ± 5 min, systems with an uncoated stent occluded after 11 ± 2 min, and systems containing a heparin-coated stent after 19 ± 8 min. In vitro systems containing no stent (control) or a heparin-coated stent showed an increase of TSO, compared to systems containing an uncoated stent ($P=0.068$). Surface expression of CD62p, CD63, and anti-fibrinogen initially decreased, then increased until stent occlusion. Flow cytometric analysis showed that an early decrease in mean channel fluorescence intensity (MCFI) of activation-dependent epitopes was accompanied by a decreased TSO.

I. Scharrer/W. Schramm (Ed.)
30th Hemophilia Symposium Hamburg 1999
© Springer-Verlag Berlin Heidelberg 2001

Conclusion

We could demonstrate that heparin coating of coronary stents increases the time until occlusion of an in vitro system, compared to systems containing an uncoated stent. Therefrom, the risk of an acute or subacute reocclusion of stented coronary vessels might be reduced by the use of heparin-coated stents.

High-Speed Detection of Human Progenitor Cells (HPC) to Support the Timing of Aphereses

M. M. Magens, M. Brockmann, I. Carrero, B. Bernien, K. Warbende, P. Kuehnl, K. Gutensohn

Introduction

The transfusion of peripheral blood progenitor cells (PBPC), autologous or alloge-neic, is increasingly being performed to provide rapid hematopoietic recovery after myeloablative high-dose chemotherapy [4, 6]. The application of G-CSF stimulates the proliferation of bone marrow stem cells so that they can be collected from peripheral blood by leukapheresis [2].

To avoid unsuccessful leukapheresis procedures, different peripheral blood parameters have been tested for their ability to predict the outcome of the stem cell harvest. The daily monitoring of the PBPC-concentration as determined by flow cytometric analysis, has turned out to be the most reliable parameter to predict the success of a stem cell harvest [1, 3].

The purpose of this study was to evaluate the Immature-Myeloid-Information Channel (IMI) of the Sysmex SE-9000 (Sysmex, Norderstedt). It provides a new non-immunologic approach for the detection of PBPC that can be performed in 90 seconds. Therefore, aliquots of the same sample were analyzed flow-cytometrically in accordance with the ISHAGE guidelines [5] and with the SE-9000, and both con-centrations were correlated in linear regression analysis. Additionally, the preaphe-resis concentrations were tested for their predictive value by correlating them with the CD34+ content of the stem-cell product.

Material and Methods

Mobilization of PBPC was achieved by the application of 2x5 µg/kg bw G-CSF (gra-nulocyte colony stimulating factor). Analyses were performed in peripheral blood samples (n=71) obtained from 13 patients with hematological and oncological diseases. From the same sample, one aliquot was taken to be analyzed with the Sysmex SE-9000, and another one to be analyzed flow cytometrically in accordan-ce with the ISHAGE guidelines.

In its IMI-channel the Sysmex SE-9000 employs a lysis reagent to destroy matu-re white blood cells which are characterized by a higher membrane-lipid concen-tration than immature white blood cells. The remaining cells are analyzed by elec-tric means and displayed in a scattergram indicating the cellular volume on the abs-cissa and the plasma-to-nucleus ratio on the ordinate. Of all the immature cells in

I. Scharrer/W. Schramm (Ed.)
30th Hemophilia Symposium Hamburg 1999
© Springer-Verlag Berlin Heidelberg 2001

the scattergram, small cells with a low plasma-to-nucleus ratio are enclosed by a predefined gate and counted as HPC (human progenitor cells).

For comparison of HPC-data, CD34$^+$ measurements were performed in accordance with the ISHAGE guidelines. Briefly, 100 µL of the same sample were incubated with CD34-PE and CD45-FITC antibodies for 15 minutes. Hereafter, red blood cells were lysed (Orthe Mune Lysing Reagent, Ortho, Neckargemünd). Before flow cytometric measurement, cells were washed twice and resuspended in 1 mL of phosphate buffered saline (Dulbecco´s PBS, Life Technology, Scotland). For data acquisition and analysis a FacsCalibur Cytometer from Becton Dickinson (San Jose, USA) with standard 488-nm laser excitation and CellQUEST-Software (BD) were applied.

Results

The correlation between peripheral blood concentrations of HPC and CD34$^+$-cells was r=0.34 (Fig. 1). In 11 out of 13 patients a peripheral blood HPC of ≤20/µL was accompanied by a flow cytometric CD34$^+$ concentration that was also below 20/µL. However, HPC values ±20/µL only showed a correlation of r=0.23 with flow cytometry.

Additionally, the quality of the respective PBPC-products (n=28) was measured by flow-cytometric determination of CD34$^+$-cells per kilogram bodyweight. The PBPC content of the product was correlated with the preapheresis CD34$^+$- and the preapheresis HPC concentration in peripheral blood (Fig. 2). The coefficient of correlation between the preapheresis concentration of the HPC cells and the CD34$^+$ content in the leukapheresis product was r=0.17, whereas the correlation of the preapheresis CD34$^+$ concentration and the CD34$^+$ yield was r=0.96.

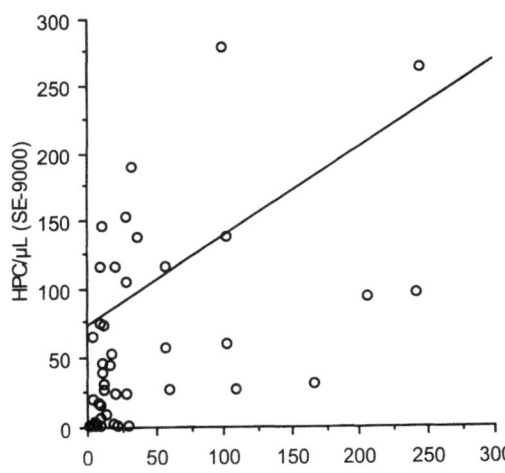

Fig. 1. Regression plot. PBPC in
peripheral blood during mobilization

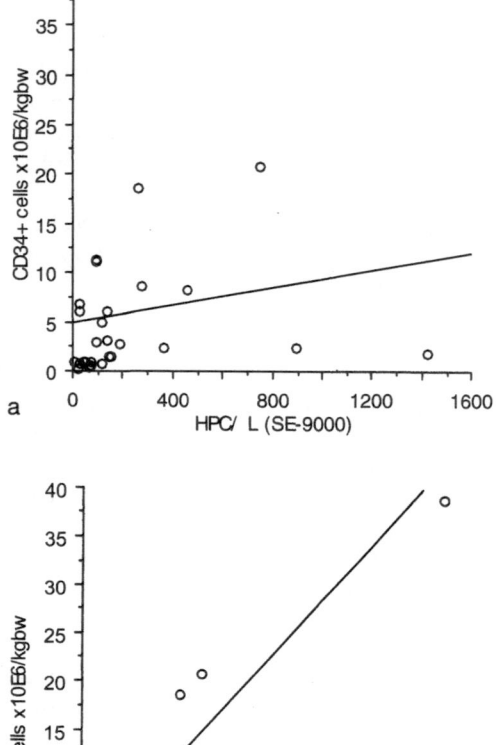

Fig. 2a,b. a Regression plot: prea-pheresis HPC in peripheral blood and CD34+-cells in the stem-cell product r=0.17
b Regression plot: preapheresis CD34+ in peripheral blood and CD34+-cells in the stem-cell pro-duct r=0.96

Discussion

The best parameter available to predict the success of a PBPC leukapheresis is the concentration of CD34-positive cells in peripheral blood as determined by flow cytometric means, as our data confirm [7, 8]. The IMI-channel measures HPC a lot faster and cheaper, but not to the same extent of accuracy. Therefore, it cannot replace the immunologic analysis.

If one considered the data of every patient separately, the concentration of peri-pheral blood HPC would correlate rather well with the CD34+ concentration in peri-pheral blood. However, the absolute HPC results obtained from different patients cannot be compared. For example, in one patient an HPC-concentration of 97/µL coincided with a $CD34^+$ concentration of 242/µL guaranteeing a very successful PBPC harvest, whereas in another patient an HPC of 116/µL corresponded with a $CD34^+$ of 10/µL resulting in a poor apheresis success.

The PBPC-cells of different patients seem to have individual properties which prevent comparable HPC results. The PBPC of different patients could be characterized by a varying sensitiveness to the lysing reagent used in the IMI-channel. Also, PBPC cells of one patient could be of a different size than those of another patient. The individual size of the cells of different patients cannot be accounted for by the application of a fixed gate to define HPC. It therefore bears the risk of either excluding PBPC from the HPC gate, or including immature cells which are not PBPC.

Conclusions

We conclude that the non-immunologic HPC analysis can be used as an additional parameter to monitor the onset of a PBPC apheresis. The method represents a fast, easy-to-perform and - regarding the single analysis - cheap approach to determine PBPC concentrations in peripheral blood. However, due to the little interindividual comparability of the HPC concentrations of different patients, the SE-9000 can only be helpful in timing the flow-cytometric measurement of $CD34^+$-cells, but not in timing the apheresis procedure. Flow cytometric analyses can be postponed until the HPC reaches 20 cells/µL.

References

1. Armitage S, Hargreaves R, Samson D, et al. (1997) CD34 counts to predict collection of adequate peripheral blood progenitor cells. Bone Marrow Transplant 20: 587-591
2. Brice P, Divine M, Marolleau JP, et al. (1994) Comparison of autografting using mobilized peripheral blood stem cells with and without granulocyte colony-stimulating factor in malignant lymphomas. Bone Marrow Transplant 14: 51-55
3. Fontao-Wendel R, Lazar A, Melges S, et al. (1999) The absolute number of circulating CD34+ cells as the best predictor of peripheral hematopoietic stem cell yield. J Hematother 8: 255-262
4. Gratwohl A, Hermans J (1994) Bone marrow transplantation activity in Europe 1992: Report from the European group for bone marrow transplantation. Bone Marrow Transplant 13: 5-10
5. Sutherland D, Anderson L, Keeney M, et al. (1996) The ISHAGE guidelines for CD34+ cell determination by flow cytometry. J Hematother 5: 213-226
6. Williams S, Zimmermann T, Grad G, Mick R (1993) Source of stem cell rescue: Bone marrow versus peripheral blood progenitors. J Hematother 2: 521-523
7. Yu L, Leisenring W, Bensinger W, et al. (1999) The predictive value of white cell or CD34+ cell count in the peripheral blood for timing apheresis and maximizing yield. Transfusion 39: 442-450
8. Zimmermann T, Lee W, Bender J, et al. (1995) Quantitative CD34 analysis may be used to guide peripheral blood stem cell harvests. Bone Marrow Transplant 9: 439-444

Semi-Automated Flow Cytometry Can Help in Timing the Onset of a Stem-Cell Leukapheresis

M. M. Magens, M. Brockmann, I. Carrero, M. Weiland, S. Schlichting, P. Kuehnl, K. Gutensohn

Introduction

To reconstitute hematopoiesis after myeloablative chemotherapy the transplantation of autologous or allogeneic peripheral blood progenitor cells (PBPC) is increasingly performed [6, 10]. Following G-CSF mobilization PBPC can be collected from peripheral blood by leukapheresis [3].

To monitor the onset of the PBPC-harvest and to determine the product quality following stem cell collection, flow cytometric analysis of CD34-positive cells is performed [1, 5]. The flow cytometric assays to quantify PBPC have been characterized by widely divergent data [2, 4]. The desire to standardize the analysis procedure has led to the development of the ISHAGE guidelines (International Society for Hematotherapy and Graft Engineering) for CD34+-cell determination published in 1996 [8]. Recently, new kits for direct quantification have been introduced.

The purpose of this study was to evaluate the latest version of a semi-automated method with associated software for flow cytometric measurement of CD34-positive cells (ProCOUNT™, Becton Dickinson).

Material and Methods

Mobilization of PBPC was achieved by the application of 2x5 µg/kgbw G-CSF (granulocyte colony stimulating factor). Analyses were performed in peripheral blood samples (n=59) and leukapheresis products (n=25), obtained from 10 patients with hematological and oncological diseases.

From the same sample, one aliquot was taken to be analyzed following the ISHAGE guidelines, and another one to be analyzed with ProCOUNT™ (PC). All measurements were performed using a FacsCalibur Cytometer from Becton Dickinson (BD, San Jose, USA) with standard 488-nm laser excitation.

For analysis, aliquots were pipetted into ready-to-use tubes (TruCOUNT™) containing a known number of beads employed to calculate the absolute concentration of PBPC/µL. The samples were incubated with antibodies (CD34, CD45) and a nucleic acid dye for 15 minutes after which a 30-minute lyse-no-wash procedure was performed. For data acquisition and analysis, PC software (version 2.0a1; 1998) was applied. The software uses valley-seeking algorithms for gating and defining cell populations. Additionally, it tests the results for reasonability and otherwise produces a warning.

I. Scharrer/W. Schramm (Ed.)
30th Hemophilia Symposium Hamburg 1999
© Springer-Verlag Berlin Heidelberg 2001

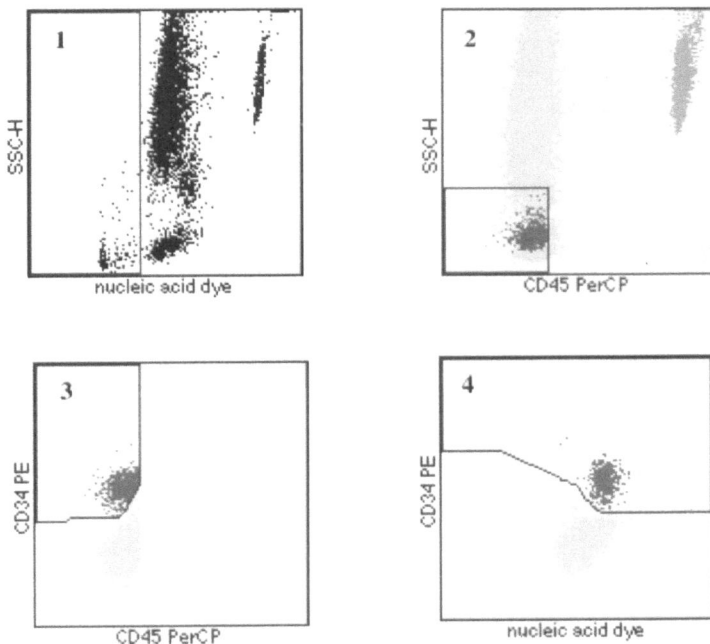

Fig. 1. Apheresis product: Four dot plots from a PC analysis. The software utilizes valley-seeking algorithms to separate different cell populations and to generate the gates. First at all, platelets, reticulocytes, and debris are referred to as events with a small uptake of nucleic acid dye and are therefore excluded (plot 1). In plot 3 and 4 the algorithm defines the CD34+ population. Next, these cells are shown and gated in plot 2. The *upper right part* of plots 1 and 2 shows the beads

For comparison of PC data, CD34+ measurements were performed in accordance with the ISHAGE guidelines. Briefly, 100 µL of the same sample were incubated with CD34-PE and CD45-FITC antibodies for 15 minutes. Hereafter, red blood cells were lysed (Orthe Mune Lysing Reagent, Ortho, Neckargemünd). Before flow cytometric measurement, cells were washed twice and resuspended in 1 mL of phosphate buffered saline (Dulbecco´s PBS, Life Technology, Scotland). For data acquisition and analysis CellQUEST-Software (BD) was applied.

Results

During monitoring of CD34-positive cells in peripheral blood, the correlation of CD34+ cells measured by ProCOUNT and the ISHAGE-protocol was r=0.993. However, in 9 out of 59 analyzed samples (15.3%) the PC-software generated a warning recommending manual reanalysis. Following manual gating, the correlation was improved to r=0.994.

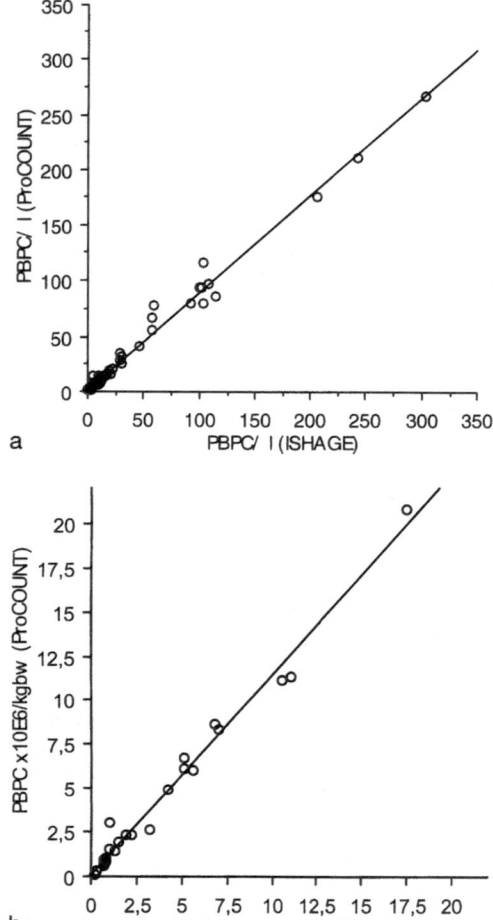

Fig. 2a,b. a CD34+ cells in peripheral blood during mobilization ($y=0.9x+1.9$; $r=0.994$). **b** CD34+ cells as 10^6 per kilogram body weight in apheresis products ($y=0.9x-0.62$; $r=0.995$)

For PBPC-apheresis products, the correlation of PC and the ISHAGE protocol was calculated to have been r=0.991. A manual reanalysis was necessary in 10 of 25 samples (40%), and hereby the correlation was improved to r=0.995.

Discussion

Flow cytometric determination of CD34-positive cells is the best way to evaluate the quality of leukapheresis products, since neither morphologic parameters nor colony-assays allow an as fast and accurate measurement of the PBPC content of the product [2, 7]. In addition, the CD34+ analysis is also applicable with peripheral blood samples to monitor the onset of PBPC apheresis [11, 12].

The flow-cytometric measurement of PBPC as suggested by the ISHAGE requires many steps including the programming of an acquisition templet before starting for the first time. PC simplifies many of these steps. The software needs only to be installed and is then ready for use. For acquisition and analysis, it tells the operator step by step what to do next and finally calculates the concentration of PBPC or the CD34+ content of a leukapheresis product [9]. Nevertheless, a careful study of the accompanying handbook is essential. In comparison to the previous PC version, the manual reanalysis has become a lot faster and easier. Compared to the ISHAGE protocol, the overall analysis time using PC is longer but gives the operator more walkaway time while providing almost the same accuracy, as our data show.

Conclusion

We conclude that the kit and semi-automated software for CD34-cell data acquisition and analysis are applicable for CD34+ measurement during monitoring and for evaluation of PBPC products. Despite the fact that only a small improvement was achieved by manual reanalysis, reviewing the plots and analysis by experienced staff is recommendable.

References

1. Armitage S, Hargreaves R, Samson D, et al. (1997) CD34 counts to predict collection of adequate peripheral blood progenitor cells. Bone Marrow Transplant 20: 587-591
2. Bender J, Lum L, Unverzagt K, et al. (1994) Correlation of colony-forming cells, long-term culture initiating cells and CD34+ cells in apheresis products from patients mobilized for peripheral blood progenitors with different regimens. Bone Marrow Transplant 13: 479-485
3. Brice P, Divine M, Marolleau JP, et al. (1994) Comparison of autografting using mobilized peripheral blood stem cells with and without G-CSF in malignant lymphomas. Bone Marrow Transplant 14: 51-55
4. Chang A, Ma DD (1996) The influence of flow cytometric gating strategy on the standardization of CD34+ cell quantitation: An Australian multicenter study. Australasian BMT Scientists Study Group. J Hematother 5: 605-616
5. Fontao-Wendel R, Lazar A, Melges S, et al. (1999) The absolute number of circulating CD34+ cells as the best predictor of peripheral hematopoietic stem cell yield. J Hematother 8: 255-262
6. Gratwohl A, Hermans J (1994) Bone marrow transplantation activity in Europe 1992: Report from the European group for bone marrow transplantation. Bone Marrow Transplant 13: 5-10
7. Serke S, Säuberlich S, Huhn D (1991) Multiparameter flow-cytometrical quantitation of circulating CD34+ cells: correlation to the quantitation of circulating haemopoietic progenitor cells by in vitro colony-assay. Br J Haematol 77: 453-9
8. Sutherland D, Anderson L, Keeney M, et al. (1996) The ISHAGE guidelines for CD34+ cell determination by flow cytometry. J Hematother 5: 213-226
9. Ward T, Grenier K, Knape C, et al. (1997) ProCOUNT™. Setting the standard for progenitor cell enumeration. San Jose, CA: Becton Dickinson Immunocytometry Systems
10. Williams S, Zimmermann T, Grad G, Mick R (1993) Source of stem cell rescue: Bone marrow versus peripheral blood progenitors. J Hematother 2: 521-3

11. Yu L, Leisenring W, Bensinger W, et al. (1999) The predictive value of white cell or CD34+ cell count in the peripheral blood for timing apheresis and maximizing yield. Transfusion 39: 442-450
12. Zimmermann T, Lee W, Bender J, et al. (1995) Quantitative CD34 analysis may be used to guide peripheral blood stem cell harvests. Bone Marrow Transplant 9: 439-444

IX.g   Poster: Diagnostic Problems

Current Topics of Official Batch Release: Determination of FXIII Activity in Fibrin Glues and FXIII Concentrates and Measurement of Heparin/AT Complexes in FVIII Products

N. Beer, A. Corda, A. Hunfeld, G. Jagarzewski, R. Seitz

Determination of FXIII Activity in Fibrin Glues and FXIII Concentrates

Background

In the scope of the official batch release of blood products, FXIII potency has to be determined in FXIII concentrates and fibrin glues. A clot lysis assay for the determination of FXIII is described in the monograph for fibrin glues. This assay is based on the different solubility of cross-linked and non-cross-linked fibrin in chloroacetic acid. However, due to the semiquantitative characteristic this method is not suitable for the determination of FXIII potency.

Therefore, we recently changed the assay system. At present, FXIII activity is estimated using a commercially available test kit (Berichrom FXIII; Behringwerke AG, Marburg, Germany), which is a coupled optical assay with the decrease of NADH as indicating reaction. This method, which is intended to determine the activity of FXIII in plasma samples, certainly renders a quantitative estimation, but cannot be transferred to concentrate samples without modifications because of different matrix conditions. Here, we present our first experience when establishing the assay for the determination of FXIII potency in fibrin glues and FXIII concentrates.

Method

Experiments were performed according to the manufacturer's instructions with slight modifications:
1. the assay was adapted for microplates;
2. the reaction time was prolonged to 1 h.
The principle of the method is shown in Figure 1.

Results

The kinetics of the FXIII activity in plasma, fibrin glue, and FXIII concentrate are different (Fig. 2). The time for reaching the linear range of the reaction and the maximum reaction velocity (V_{max}) is clearly delayed in the fibrin glue and con-

I. Scharrer/W. Schramm (Ed.)
30th Hemophilia Symposium Hamburg 1999
© Springer-Verlag Berlin Heidelberg 2001

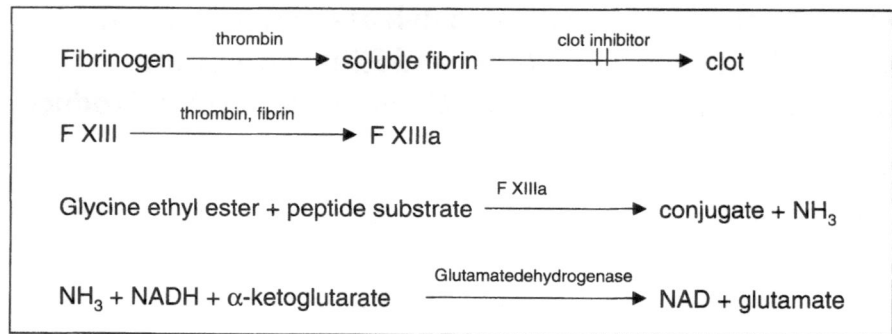

Fig. 1. Principle of the method

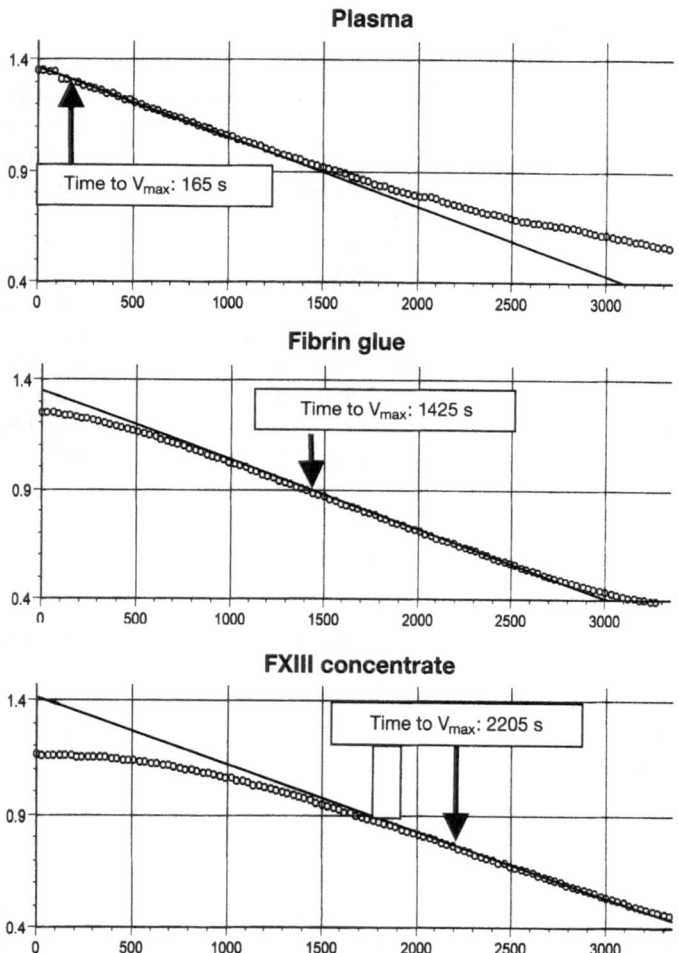

Fig. 2. Kinetic of FXIII activity in plasma, fibrin glue, and FXIII concentrate

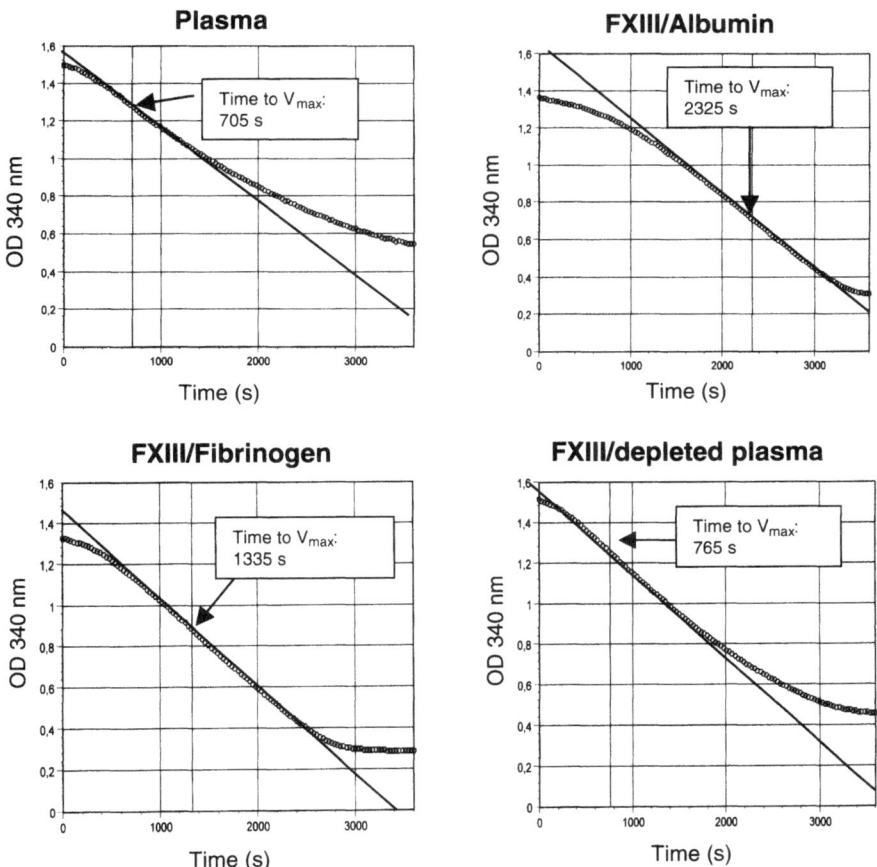

Fig. 3. Kinetic measurement of FXIII in normal plasma and in concentrates after addition to albumin, fibrinogen, or FXIII-deficient plasma

centrate when compared to the plasma sample. This observation is particularly evident in the concentrate sample with more than 30 min elapsed time until reaching V_{max}. An evaluation according to the manufacturer's instructions (period for evaluation: 5–10 min after start of the reaction) would therefore consequently lead to false low values. It is well known that activation of FXIII to FXIIIa by thrombin is accelerated in the presence of fibrin. The strong prolongation of the activation phase of the concentrate sample, which does not contain any fibrinogen in contrast to plasma or fibrin glue, is therefore not surprising.

Dilution of the FXIII concentrate with a solution containing fibrinogen (2.5 mg/ml) instead of albumin (1%) consequently leads to a shortening of the activation period (from about 40 min to approximately 20 min). However, the reaction is still delayed when compared to plasma (Fig. 3). Only when the concentrate is diluted with FXIII-deficient plasma (kindly provided by Centeon Pharma GmbH)

Table 1. Recovery of FXIII after substitution of depleted plasma with FXIII concentrate

Sample	Theoretical	Estimated
Normal plasma	100%	108%
50% plasma + 50% FXIII concentrate	100%	103%

Table 2. Theroretical and estimated FXIII content of several standard plasmas

Sample	Theoretical	Estimated
Normal control plasma	110%	123%
Pathological control plasma	33%	45%
Pooled plasma of 10 donors	100%	140%

is the activation process similar to the kinetic of FXIII activation in normal human plasma.

Nevertheless, the slope in the linear range of the reaction is nearly identical in all of the different reaction mixtures. Therefore, the evaluation reveals similar FXIII concentrations if the period for the estimation of V_{max} is set at 1 h (0.91 U/ml in the presence of albumin, 1.03 U/ml in the presence of fibrinogen, 1.01 U/ml in FXIII-deficient plasma).

The accuracy of the results was proved by an experiment in which normal plasma was first diluted twofold with saline and then substituted by addition of FXIII concentrate. The amount of concentrate added to the diluted plasma to give a final FXIII content of 100% was calculated based on the estimations shown above (1 U/ml; Table 1).

A general problem of the FXIII determination regarding batch release is the lack of a common standard. Table 2 shows the stated FXIII content of several standard plasmas with a defined FXIII activity compared to apparent values, which were estimated using a standard curve of plasma with a FXIII activity of 90%. It is evident that the result of the estimation is considerably dependent on the selection of the standard material.

Conclusion

A quantitative determination of FXIII activity in concentrates using the Berichrom FXIII test kit can be achieved by slight modifications of the assay.

The establishment of a common standard for FXIII is an urgent necessity with regard to official batch release.

Measurement of Heparin in Complex with AT

Background

Heparin is widely used for the production of blood products, either applied as excipient in order to prevent the product from generation of activated clotting factors together with AT or coupled as ligand to a matrix for an affinity chromatography step. Hence, many blood products contain AT and heparin in varying concentrations.

An often-used method to determine AT activity is the chromogenic measurement of the inhibition of FXa. This assay is usually performed in the presence of an excess of heparin, since heparin strongly accelerates the formation of the inactive complex between FXa and AT without interfering with the FXa activity by itself.

Another situation arises when estimating heparin in samples, which additionally contain AT, because on the one hand heparin is only active in complex with AT, and on the other hand AT alone is able to inhibit FXa. Therefore, an exact determination of heparin requires that the interference of AT is taken into consideration.

We describe an assay, which was developed for the determination of heparin in FVIII concentrates in consideration of the above-mentioned problem.

Method

The heparin determination consists of two independent assays. First, the AT content of the FVIII concentrate is determined using a chromogenic anti-FXa assay. Based on this estimation the concentrate is then diluted to give an AT concentration of 50 mIU/ml. 50 μl of the dilution are incubated with 100 μl Tris-buffered FXa solution in a microplate well for 10 min before the reaction is started by addition of 50 μl chromogenic substrate (S2765) solution. The heparin concentration of the sample can be calculated using a heparin standard curve, which of course has to be prepared in the presence of the same AT concentration (12.5 mIU/ml final test concentration).

Results

In order to define the linear range, FXa activity was estimated in the presence of 12.5 mIU AT/ml and heparin in the range of 0.5–20 mU/ml (final test concentration). Linearity was observed for concentrations up to 2.5 mU heparin/ml, whereas higher concentrations of heparin led to a flattening of the curve (Fig. 4).

Figure 5 shows the mean results and standard deviations of six independent assays, and demonstrates the good reproducibility of the test. The intra-assay CV in the linear range is usually below 3%. The detection limit amounts to about 0.3 mU heparin/ml (final test concentration); the limit of determination is in the range of 1 mU/ml.

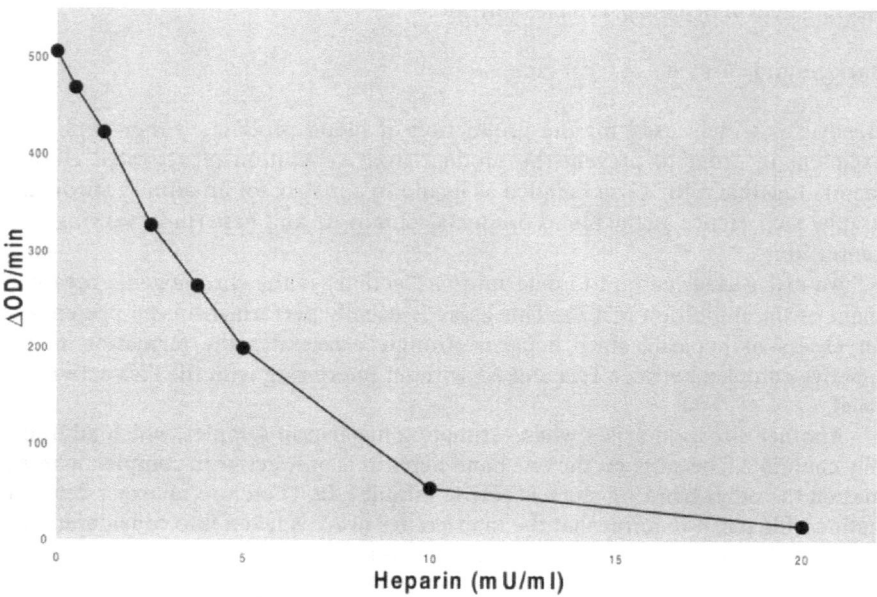

Fig. 4. Estimation of FXa activity in the presence of 12.5 mIU AT/ml and heparin in the range of 0.5–20 mU/ml (final test concentration)

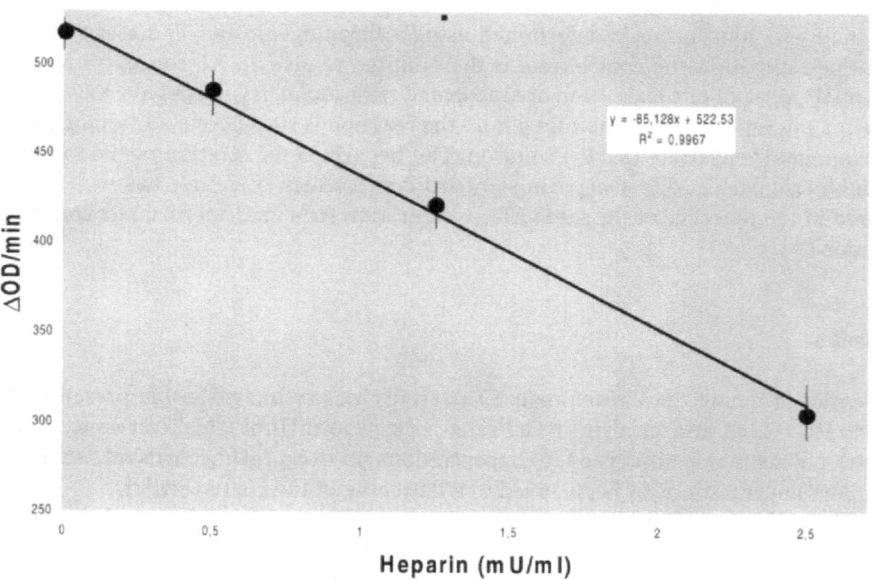

Fig. 5. Mean results and standard deviations of six independent assays demonstrating the good reproducibility of the test

Discussion

This assay was developed in order to detect heparin, which was added during the production of a certain FVIII preparation, in the finished product. This specific FVIII product has an average AT content of 0.55 ± 0.09 IU/ml ($n=7$ batches) and contains 21 ± 8 mIU heparin/ml. Taking into consideration that the preparation had to be diluted due to the AT content, this result lies below the determination limit which amounts to 40 mIU/ml for the reconstituted product, but is clearly above the detection limit of 13 mIU/ml.

In general, the assay described here can be applied to other preparations, too. However, a suitable ratio between the concentrations of AT and heparin is a prerequisite for the suitability of the test. For instance, if the AT content exceeds a certain limit, a determination of heparin becomes impossible because the required dilution of the samples leads to a heparin concentration below the detection limit. In such a case, a variation of the AT test concentration could solve the problem.

Thus, the suitability of the assay must be considered case by case and, if the test is possible at all, it may require further adaptation to certain conditions.

Comparison of BVDV and SFV Used as Models for Hepatitis C Virus in Virus Validation Studies

H. Seitz, J. Blümel, H. Scheiblauer, A. Scheidler, I. Schmidt, J. Löwer, H. Willkommen

Introduction

It has been shown that plasma-derived products transmitted viruses in the past, even when the starting material was controlled for viral contamination in accordance with the state-of-the-art procedure [1]. This indicates that donor selection and control of source material is insufficient to ensure the viral safety of plasma-derived products. The manufacturing process itself plays a central role in making the products as safe as possible.

In order to guarantee a high level of product safety, manufacturing processes for plasma derivatives have, therefore, to be highly effective in inactivating and/or removing viruses. The capacity of the process for each individual product has to be investigated in order to show inactivation and/or removal of a broad range of viruses [2]. Virus validation studies are designed to test this capacity under conditions comparable to the manufacturing process using appropriate in vitro virus assays.

For hepatitis C virus (HCV), which is of much concern regarding the safety of plasma derivatives, no efficient in vitro infection system is available at present. Consequently, virus validation studies have to be carried out with appropriate model viruses to demonstrate the virus safety with respect to HCV. Bovine viral diarrhea virus (BVDV) is preferentially used as a model virus, but togaviruses, such as Semliki Forest virus (SFV), are also discussed to be appropriate because high physiochemical similarities to HCV have been postulated [3, 4].

The objective of this study was to compare the model viruses for HCV, BVDV, and SFV. A virus partitioning step, e.g., Cohn-Oncley ethanol fractionation (precipitation and removal of paste III), and the inactivation kinetics of BVDV and SFV by solvent/detergent and heat treatment were analyzed.

Material and Methods

Virus and Cells

BVDV obtained from G. Pauli (Robert-Koch-Institute, Berlin) was propagated and titrated on MDBK cells (ATCC CCL-22). SFV was provided by J. Thiel (Institute of Virology, Giessen) and cultivated on Vero cells (ATCC CCL-81). Cells were grown in DMEM supplemented by 10% fetal calf serum (FCS). Virus stocks for spiking experiments were obtained from supernatant of cells cultivated in DMEM containing 1% FCS.

I. Scharrer/W. Schramm (Ed.)
30th Hemophilia Symposium Hamburg 1999
© Springer-Verlag Berlin Heidelberg 2001

Virus Titration

Virus titers were quantified by estimation of the tissue culture infectious dose (TCID$_{50}$). Serial threefold sample dilutions were prepared in DMEM and eight replicates per dilution were tested on 96-well microtiter plates. Cytopathic effects of SFV and BVDV were checked on days 3–5. Infectivity (TCID$_{50}$) was calculated according to the maximum likelihood method.

Cohn-Oncley Fractionation

Cohn-Oncley fractionation of resolved precipitate II/III into supernatant and precipitate III has been described in detail by Scheiblauer et al. [5]. Briefly, the resolved precipitate II/III W was spiked 1/10 with BVDV or SFV and adjusted to pH 5.4. After adding ethanol (final concentration: 17%) the solution was stirred at –5°C for 2 h. Separation into supernatant III and precipitate III was performed by centrifugation (10,000xg, 15 min, –5°C). All samples (sample before separation, precipitate and supernatant III) were immediately drawn and titrated as described above.

Solvent/Detergent Treatment

A 5% albumin solution was mixed with 0.3% tri-n-butyl phosphate (TNBP) and 1% polysorbate 80 of bovine or plant origin. 225 ml was spiked with 25 ml of each virus (BVDV or SFV) and incubated at 27°C for at least 1 h. Samples drawn at various times were immediately diluted 1/100 with DMEM and titrated as described above. Solvent/detergent treatment was reevaluated at 16°C and 6°C. Additionally, inactivation of BVDV and SFV was studied using various solvent/detergent concentrations (75%, 50%, 25% of the 0.3% TNBP and 1% polysorbate 80 solution).

Pasteurization

A 5% IgG solution buffered with 2 g/l NaCl and 150 g/l glycine was supplemented without and with saccharose (588 g/l, 1000 g/l, or 1500 g/l). Each mixed solution (225 ml) was spiked with 25 ml of BVDV or SFV. Afterwards, spiked material was treated at 60°C for 10 h. Samples were drawn at different times and titrated as described above.

Results

The Cohn-Oncley fractionation step was investigated under standard conditions, the inactivation procedures (solvent/detergent and heat treatment) were studied at various process conditions in order to consider the influence of critical process parameters.

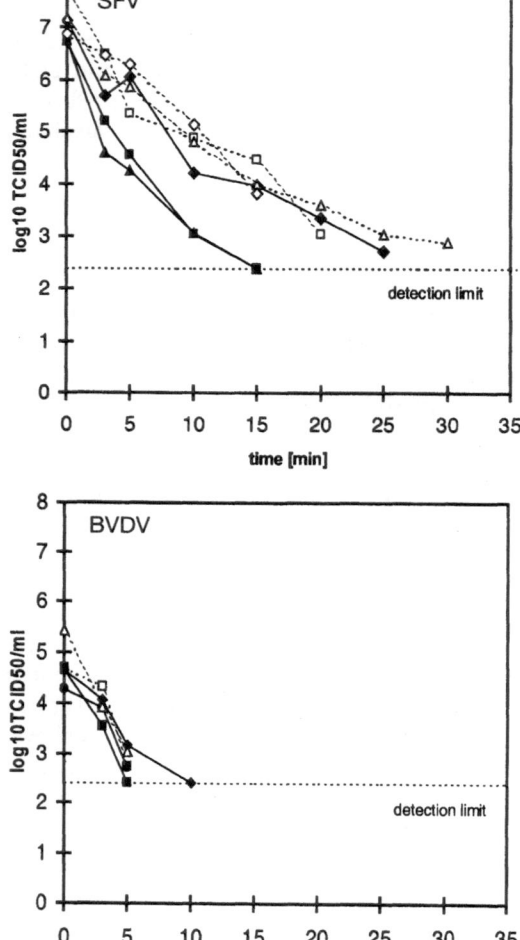

Fig. 1. Inactivation kinetics of SFV and BVDV using 0.3% (v/v) TNBP, 1% (v/v) polysorbate 80. Parallel runs are expressed by several symbols (■, ▲, ◆). *Open symbols* indicate inactivation kinetics using polysorbate 80 of plant origin, while *closed symbols* indicate kinetics dependent on using bovine polysorbate 80

Solvent/Detergent Treatment

Temperature, origin of S/D (plant or animal derived), and S/D concentration were varied and the influence of these parameters on the inactivation kinetics investigated. Both, SFV and BVDV were effectively inactivated below the limit of detection when 0.3% TNBP and 1% polysorbate 80 were used. However, inactivation of SFV was delayed in comparison to BVDV under these conditions (Fig. 1).

Process variations (lower temperature, solvent/detergent concentration reduced to 50%) had only a minor effect on inactivation of BVDV, but the inactivation of SFV was significantly impaired at lower temperatures and lower solvent/

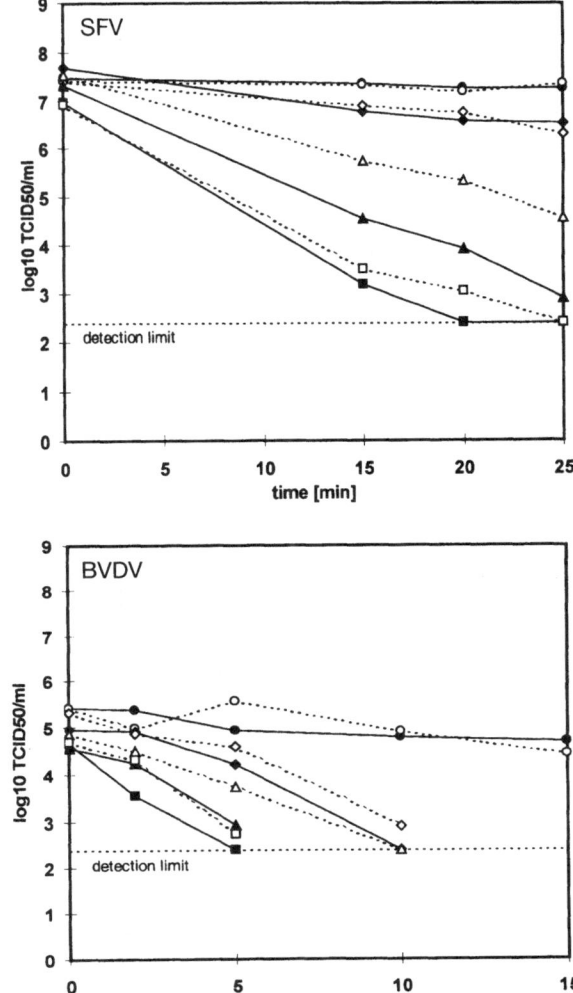

Fig. 2. The influence of various solvent/detergent concentrations on the inactivation kinetics of SFV and BVDV was investigated. Studies were performed with: ■, 100% (0.3% TNBP, 1% polysorbate 80); ▲, 75% (0.23% TNBP, 0.75% polysorbate 80); ◆, 50% (0.15% TNBP, 0.5% polysorbate 80); ●, 25% (0.08% TNBP, 0.25% polysorbate 80). *Open symbols* indicate kinetics using plant polysorbate 80, *closed symbols* indicate kinetics dependent on using bovine polysorbate 80

detergent concentrations (Figs. 2, 3). The origin of solvent/detergent (bovine or plant) did not affect the inactivation kinetics of both viruses at any variations.

Incomplete inactivation of SFV was observed in some samples after 6 h if the S/D treatment was performed at 16 and 6°C, and higher sample volumes were tested. BVDV, however, was completely inactivated within 5 min (Table 1).

Pasteurization

Pasteurization was investigated with both viruses and the stabilizer concentration (saccharose) varied in these experiments (Fig. 4). It was demonstrated that BVDV

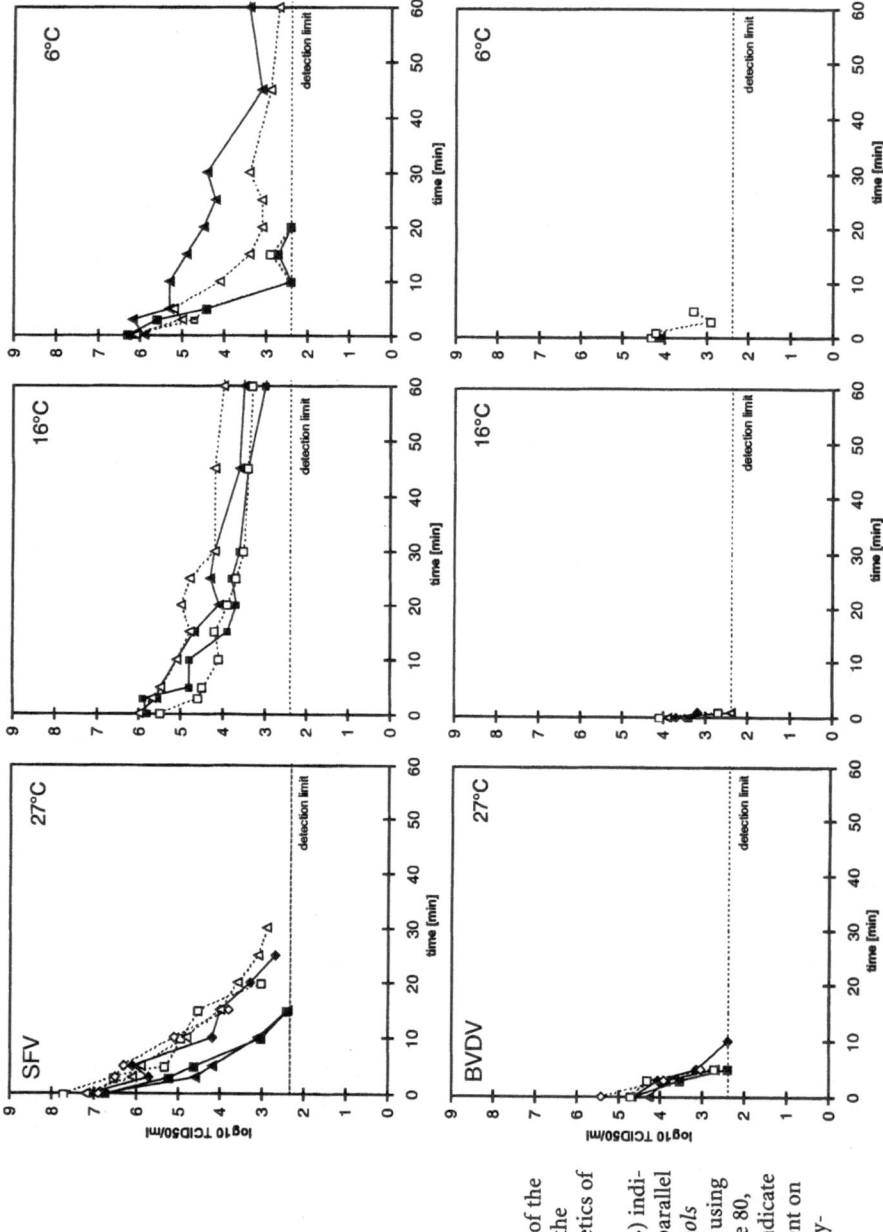

Fig. 3. Influence of the temperature on the inactivation kinetics of SFV and BVDV. Symbols (■, ▲, ◆) indicate kinetics of parallel runs. *Open symbols* indicate kinetics using plant polysorbate 80, *closed symbols* indicate kinetics dependent on using bovine polysorbate 80

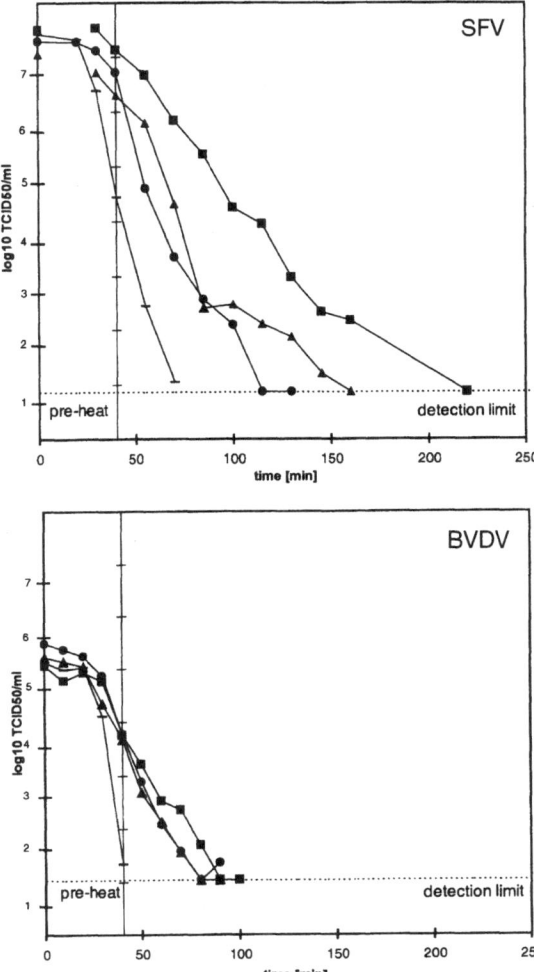

Fig. 4. Inactivation of SFV and BVDV was studied during pasteurization at 60°C. The influence of saccharose on the inactivation kinetics was determined. Studies were performed with (■) 1500 g/l, (▲) 1000 g/l, and (●) 588 g/l saccharose and without the addition of saccharose

and SFV were effectively inactivated below the detection limit. However, BVDV was inactivated faster than SFV and BVDV inactivation was not markedly affected if the saccharose concentrations varied between 588 and 1500 g/l. In contrast, inactivation of SFV was markedly delayed at increased saccharose concentrations.

Cohn-Oncley Fractionation

BVDV and SFV were distributed differently into supernatant and paste III during the Cohn-Oncley ethanol fractionation of re-solubilized precipitate II/III W (Fig. 5). While SFV was highly removed from supernatant III, the BVDV content was not markedly reduced in supernatant III.

Table 1. Titration of higher sample volumes

	S/D origin	Temperature	Time	Pos. flask	Cytotoxicity
SFV virus	Bovine	16°C	5 h	2/5	Negative
		16°C	6 h	5/5	Negative
	Plant	16°C	6 h	5/5	Negative
		16°C	6 h	5/5	Negative
	Bovine	6°C	6 h	5/5	Negative
		6°C	6 h	5/5	Negative
	Plant	6°C	6 h	5/5	Negative
		6°C	6 h	5/5	Negative
BVDV virus	Bovine	16°C	1 min	0/5	Negative
	Plant	16°C	1 min	0/5	Negative
	Bovine	6°C	5 min	2/5	Negative
	Plant	6°C	15 min	5/5	Negative

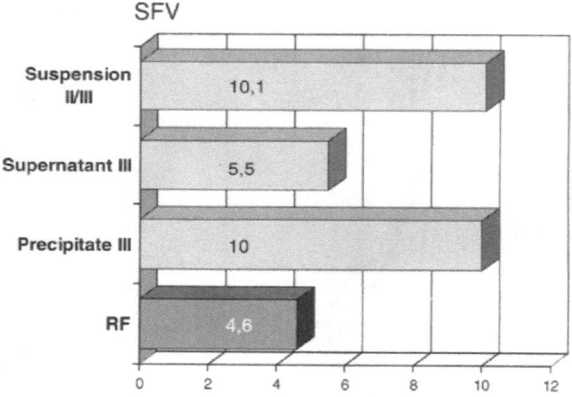

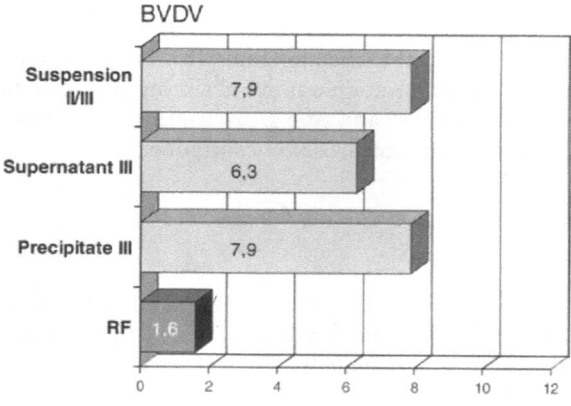

Fig. 5. Removal of SFV and BVDV during a specific step of the Cohn-Oncley fractionation: precipitation of fraction III from suspension II/III. RF, reduction factor

Discussion

There is no doubt that solvent/detergent treatment and pasteurization are effective in inactivating enveloped viruses and therefore are appropriate to support the virus safety of plasma-derived products. This has been demonstrated for BVDV and SFV, and corresponds with a series of previously published data [6, 7, 8].

However, the results also demonstrate a different behavior of BVDV and SFV in these inactivation procedures. This has been shown when temperature and solvent/ detergent concentration were varied (solvent/detergent treatment). Inactivation kinetics of BVDV were not affected at lower solvent/detergent concentrations (up to 50%) and at lower treatment temperatures (16°, 6°C). In contrast, inactivation of SFV was markedly delayed under these conditions.

The different behavior was more significant when higher sample volumes were analyzed after S/D treatment at 16°C and 6°C: no infectious BVDV was detected after 5 min treatment when 1.25 ml (5 x 0.25 ml per cell culture flask) instead of 0.4 ml (microtiter plate) were titrated. In contrast, residual infectivity was detected for SFV in some 0.25 ml samples after the full inactivation time of 6 h. This is remarkable because solvent/detergent is known to be very effective in inactivating enveloped viruses.

Comparable results were observed for inactivation by heat treatment. SFV markedly lost its sensitivity to heat inactivation at increasing saccharose concentrations, whereas the inactivation of BVDV was not affected at higher saccharose concentrations (588–1500 g/l).

The results of solvent/detergent and heat inactivation studies show that SFV was of higher physicochemical resistance under the conditions tested. In these cases, it may be a more appropriate model for HCV. As long as the sensitivity of HCV against these treatments is not known, the most resistant virus should be used as a model virus in order to avoid an overestimation of the inactivation capacity.

However, this is completely in contrast to the results obtained for the Cohn-Oncley fractionation: during precipitation of the re-solubilized precipitate II/III W into precipitate III and supernatant III, SFV was highly removed ($\sim$4.6 $\log_{10}$). BVDV, however, was only slightly eliminated from the supernatant ($\sim$1.6 $\log_{10}$) and was partitioned to almost equal parts into supernatant and precipitate. This result corresponds with other reports [9, 10, 11].

The results obtained with BVDV and SFV show that BVDV was more appropriate to studying a partitioning process like the Cohn-Oncley fractionation in order to estimate the lowest potential safety margin with respect to HCV. BVDV has, therefore, been recommended for use in studying ethanol fractionation processes [12].

Differences in the sensitivity of SFV and BVDV have been observed in each procedure (solvent/detergent and heat treatment, cold ethanol fractionation). Although both viruses are of similar structure, differences exist in the physicochemical behavior of both viruses. These differences can influence the outcome of individual virus validation studies depending on the method investigated.

In general, model viruses can only give an indication of the real physicochemical behavior of the relevant virus. Selection of model viruses and the interpretation of study results should, therefore, be carefully handled referring to the capacity of a process step in removal and/or inactivation of the relevant virus.

References

1. Willkommen H. (1997): Virus transmission by virus inactivated plasma products. In: Kretschmer V., Blauhut B. (ed.) Baillière's clinical Anaesthesiology, vol. 11. Blood, blood products and blood saving techniques, London
2. European guidelines: CPMP/BWP/268/95, CPMP/BWP/269/95 (http://www.eudra.org/emea.html)
3. Weiner AJ., Brauer MJ., Rosenblatt J., et al. (1991): Variable and hypervariable domains are found in the regions of HCV corresponding to the flavivirus envelope and NS1 proteins and the pestivirus envelope glycoproteins. Virology 180: 842–848
4. Murphy FA., Fauquet CM., Bishop DHL., Ghabrial SA., Jarvis AW., Martelli GP., Mayo MA., Summers MD. (1995): Virus Taxonomy – Classification and nomenclature of viruses. Arch. of Virol., suppl. 10
5. Scheiblauer H., Nübling M., Willkommen H., Löwer J. (1996): Prevalence of Hepatitis C Virus in Plasma Pools and the Effectiveness of cold Ethanol Fractionation. Clinical Therapeutics, 18 suppl. B: 59–70
6. Ben-Hur E. and Horowitz B. (1996): Virus inactivation in blood. AIDS 10: 1183–1190
7. Horowitz B., Prince AM., Hamman J., Watklevicz C. (1994): Viral safety of solvent/detergent-treated blood products. Blood Coagul. Fibrinol., 5 (suppl.): 21–28
8. Biescas H., Gensan M., Fernández J., et al. (1998): Characterisation and viral safety validation study of a pasteurized therapeutic concentrate of antithrombin III obtained through affinity chromatography. Haematologica, 83: 305–311
9. Bos OJM., Sunyé DGJ., Nieweboer CEF., et al. (1998): Virus validation of pH 4-treated human immunoglobulin products produced by Cohn fractionation process. Biologicals 26: 267–276
10. Dichtelmüller H., Rudnick D., Breuer B., et al. (1993): Validation of virus inactivation and removal for the manufacturing procedure of two immunoglobulins and a 5% serum protein solution treated with β-propriolactone. Biologicals 21:259–268
11. Yei S., Yu MW., Tankersley DL. (1992): Cohn-Oncley fractionation of plasma. Transfusion 32: 824–828
12. European guidelines: CPMP/BWP/269/95 (http://www.eudra.org/emea.html)

Preoperative Coagulation Screening in Children Focused on PTT Elevation

C. LEX, H. IRSFELD, G. JANSSEN, U. GÖBEL

Introduction

The usefulness of preoperative screening for coagulation disorders has been controversially discussed for years [1, 2, 3, 5]. Some authors have stated that preoperative prothrombin time (PTT) provides no further information in addition to the evaluation of the bleeding history [2, 3].

The present study attempted to elucidate the clinical relevance of PTT in children who had shown elevated PTT values during presurgical routine screening.

Patients

In our outpatient clinic, 62 children were presented between April 1997 and September 1999 for further elucidation of elevated PTT values which had been found during presurgical routine laboratory screening. Patients' characteristics including surgical procedures that were going to be performed are listed in Table 1.

Table 1. Patients' characteristics

Patient numbers:	62 children (37 male, 25 female patients)
Age range:	3 months to 15 years (mean age 5.5 ± 3.5 years)
Planned surgical procedures	55 otolaryngological surgeries including adenotomy, tonsillectomy, myringotomy with insertion of ventilation tubes 4 oral surgeries 2 herniotomies 1 circumcision

Methods

The bleeding history and comprehensive analysis of coagulation parameters were evaluated retrospectively. Coagulation parameters with underlying assays are listed in Table 2.

I. Scharrer/W. Schramm (Ed.)
30th Hemophilia Symposium Hamburg 1999
© Springer-Verlag Berlin Heidelberg 2001

418   C. Lex et al.

Table 2. Coagulation parameters with underlying assays

Standardized bleeding history

Bleeding time according to Ivy (normal value: up to 6 min)

PTT (reagent: Dapptin from Progen Immuno-Diagnostika, Heidelberg, Germany; normal value: 27–42.9 s)

Factor VIII (reagents: factor VIII deficiency plasma, Dapptin, calcium chloride from Progen Immuno-Diagnostika, Heidelberg, Germany)

Factors XI and XII (chromogenic assay, factor XI and XII deficiency plasma, APTT silica, calcium chloride from Instrumentation Laboratory, Kirchheim, Germany)

von Willebrand factor (von Willebrand antigen ELISA from Boehringer, Mannheim, Germany; von Willebrand multimere analysis performed by Prof. Budde, Hamburg, Germany)

Lupus antibodies (lupus anticoagulation test from Progen Immuno-Diagnostika)

Anti-cardiolipin/anti-phosphatidylserine antibodies (ELISA from Euroimmun, Lübeck, Germany)

Results

Repeated controls of PTT still revealed elevated values in 36 of the initial 62 patients. The most frequent cause for PTT prolongation in the remainder patients was found to be factor XI or XII deficiency (Fig. 1), which was demonstrated in 27 patients. Five of these patients had shown a positive bleeding history. In five patients, the underlying cause for PTT elevation appeared to be von Willebrand's disease. Four of these patients belonged to type I, one patient to type IIA. One of the patients with von Willebrand's disease also showed an additional factor XII deficiency. No patient with von Willebrand's disease reported a positive bleeding history. In two patients, the surgical procedure (adenotomy) was canceled after diagnosis. In one patient, lupus antibodies were additionally demonstrated. Bleeding time was not prolonged in any of the cases. Detailed results of elevated PTT with other pathological findings of coagulation parameters are listed in Table 3.

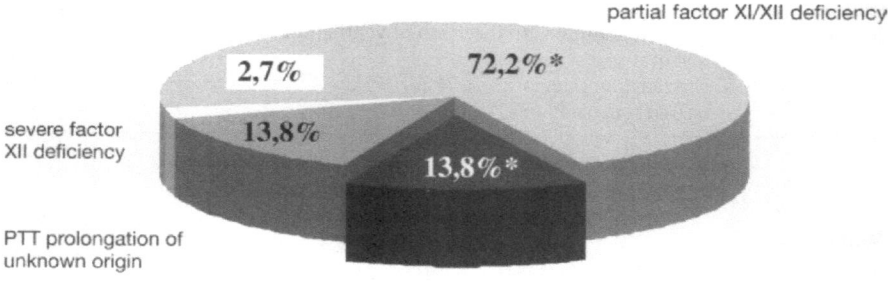

*One patient suffered from von Willebrand disease as well as partial factor XII deficiency

Fig. 1. Causes for PTT prolongation among 36 children

Table 3. Elevated PTT values in correlation to other pathological coagulation parameters

PTT (s)	27–42.9	43–49.9	50–59.9	≥60
Patients total (n)	26	27	7	2
Factor VIII <50%		3	1	1
Factor XI <67%	4	12	3	1
Factor XII <52%	8	14	6	1
Factor XII <1%				1
von Willebrand factor <60%		4	1	
Lupus antibodies				1

Conclusions

1. In approximately 40% of the patients, PTT values found during presurgical routine laboratory screening normalized after control in our laboratory. This is in accordance with Watel et al. [4], who found a persistence of PTT elevations only in 37/134 patients after first control. Extensive and detailed laboratory analysis is more expensive than a simple PTT control. This has to be taken into account when analyzing costs and efficiency.
2. Further evaluation of elevated PTT values revealed von Willebrand's disease in five patients. Factor XI/XII deficiency was the most frequent cause of randomly found PTT elevation in our patients.
3. The bleeding history of all patients did not correlate with bleeding relevant co-agulation disorders, such as von Willebrand's disease.

Acknowledgements. We would like to thank Mrs. E. Oellers, Mrs. U. Morgenrot and Mrs. H. Seliger for the performance of the laboratory assays. The Hemostasis Program of the Children's Hospital, Heinrich Heine University, is supported by the Elterninitiative Kinderkrebsklinik e.V. Duesseldorf.

References

1. Burk CD, Miller L, Handler SD, Cohen AR. Preoperative history and coagulation screening in children undergoing tonsillectomy. Pediatrics 1992; 89:691–5.
2. Close HL, Krytzer TC, Nowlin JH, Alving BM. Hemostatic assessment of patients before tonsillectomy: a prospective study. Otolaryngol Head Neck Surg 1994; 111:733–8.
3. Howells RC 2nd, Wax MK, Ramadan HH. Value of preoperative prothrombin time/partial thromboplastin time as a predictor of postoperative hemorrhage in pediatric patients undergoing tonsillectomy. Otolaryngol Head Neck Surg 1997; 117.628–32.
4. Watel A, Jude B, Caron C, Vandeputte H, Gaeremynck E, Cosson A. Successes and failure of the activated partial thromboplastin time in the preoperative evaluation. Ann Fr Anesth Reanim 1986; 5:35–9.
5. Zwack GC, Derkay CS. The utility of preoperative hemostatic assessment in adenotonsillectomy. Int J Pediatr Otorhinolaryngol 1997; 39:67–76.

Resonance Thrombographic Analysis of Coagulation Status after Transfusion of Platelet Concentrates with Different Storage Times

K. Geidel, M.A. Brockmann, A. Alisch, M. Weilandt, S. Schlichting,
P. Kühnl, K. Gutensohn

Introduction

High-dose chemotherapy usually results in bone marrow aplasia. As a result, patients become thrombocytopenic and have an increase of bleedings. In this study, we investigated the coagulation status of aplastic patients following bone marrow transplantation before and after transfusion of platelet concentrates (PCs) using resonance thrombography.

Material and Methods

Eleven patients (7 male, 4 female) suffering from CML and being in the aplastic phase were included in this study. All patients underwent a standardized chemo-therapeutic regimen. Patients received a PC when their platelet count dropped below $20x10^3/\mu l$. Every patient received two »fresh« and two »stored« PCs within 1 week. Average storage time of the fresh PCs was 1.14 ± 0.35 days, storage time of stored PCs was 3.5 ± 0.74 days.

For RTG analysis (CM-3; Amelung, Hamburg, Germany), blood samples were obtained from the patient via a Quinton catheter directly before, 1 h and 24 h after PC application. Samples were anticoagulated with sodium citrate 1:10. Blood was filled into test tubes, recalcified, and measurement started. The time during which contact activation took place [r-time (s)] and the period until maximum fibrin formation [f-time (s)] were recorded. The maximum amplitude [M (%)], which mainly reflects fibrinogen, and platelet function and p-time (s), which mainly reflect platelet function, were also assessed. Measurement was terminated after 60 min.

Results

In the group of fresh PCs, a significant ($P<0.05$) decrease of r-time, f-time, and p-time was observed 1 h after transfusion (compared to values before transfusion). Furthermore, a significant reduction of all three measured values could still be observed 24 h after transfusion, compared to values before transfusion. Within the group of stored PCs, a significant decrease of p-time 1 h after, compared to p-time

I. Scharrer/W. Schramm (Ed.)
30th Hemophilia Symposium Hamburg 1999
© Springer-Verlag Berlin Heidelberg 2001

before, transfusion of PCs could be measured. Comparing stored and fresh concentrates, a significantly increased r-time could also be monitored for stored PCs 1 and 24 h after administration of PC. However, f-time and r-time were not significant for stored PCs. M (%) was significantly higher for fresh concentrates than for stored concentrates ($P<0.05$).

Conclusion

Patients seem to have a greater benefit from receiving fresh PCs than stored PCs. Furthermore, an improved coagulation status is still present 24 h after receiving a capacity of fibrinogen quantity which seems to be affected negatively by storage of PCs. Therefore, RTG may be useful in assessing hemostatic capacity in aplastic patients.

Subject Index